Teaching Cultural Competence
in Nursing and Health Care

Dr. Marianne R. Jeffreys' grant-funded research, consultations, publications, and professional presentations encompass the topics of cultural competence, nontraditional students, student retention and achievement, self-efficacy, teaching, curriculum, and psychometrics. The first edition of her book *Teaching Cultural Competence in Nursing and Health Care: Inquiry, Action, and Innovation* received the AJN Book of the Year Award; she is also author of *Nursing Student Retention: Understanding the Process and Making a Difference*, articles, book chapters, and videos. Her conceptual models and questionnaires have been requested worldwide and in various disciplines. She is currently a professor of nursing at the City University of New York (CUNY) Graduate College and at CUNY College of Staten Island.

Dr. Jeffreys received a B.S. in nursing from the State University of New York College at Plattsburgh and M.A., M.Ed., and Ed.D. degrees in nursing education from Teachers College, Columbia University. She is a Fellow of the New York Academy of Medicine. Her awards include the international *Leininger Award* for Excellence in Transcultural Nursing, Columbia University's Teachers College Award for Scholarship and Research, and the Mu Upsilon Chapter of Sigma Theta Tau Excellence in Professional Nursing Award. She was named Consultant of the Month (December 2007) by the National Center for Cultural Competence. Her expertise has been requested for grant-funded projects (HRSA, Kellogg), as well as for institutional and departmental workshops. Professor Jeffreys may be reached at marianne.jeffreys@csi.cuny.edu.

Teaching
Cultural Competence
in Nursing and Health Care
Inquiry, Action, and Innovation

2nd Edition

Marianne R. Jeffreys, EdD, RN

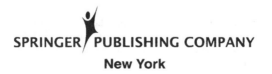

SPRINGER PUBLISHING COMPANY
New York

Springer Publishing Company, LLC
11 West 42nd Street
New York, NY 10036
www.springerpub.com

Acquisitions Editor: Allan Graubard
Project Editor: Peter Rocheleau
Project Manager: Sweety Singh
Cover Design: Mimi Flow
Composition: Aptara, Inc.

ISBN: 978-0-8261-1787-8
E-book ISBN: 978-0-8261-1788-5

10 11 12 13 / 5 4 3 2 1

Printed in the United States of America by Bang Printing

Cataloging-in-Publication Data are on file at the Library of Congress.

The author and the publisher of this Work have made every effort to use sources believed to be reliable to provide information that is accurate and compatible with the standards generally accepted at the time of publication. Because medical science is continually advancing, our knowledge base continues to expand. Therefore, as new information becomes available, changes in procedures become necessary. We recommend that the reader always consult current research and specific institutional policies before performing any clinical procedure. The author and publisher shall not be liable for any special, consequential, or exemplary damages resulting, in whole or in part, from the readers' use of, or reliance on, the information contained in this book. The publisher has no responsibility for the persistence or accuracy of URLs for external or third-party Internet Web sites referred to in this publication and does not guarantee that any content on such Web sites is, or will remain, accurate or appropriate.

To my son, Daniel W. Edley

Contents

Contributors

Theresa M. Adams, MSN, RN, CSN
Assistant Professor of Nursing
Doctoral Student, PhD in Leadership
Alvernia University
Reading, PA

Roxanne Amerson, PhD, RN, BC, CTN-A
Instructor
Clemson University
Clemson, SC

Kevin Antoine, J.D.
Attorney/Chief Diversity Officer
State University of New York (SUNY) Downstate
Brooklyn, New York
Former Fellow, Harvard School of Public Health

Phyllis D. Barham, RN, MS
Senior Lecturer and Chief Academic Advisor
BSN Program
Old Dominion University
Norfolk, VA

Patricia Bartley-Daniele, MSN, FNP-BC, CCRN, CNRN, CAPAN, CAPA
Nurse Practitioner
Department of Advanced Practice Nursing
Department of Anesthesia
NYU Langone Medical Center
New York, NY

Richardean Benjamin, PhD, PMHCNS-BC, MPH, ANEF, FAAN
Associate Dean
College of Health Sciences
Old Dominion University
Norfolk, VA

Lenore Bertone, MS, RN
Registered Professional Nurse
Treatment Team Leader
South Beach Psychiatric Center
Staten Island, NY

Patricia Burrell, PhD, APRN, APMHCNS-BC, CNE
Interim Department Chair for Graduate and Post-Baccalaureate Programs
Evaluation & Research Director, Transcultural Nursing Center
Professor of Nursing
College of Nursing and Health Sciences
Hawaii Pacific University
Kaneohe, HI

Karen Costello, BSN, RN, OCN
Staff Nurse
Bone Marrow Transplant Unit
Hackensack University Medical Center
Hackensack, NJ

Jo-Ann Douglas, MS, RN
Staff Nurse
Beth Israel Medical Center
New York, NY

Phyllis M. Eaton, PhD, RN, PMHCNS-BC
Lecturer
Old Dominion University
Norfolk, VA

Cynthia Karczewski, MS, RN
Manhattan Borough Nursing Director
New York City Department of Health and Mental Hygiene
Office of School Health
New York, NY

Rachelle Larsen, PhD, RN
Associate Professor
College of St. Benedict/St. John's University
St. Joseph, MN

Rona F. Levin, PhD, RN
Professor and Chair
Department of Graduate Nursing
Lienhard School of Nursing
Pace University
New York, NY

Vivien Li, BS, RN
Registered Nurse
Lutheran Medical Center
Brooklyn, NY

Stephen R. Marrone, EdD, RN-BC, CTN-A
Deputy Nursing Director
Institute of Continuous Learning
State University of New York (SUNY)
SUNY Downstate Medical Center
Clinical Assistant Professor of Nursing
SUNY Downstate College of Nursing
Brooklyn, NY
Clinical Associate Professor of Nursing
Case Western Reserve University
Cleveland, OH
Adjunct Assistant Professor of Nursing Education
Teachers College Columbia University
New York, NY

Kathleen M. Nevel, MEIE, BA
Doctoral Student, PhD in Leadership
Alvernia University
Reading, PA

Sara Newman, MS, CNS, ANP-C
Home Care Consultant
Visiting Nurse Service of New York
New York, NY

Mary O'Donnell, PhD, RN
Associate Professor and Chair
Nursing Department
The City University of New York (CUNY) College of Staten Island
Staten Island, NY

Kay Palmer, MSN, RN, CRRN
Undergraduate Program Director
Old Dominion University
Norfolk, VA

Rachelle Parsons, PhD, RN
Associate Professor
College of St. Benedict/St. John's University
St. Joseph, MN

LuAnn Reif, PhD, RN
Associate Professor
College of St. Benedict/St. John's University
St. Joseph, MN

Carolyn M. Rutledge, PhD, FNP-BC
Associate Professor
Co-Director of the DNP Program
Old Dominion University
Norfolk, VA

Joanne K. Singleton, PhD, RN, FNP-BC, FNAP
Family Nurse Practitioner, and Doctor of Nursing Practice
    Program Director
Department of Graduate Studies
Lienhard School of Nursing
Pace University
New York, NY

Jeanette Velez, MA, CDP
Administrative Program Manager/Physician Liaison
Huron, a Cleveland Clinic Hospital
East Cleveland, OH

Lynn Wiles, RN, PhD(c), CEN
Senior Lecturer
School of Nursing
Old Dominion University
Norfolk, VA

Judy Xiao, MA, MS
Assistant Professor
Coordinator of Periodicals Services
Library
The City University of New York (CUNY) College of Staten Island
Staten Island, NY

Preface

Preparing nurses and other health professionals to provide quality health care in the increasingly multicultural and global society of the 21st century requires a comprehensive approach that emphasizes cultural competence education throughout professional education and professional life. Nurses and other health care providers, educators, administrators, professional association leaders, managers, and researchers are called upon to:

- Provide optimal care for the large number of culturally diverse patient populations
- Implement cultural competence education strategies in academic and hospital settings for diverse learners
- Evaluate outcomes of cultural competence education
- Prevent multicultural workplace conflict and promote multicultural workplace harmony
- Personally engage in lifelong cultural competence education

These tasks can seem daunting and overwhelming without appropriate resources. If you want to develop *optimal cultural competence* in yourself and others, *Teaching Cultural Competence in Nursing and Health Care, 2nd Edition*, and the *Cultural Competence Education Resource Toolkit* are the how-to resources for you. These hands-on, user-friendly resources reveal a systematic 7-step approach that takes nurses, educators, administrators, professional association leaders, managers, educators, students, and other health care providers from their own starting points toward the pinnacle—*optimal cultural competence*. Appropriate for all levels and settings (academic, health care institutions, employee education, professional associations, and continuing education), the book and toolkit end the struggle to find ready-to-use materials for planning,

implementing, and evaluating cultural competence education strategies
and programs. Users of the book and toolkit will find the following:

- A model to guide cultural competence education
- Questionnaires for measuring and evaluating learning and performance
- A guide for identifying at-risk individuals and avoiding pitfalls
- A wide selection of educational activities
- Techniques for diverse learners
- Chapters detailing employee orientation, inservices, and continuing education
- Chapters detailing multidimensional strategies for undergraduates and graduates
- Vignettes, case examples, illustrations, tables, and assessment tools
- Abstracts and sample research reports from researchers evaluating strategies

Based on the results of several post-doctoral grant-funded studies, practical teaching experience with academically and culturally diverse learners across all levels, and multidisciplinary literature, the book and toolkit provide resources and a wealth of information for all user groups.

The book is divided into three parts: Part I, Getting Started; Part II, Tools for Assessment and Evaluation; and Part III, Educational Activities for Easy Application.

Part I is comprised of three chapters filled with resources to help educators begin teaching cultural competence. Essential background information about the multidimensional process of teaching cultural competence offers a valuable guide for educators at all levels who are planning, implementing, and evaluating cultural competence education.

Educators and researchers are continually challenged to measure outcomes following educational interventions. Part II addresses this challenge by introducing several quantitative questionnaires and assessment tools [to be found in the toolkit] and discussing implementation and data interpretation strategies in a detailed, user-friendly approach that is easily adapted by novice and advanced researchers. Questionnaires, assessment tools, a cultural competence documentation log, and a research report template are easily accessed in the accompanying *Cultural Competence Education Resource Toolkit*. (See details concerning toolkit access in the final section of the preface.)

Part III offers a wide selection of educational activities that can easily be applied by educators everywhere. Three chapters (6, 10, and 13) provide a general overview and a menu of activities and strategies for use in three areas: the academic setting, the health care institution, and professional associations. Chapter discussions, supplementary diagrams, and descriptions of toolkit items explore the 7 steps essential for optimal cultural competence development:

- Self-assessment
- Active promotion
- Systematic inquiry
- Decisive action
- Innovation
- Measurement
- Evaluation

Five chapters (7, 8, 9, 11, and 12) in Part III creatively link strategies via detailed case exemplars that spotlight various populations and settings.

The book's final chapter (Chapter 14) presents important implications for educators everywhere. Educators are challenged to commit to a focused and transformational change that will not only advance the science and art of cultural competence education, but will also result in culturally congruent care, ultimately benefiting health care consumers worldwide. The urgent expansion of educational research specifically focused on the teaching and learning of *optimal* cultural competence is emphasized, and areas for further inquiry and research, and future goals are proposed. Extensive references are provided at the end of the book.

Unquestionably, implementing creative, evidence-based educational activities that promote positive cultural competence learning outcomes for culturally diverse students and health care professionals continues to be a challenge. A new challenge is to reach beyond competence (a minimum expectation) toward *optimal cultural competence*. This new quest recognizes that all individuals, groups, and organizations have the potential for "more." Optimal cultural competence embraces the diversity of diversity, requires ongoing active learning, fosters multicultural workplace harmony, and promotes the delivery of the highest level of culturally congruent patient care.

Why *optimal cultural competence*?

First, culture is a crucial factor in promoting wellness, preventing illness, restoring health, facilitating coping, and enhancing quality of life for all individuals, families, and communities. Unfortunately, the two main goals of the U.S. Department of Health and Human Services report *Healthy People 2010* have not been met. The first goal—to increase quality and years of healthy life for all—can only be achieved when an examination of "quality of life" and the meaning of "health and well-being" within a cultural context are put into service. The second goal was to eliminate health disparities among different segments of the population, which necessitated culture-specific and competent actions designed to eliminate disparities; however, health disparities remain overwhelming. As such, customized health care that responds to a client's cultural values, beliefs, and traditions (culturally congruent care) remains urgent (Giger et al., 2007; Leininger, 2002a, 2002b; Rosal & Bodenlos, 2009; Whitt-Glover et al., 2009). For health care professionals with some cultural competence skills, the challenge now is to go beyond mere cultural competence toward optimal cultural competence. It is also imperative that health professionals without cultural competence education actively begin their journey to develop optimal cultural competence.

Second, culturally congruent health care is a basic human right, not a privilege, and therefore every human is entitled to it. The International Council of Nurses (ICN) *Code for Nurses* (ICN, 1973), the American Nurses Association (ANA) *Code of Ethics* (ANA, 2001), and the *National Standards for Culturally and Linguistically Appropriate Services in Health Care* (Office of Minority Health, 2001) are important documents that serve as reminders. Criteria devised by accreditation and credentialing agencies such as the Joint Commission on Accreditation of Healthcare Organizations, the National Committee on Quality Assurance, the American Medical Association, and the National League for Nursing strive to ensure that culturally competent health care series and education are provided. The essential inclusion of cultural competence as viewed from an ethical and legal standpoint is addressed on varying levels within the disciplines of physical therapy, occupational therapy, speech-language pathology, dentistry, medicine, psychology, and social work (AAMC, 2005; ADA, 2005, 2007; APA, 1994; APTA, 2008; Lubinski & Matteliano, 2008; NASW, 2001, 2007, 2009; Nochajski & Matteliano, 2008; Panzarella & Matteliano, 2008). Not only are nurses, physicians, other health care providers, and institutions ethically and morally obligated to provide the best culturally congruent care possible (optimal cultural competence), they are also legally mandated to do so. Within the scope of professional practice, nurses and other health professionals are expected to actively seek out ways to promote culturally congruent care at optimal levels.

The *AJN* award-winning first edition of *Teaching Cultural Competence in Nursing and Health Care* introduced readers to easy-to-use teaching–learning strategies for cultural competence education. Positive comments about the first edition, along with a surge of requests for "more" from academic and employee educators, researchers, practicing health professionals, and students from around the world and in various disciplines, inspired the writing of the expanded second edition and the creation of the *Cultural Competence Education Resource Toolkit*. The ideas and suggestions presented here are not meant to be exhaustive, but are offered to stimulate new ideas and invite health professionals to explore new paths on the journey to developing cultural competence in oneself and others. Readers are encouraged to pause, reflect, and question throughout the book in order to gain new insights and perspectives. Everyone is empowered to contribute to a transformational change in health care that prioritizes *optimal cultural competence* development and embraces diversity.

About the Cultural Competence Education Resource Toolkit

As mentioned previously, this book includes a valuable and ready-to-use Cultural Competence Education Resource Toolkit. The Toolkit consists of three sets of tools and a total of 21 distinct tools. The three sets of tools are: Resources for Academic Settings; Resources for Health Care Institutions; and Resources for Professional Associations. Taken together, the tools provide a comprehensive set of materials for planning, implementing, and evaluating cultural competence education strategies and programs. These tools may be used alone or in conjunction with other tools and will be of use to a broad range of readers at all levels: nurses, educators, administrators, association leaders, managers, researchers, students, and other health care providers. The tools and this book will enable you to achieve optimal cultural competence.

All of these tools are to be found on a special website. The address of the website is springerpub.com/jeffreystoolkit. You can download and print the tools from this website and you can also distribute them electronically.

An important note: As a purchaser of this book you are entitled to employ these tools for individual use without extra charge. Any use of the toolkit or portions of the toolkit beyond individual, personal use (such as within an institutional setting and/or in a research study) will require a license from Springer Publishing Company and payment of a modest fee for a one year unlimited use license.

To obtain more information regarding such an institutional license including terms and fees please contact Springer Publishing Company at any one of the following:

Phone: 212 431 4370 or toll-free at 877 687 7476
Fax: 212 941 7842
Email: customerservice@springerpub.com
Mail: Springer Publishing Company
      Customer Service
      11 West 42nd Street
      New York, New York 10036

We thank you for your adherence to these terms of use.

Acknowledgments

Partial funding for previous research on the Transcultural Self-Efficacy Tool (TSET) and the assessment of students' transcultural self-efficacy perceptions was obtained from the Nursing Education Alumni Association (NEAA) of Teachers College, Columbia University Postdoctoral Research Fellowship Award; The Research Foundation of the City University of New York PSC-CUNY Research Award Program; The City University of New York College of Staten Island Division of Science and Technology Research Award; and the Mu Upsilon Chapter of Sigma Theta Tau International Honor Society in Nursing.

Teaching Cultural Competence in Nursing and Health Care

PART I

Getting Started

Part I, Getting Started, contains three chapters filled with resources and tools to help educators begin teaching cultural competence. Essential background information about the multidimensional process of teaching cultural competence offers a valuable guide for educators at all levels when planning, implementing, and evaluating cultural competence education.

Chapter 1 overviews key issues, concerns, and new challenges facing health care consumers, professionals, and educators. Professional goals, societal needs, ethical considerations, legal issues, changing demographics, and learner characteristics are highlighted. Select cultural values and beliefs are vividly compared and contrasted in a supplementary table that enhances the text. The chapter concludes with a discussion of factors influencing cultural competence development among culturally diverse learners and proposes that confidence, or in the context of this book transcultural self-efficacy (TSE), is a major component in cultural competence development and a strong influencing factor in achieving culturally congruent care.

Creating environments that embrace diversity, meeting the culture-specific needs of patients, preventing multicultural workplace conflict, and promoting multicultural workplace harmony are portrayed in Chapter 2. These endeavors begin with diversity awareness of self and others, with each defined at the beginning of the chapter. Several poignant clinical and workplace examples illustrate the significance of actively weaving cultural competence throughout all aspects of health care settings. The acronym "COMPETENCE" assists health care professionals in remembering essential elements for optimal cultural competence development.

Chapter 3 introduces a model to guide cultural competence education—the Cultural Competence and Confidence (CCC) model. The underlying assumptions, principles, concepts, and terms associated with the model's development are concisely presented. A unique feature of the model (and the book) is that its major concepts, propositions, and constructs are supported by several quantitative studies using a questionnaire also discussed in this book and available in the Jeffreys Cultural Competence Education Resource Toolkit (Jeffreys, 2010). The visual illustration of the model enhances understanding of the text. A second illustration expands on the CCC model illustration by tracing the proposed influences of TSE (confidence) on a learner's actions, performance, and persistence for learning associated with cultural competency development and culturally congruent care. The model has relevance to other disciplines recognizing the essential inclusion of cultural competence within clinical practice and in initial and/or ongoing educational preparation, such as physical therapy, occupational therapy, speech-language pathology, dentistry, medicine, psychology, and social work. The model is brought to life through a realistic "Educator-In-Action" vignette featuring cultural competence education in the health care institution (hospital setting).

CHAPTER 1

Overview of Key Issues and Concerns

Marianne R. Jeffreys, EdD, RN

Meeting the health care needs of culturally diverse clients has become even more challenging and complex. In addition to acknowledging the cultural evolution (growth and change) occurring in the United States (and other parts of the world), it is imperative that nursing and other health care professions appreciate and understand the impending cultural revolution. The term *cultural revolution* implies a "revolution of thinking" that seeks to embrace the evolution of a different, broader worldview (Jeffreys & Zoucha, 2001). Both cultural evolution and cultural revolution have the potential to bring about a different worldview regarding cultural care and caring by including key issues previously nonexistent, underrepresented, or invisible in the nursing and health care literature. This new vision challenges all health care professionals to embark upon a new journey in the quest for cultural competence and culturally congruent care for all clients (Jeffreys & Zoucha, 2001). This new journey also challenges health care professionals and organizations to go beyond the goal of achieving "competence" (minimum standard) toward the goal of achieving "optimal" cultural competence (standard of excellence). Educators everywhere are additionally challenged to learn how to lead the quest for culturally congruent health care by implementing creative, evidence-based educational activities that promote positive cultural competence learning outcomes for culturally diverse students and health care professionals, aiming to reach beyond minimal competence to the achievement of optimal cultural competence.

This transformational journey begins by seeking to understand the key issues, concerns, and new challenges facing health care consumers and professionals today and in the future. This chapter evokes professional awareness, sparks interest, stimulates revolutionary thought, highlights vital information, and shares new ideas concerning the health care needs of culturally diverse clients and the development of cultural competence among culturally diverse health care professionals. *Cultural competence* has been described as a multidimensional process that aims to achieve culturally congruent health care (Andrews & Boyle, 2008; Campinha-Bacote, 2003; Leininger, 1991a; Purnell & Paulanka, 2008). Culturally congruent health care refers to health care that is customized to fit with the client's cultural values, beliefs, traditions, practices, and lifestyle (Leininger, 1991a). It is beyond the scope of this chapter to provide a summary review of the existing literature concerning cultural competence and health care. Rather, this chapter emphasizes select points from the literature, identifies future complexities and challenges in health care, discusses factors influencing cultural competency development, and proposes a construct involved in the process of cultural competence development and education.

COMPLEXITIES, CHANGES, AND CHALLENGES IN HEALTH CARE

Rapid growth in worldwide migration, changes in demographic patterns, varying fertility rates, increased numbers of multiracial and multiethnic individuals, and advanced technology contribute to cultural evolution. For the purpose of this book, *cultural evolution* refers to the process of cultural growth and change within a society (Jeffreys & Zoucha, 2001). Within the nursing literature, cultural growth, change, and the need for culturally congruent nursing care have been frequently reported in various countries outside the United States including Australia, Canada, Israel, Sweden, South Africa, and the United Kingdom (Cowan & Norman, 2006; Davidson, Meleis, Daly, & Douglas, 2003 Douglas, 2000; Douglas et al., 2009; Glittenberg, 2004; Holtz, 2008). Although this book addresses cultural changes in the United States, readers should recognize that globalization is a worldwide phenomenon, with populations now moving more frequently than ever before. Because more people are migrating to several different places, the acculturation experience may include cultural values and beliefs (CVB) assimilated from more than one source, resulting in new ways of expressing traditional CVB and/or resulting in new cultural values and belief patterns. Consequently, health care professionals are challenged to meet the needs of changing societies in new and different ways.

The United States Census (U.S. Census Bureau, 2002) and Healthy People 2010 (DHHS, 2000) provide valuable data about select population characteristics; however, they are limited in providing information about cultural values, beliefs, behaviors, and practices associated with the many diverse cultural groups existing within the United States. For example, it is helpful to know that minority populations are increasing more rapidly than white non-Hispanic, nonimmigrant populations (as determined by such variables as age and fertility rates), further justifying and demanding increased population-specific resource allocation (Kosoko-Lasaki, Cook, & O'Brien, 2009). It is also crucial to have identified health dispari-ties, high priority areas, goals, and proposed strategies for improvement; however, nurses and other health care professionals must become actively aware of the diverse cultural groups comprising each designated minority category if Healthy People 2010 and 2020 goals are to be met (de Chesnay & Anderson, 2008). For example, the "Hispanic" category may include individuals whose heritage may be traced to Cuba, Nicaragua, Mexico, Puerto Rico, Peru, Spain, and/or other countries, each also representing much diversity within and between groups. Diversity may exist based on birthplace, citizenship status, reason for migration, migration history, food, religion, ethnicity, race, language, kinship and family networks, educational background and opportunities, employment skills and op-portunities, lifestyle, gender, socioeconomic status (class), politics, past discrimination and bias experiences, health status and health risk, age, insurance coverage, and other variables that go well beyond the restrictive labels of a few ethnic and/or racial groups.

The projected increase of multiracial and multiethnic (multiple her-itage) individuals in the United States (Glittenberg, 2004; Johnson, 1997; Lee & Fernandez, 1998; Perlmann, 1997; Sands & Schuh, 2004; Spickard & Fong, 1995) and throughout the world demonstrates a growing change in demographic patterns, adding to this new cultural evolution. Forced single category choices and/or the "other" category make the unique cul-ture of the multiracial and multiethnic individual invisible (Jeffreys, 2005; Jeffreys & Zoucha, 2001). Although the 2000 U.S. Census permitted in-dividuals to select more than one racial/ethnic category, the lateness of this option demonstrates the reluctance of society to acknowledge and appreciate the existence of mestizo (mixing) in the United States (Nash, 1995). The late repeal of the last laws against miscegenation (race mixing) in the 1970s attests not only to societal reluctance, but also to political resistance reflecting racial ideologies of some white Americans (Pascoe, 1996).

Inconsistent use of the data from individuals selecting more than one census category is confusing and typically favors the antiquated process of assigning individuals to one category only; usually the minority sta-tus or politically advantageous category is selected. For example, when reporting the number of "minority" individuals within a public school system for the purpose of demonstrating integration within a predominantly white school, someone selecting "black" and "white" would be assigned as being "black." In reality, it may be impossible for a multiethnic and/or multiracial individual to choose one ethnic or racial identity over the other (Hall, 1992; Pinderhughes, 1995). Multiple heritage identity can include membership within one select group, simultaneous membership with two or more distinct groups, synthesis (blending) of cultures, and/or fluid identities with different groups that change with time, circumstance, and setting (Daniel, 1992; Root, 1992; Spickard & Fong, 1995). Moreover, multiple heritage individuals often describe being "multiracial" or "multiethnic" as a separate and unique culture (Root, 1997; Spickard, 1997). Culturally congruent health care for the 6,826,228 individuals who identified as being of more than one race in the 2000 Census (U.S. Census Bureau, 2002) must begin with openly acknowledging the uniqueness of multiple heritage individuals and seeking to learn about their lived experience. Multiple heritage individuals present unique concerns and challenges for transcultural nurses and other health care professionals because of the lack of research and published studies in nursing and health care (Jeffreys, 2005; Jeffreys & Zoucha, 2001).

Similarly, other underrepresented, invisible, unpopular, or new issues present complexities and challenges to health care professionals because of the lack of substantive research, resources, and expertise specifically targeting such topics related to culture and changing populations (cultural evolution). With the rapid changes and influx of new populations from around the world, nurses are, more than ever before, faced with the challenge of caring for many different cultural groups. Changes are occurring more rapidly in urban, suburban, and rural areas, often with cultural groups clustering together in ethnic neighborhoods. This means that there is less time for nurses to learn about and become accustomed to new cultural groups. Lack of nurses with transcultural nursing expertise presents a severe barrier in meeting the health care needs of diverse client populations (Leininger & McFarland, 2002).

Political changes throughout the world have resulted in large migration waves from former socialist, communist, monarchal, and dictatorship nations. Too many choices (in health care planning options) may overwhelm individuals who are not used to such freedoms (Miller, 1997). Mismatches in expectations between health care professional and client can cause poor health outcomes, stress, and dissatisfaction. Nurses unfamiliar with various political systems and the potential impact on clients' perceptions may be unprepared to provide culturally congruent care for these clients. Understanding the ethnohistory, especially the influence of politics, economics, discrimination, intergroup and intragroup conflicts, is an important cultural dimension that warrants further attention (Davidson, Meleis, Daly, & Douglas, 2003 Glittenberg, 2004; Leininger & McFarland, 2002, 2006; Miller, 1997). Despite the commonality of national origin, cultural experiences may be quite different for persons seeking asylum, refugees, and immigrants, and may vary at different points in history, necessitating an accurate and individualized appraisal.

Health care professionals are also challenged to differentiate between numerous minority groups around the world (who may have been victims of overt and/or covert stereotyping, prejudice, discrimination, and racism) and dominant groups. Within the United States, it has been well documented that discrimination, stereotyping, prejudice, and racism exist in nursing and health care (Abrums & Leppa, 2001; ANA, 1998b; Barbee & Gibson, 2001; Bolton, Giger, & Georges, 2004; Bosher & Pharris, 2009; Farella, 2002; Huff & Kline, 1999; Kosoko-Lasaki et al., 2009; Porter & Barbee, 2004; Wilson, 2007). This unpopular topic has not gained the sufficient attention and action necessary to actively dismantle stereotyping, prejudice, discrimination, and racism. Raising awareness is insufficient; taking appropriate and definitive action through well-planned positive innovative interventions followed by evaluation strategies will move beyond complacent "passive advocacy" to positive "active innovative advocacy." Such innovative actions require development of cultural competence and sincere commitment on the part of health care professionals.

Groups identified as "subcultures" have been identified as "vulnerable populations"; such populations present complex scenarios to health care professionals today and will do so in the future (de Chesnay & Anderson, 2008; Giger et al., 2007; Kosoko-Lasaki et al., 2009). For example, illegal immigrants, migrant workers, tenant farmers, and the homeless often present unique health care challenges due to lack of health insurance, illiteracy, poverty, and fear. In addition, tenant farmers and migrant workers may be grouped together under the heading of "rural health"; thus, the truly unique culture(s) and needs within and between groups across various geographic regions may remain undiscovered. Because tenant farmers may receive food and housing as part of their wages, they may not be eligible for food stamps; Medicaid; Women, Infants, and Children; public assistance; or other social services. Employee benefits such as health insurance and dental insurance are usually nonexistent. Funds for clothing, soap, toothpaste, toothbrushes, and other toiletries may be scarce, making tenant farmers susceptible to preventable diseases. Geographic isolation and lack of transportation are barriers encountered within rural communities, thus presenting another barrier to health care access. Within the United States, health insurance diversity presents inconsistencies in health care, especially in health promotion and illness prevention. Consequently, primary care for treatment of acute and advanced problems is not routinely accessible with delayed entry into the health care system occurring.

The global economic crisis, rising unemployment rates, loss of health insurance coverage, job and retirement uncertainty, increased housing foreclosures, and general economic unrest present multifaceted problems that political leaders, financial advisers, and the general public are poorly equipped to address effectively and with which they are inexperienced. Within a multicultural society, different CVB concerning economic stability, lifestyle expectations, acceptance of charity, debt, and profit further complicate these problems. Stress associated with periods of economic uncertainty and doubt may present greater numbers of individuals seeking and/or needing mental health services and/or other health services for diseases often triggered or exacerbated by stress. Inability to pay for medical services, drugs, housing, and food may aggravate health and social problems as well as intensify personal debt, thereby broadening deficits in the overall economy. The global economic crisis has spurred the forced, rapid movement and lifestyle changes of individuals, families, and even whole communities.

Rapidly moving populations bring unfamiliar diseases, new diseases, treatments, and medicines, challenging health care professionals to become quickly proficient in accurate diagnosis, treatment, and prevention. For example, nurses unfamiliar with malaria may be suddenly faced with several refugees from Africa who require treatment for malaria. Newer diseases, such as severe acute respiratory syndrome (SARS) and swine flu, can cause epidemics if not identified early and then properly controlled. Medicines and treatments considered "alternative" or "complementary" within the culture of Western medicine may actually be considered "routine" in other cultures. Medicines considered "routine" within the culture of Western medicine may have varying and adverse effects with different ethnic or racial groups due to health beliefs and/or due to genetic differences in body processes (e. g., metabolism) and/or anatomical characteristics (e. g., sun absorption based on skin color). The growing new field of ethnopharmacology attests to the urgent need to investigate the pharmacokinetics, pharmacodynamics, and overall pharmacological effects of drugs within specific cultural groups. Unfortunately, insurance company approval for drug therapy regimen is often guided by drug studies among primarily homogeneous populations, rather than taking into account new, however sparse empirical evidence provided by ethnopharmacological studies.

Inconsistencies in the expected roles of the nurse may vary from culture to culture, therefore confounding the therapeutic nurse–client interaction, nurse–nurse interaction, nurse–physician interaction, and nurse–family interaction. Differences in nursing practice throughout the world influence how the nurse views power, autonomy, collaboration, and clinical judgments (Sherman & Eggenberger, 2008; Zizzo & Xu, 2009). Whether the nurse is viewed as a well-educated professional, vocational service provider, paraprofessional, uneducated worker, or servant will impact greatly on the therapeutic and working relationship (Purnell, 2008). Furthermore, whether the nurse is viewed as an outsider, "stranger," "trusted friend," or insider will significantly influence the nurse–client relationship, the achievement of culturally congruent care, and optimal health outcomes (Leininger, 2002c). The mismatch between the diversity of registered nurses and U.S. populations presents one large barrier to meeting the needs of diverse populations. For example, white nurses of European-American heritage represent approximately 90% of all registered nurses (Barbee & Gibson, 2001; Bosher & Pharris, 2009; Kimball & O'Neill, 2002).

Expected roles and perceptions about other health care professionals will also vary from culture to culture, thus necessitating an accurate appraisal of clients' baseline knowledge, beliefs, and expectations, if culturally congruent care is to be achievable by the multidisciplinary health care team. Gender roles and expectations about members of the health care team are variable. Within certain cultures, it may be unacceptable for women to become physicians and provide care for male patients; conversely, it may be unacceptable for men to become nurses and provide care for female patients (Purnell & Paulanka, 2008; St. Hill, Lipson, & Meleis, 2003). In some cultures there may not be a word or concept for "psychologist," "psychiatrist," "dietician," "social worker," "physical therapist," "occupational therapist," "respiratory therapist," or "recreational therapist," thus presenting new challenges for health care professionals in Western society. For example, there is no word in Korean for psychologist or psychiatrist; mental illness is highly stigmatized, with clients and families encountering great difficulties when mental illness occurs (Donnelly, 1992, 2005). In some countries, nurses may be trained to perform radiologic procedures and physical therapy interventions (Lattanzi & Purnell, 2006). This broad diversity calls for students, nurses, the nursing profession, and other health care professionals to become active participants (and partners) in the process of developing cultural competence and actively seek and embrace a broad (even revolutionary) worldview of diversity.

ETHICAL AND LEGAL ISSUES

Culturally congruent health care is a basic human right, not a privilege (ANA, 1985, 1998a, 2001; Cameron-Traub, 2002; Douglas et al., 2009; International Council of Nurses, 1973; Leininger, 1991a, 1991b; UN,

1948; WHO, 2002, 2006); therefore every human should be entitled to culturally congruent care (see Exhibit 1.1). In addition, empirical findings clearly document the strong link between culturally congruent care and the achievement of positive health outcomes. Increasing numbers of lawsuits with clients claiming that culturally appropriate care was not rendered by hospitals, physicians, nurses, and other health care providers attest to the complicated legal issues that may arise from culturally incongruent care. Furthermore, clients are often winning their cases in court (Leininger & McFarland, 2002). The ICN *Code for Nurses* (1973), the ANA *Code of Ethics* (1985, 2001), and the *National Standards for Culturally and Linguistically Appropriate Services in Health Care* (Office of Minority Health [OMH], 2001), are several important documents that serve as direct reminders and provide guidance to health professionals. Not only are nurses and other health care providers ethically and morally obligated to provide the best culturally congruent care possible but nurses and health care providers are legally mandated to do so. Within the scope of professional practice, nurses and other health professionals are expected to actively seek out ways to promote culturally congruent care as an essential part of professional practice. For example, the discipline of social work recognizes that the "shifts in the ethnic composition of American society in the coming 45 years (U.S. Census Bureau, 2004) and the realities of racism, discrimination, and oppression combine to make cultural competence essential to effective social work practice, and thus to social work education" (Krentzman & Townsend, 2008). The essential inclusion of cultural competence from an ethical and a legal standpoint is addressed on varying levels within the disciplines of physical therapy, occupational therapy, speech-language pathology, dentistry, medicine, psychology, and social work (AAMC, 2005; ADA, 2005, 2007; APA, 1994; APTA, 2008; Gerstein et al., 2009; Lubinski & Matteliano, 2008; NASW, 2001, 2007, 2009; Nochajski & Matteliano, 2008; Panzarella & Matteliano, 2008; Ponterotto et al., 2010; Suh, 2004).

Exhibit 1.1   Tracing the legal right to healthcare: International and U.S. law

Kevin Antoine, J.D.
Chief Diversity Officer
State University of New York (SUNY) Downstate
Brooklyn, New York

Sixty years ago the United States ratified the constitution of the World Health Organization (WHO), which recognized healthcare as a fundamental right.[1] Emerging from the end of World War II as the leader of the free world, the United States was the driving force in drafting the constitution of the WHO, the United Nations Charter (UN Charter), and the Universal Declaration of Human Rights (UDHR). Each of these documents recognizes a legal right to healthcare and advocates the involvement of many sectors of society in removing barriers to healthcare access and treatment.[2]

Ratification of an international treaty is the only act under the American constitution that gives an international treaty legal status in the United States. The American constitution requires that the Senate ratify (give its advice and consent) an international treaty with a two-thirds vote.[3] Once the Senate ratifies an international treaty, that treaty becomes national law in the United States, equivalent to a federal statute.[4]

The American Senate ratified the UN Charter in 1945[5] (giving legal effect also to the UDHR and the WHO Constitution, both of which are authorized by the UN Charter), and the United States was one of the original countries to sign the UDHR and the WHO Constitution in 1948. In 1992, the American Senate also ratified the International Covenant on Civil and Political Rights (ICCPR), which establishes universal standards for the protection of basic civil and political liberties and a fundamental right to health care.[6]

Arguably, the UN Charter, the WHO constitution, and the UDHR have been the law in the United States since at least the 1940s, and the ICCP has been law since 1992. Under the *last in time rule,* only a later enacted federal statute can supercede them.[7] The last in time rule was established by the U.S. Supreme Court in the case of *Ping v U.S. (1889).* In 1858, the United States and China ratified a treaty addressing immigration between the two countries, granting reciprocal rights of unrestricted travel between them. In 1888, subsequent to the discovery of gold in California, the United States Congress enacted a federal statue severely limiting Chinese laborers from entering the United States, which violated the terms of the 1858 treaty.

In upholding the federal statute, the U.S. Supreme Court held that a federal statute could supercede a treaty if enacted after ratification of the treaty, and a treaty could supercede a federal statute if ratified after the enactment of a federal statute.[8] There have been no later enacted federal statutes that repealed the U.S. Senate ratification of the United Nations Charter. Therefore, Americans have had a right to health care since 1948.

With the right to healthcare established as a fundamental right in 1948, healthcare delivery must comply with the American Constitution's equal protection clause of the Fourteenth Amendment.[9] Whether a private provider or a single payer public system provides health care, compliance with the Fourteenth Amendment's equal protection clause would uniformly address the unfair, unjust, and avoidable causes of ill health.

A reconstituted Department of Health and Human Services could regulate oversight of the process. It would be able to address issues of health inequity in a way similar to how the U.S. International Trade Commission (ITC) monitors international and national compliance with American intellectual property law[10] and the Equal Employment Opportunity Commission's power to prohibit discrimination in both private and public employment.

The United States recognized a legal right to healthcare when it ratified the World Health Organization's constitution, the United Nations' Charter, and the Universal Declaration of Human Rights more than sixty years ago. The Obama administration must muster the political will necessary to implement healthcare as a fundamental right into the national policy of the United States.

---

[1] World Health Organization's Constitution.
[2] Articles 55 and 56 of the UN Charter, Article 25 of the UDHR, Article 1 of the WHO Constitution.
[3] Article 2 Section 2 of the U.S. Constitution.
[4] Article 6 of the U.S. Constitution.
[5] Office of the Historian, U.S. State Department.
[6] Jimmy Carter, *U.S. Finally Ratifies Human Rights Covenant*. The Carter Center (1992).
[7] Ping v US, 130 US 581 (1889).
[8] Martin, Schnably, Wilson, Simon, Tushnet. *International Human Rights and Humanitarian Law: Treaties, Cases and Analysis* (2006).
[9] The laws of a state must treat an individual in the same manner as others in similar conditions and circumstances.
[10] International Trade Commission Web site.

To "assist, support, facilitate, or enhance" culturally competent care, Leininger (1991a) proposed three modes for guiding nursing decision and actions: (a) culture care preservation and/or maintenance; (b) culture care accommodation and/or negotiation; and (c) culture care repatterning and/or restructuring that also have multidisciplinary relevance. Because culturally congruent care can only occur when culture care values, expressions, or patterns are known and used appropriately (Leininger, 1995a), a systematic, thorough cultural assessment is a necessary precursor to planning and implementing care (AACN, 2008, 2009; AAMC, 2005; Andrews, 1992; Andrews & Boyle, 2008; APA, 1994; APTA, 2008; Campinha-Bacote, 2003; Giger & Davidhizar, 2008; JCAHO, 2008; Lattanzi & Purnell, 2006 Leininger, 2002a, 2002c; Lubinski & Matteliano, 2008; NASW, 2001, 2007, 2009; Nochajski & Matteliano, 2008; Panzarella & Matteliano, 2008; Purnell & Paulanka, 2008; Spector, 2009). Assessment, planning, implementing, and evaluating culturally congruent care requires active, ongoing learning based on theoretical support and empirical evidence. The goal of culturally congruent care can only be achieved through the process of developing (learning and teaching) cultural competence (Jeffreys, 2006).

BARRIERS

Professional goals, societal needs, ethical considerations, and legal issues all declare the need to prioritize cultural competence development, necessitating a conscious, committed, and transformational change in current nursing practice, education, and research (Jeffreys, 2002). Although nursing and other health care professions can be transformed through the teaching of transcultural nursing (Andrews, 1995; Leininger, 1995a, 1995b; Leininger & McFarland, 2002, 2006), two major barriers prevent a rapid effective transformation. One major barrier is the lack of faculty and advanced practice nurses formally prepared in transcultural nursing and in the teaching of transcultural nursing (AACN, 2008, 2009; Andrews, 1995; Jeffreys, 2002; Leininger, 1995b; Ryan, Carlton, & Ali, 2000). The second major barrier is the limited research evaluating the effectiveness of teaching interventions on the development of cultural competence (Jeffreys, 2002). These two barriers are further complicated by the (a) changing demographics of students and health care professionals and (b) severe shortage of nurses and nursing faculty. Other health professions have also acknowledged the lack of diversity within their respective fields as well as the lack of faculty prepared to incorporate substantive cultural competence education within professional education as severe barriers to effective transformation (AAMC, 2005; ADA, 2007; APA, 1994; APTA, 2008; Gerstein, et al., 2009; Kazdin, 2008a, 2008b; Lubinski & Matteliano, 2008; NASW, 2001, 2007; Nochajski & Matteliano, 2008; Panzarella & Matteliano, 2008; Ponterotto, et al., 2010; Rosenkoetter & Nardi, 2007). Several of these factors are highlighted in the following sections.

Parts II and III of this book present action strategies, innovations, and practical examples for cultural competence education and evaluation aimed at overcoming barriers and invigorating an effective transformation that reaches beyond competence to "optimal" cultural competence. The goal of optimal cultural competence recognizes that cultural competence is not an end product, but an ongoing developmental process; therefore individuals, groups, and organizations can continually "improve," striving for "peak performance" outcomes or standards of excellence. Steps essential for optimal cultural competence development include: self-assessment, active promotion, systematic inquiry, decisive action, innovation, measurement, and evaluation.

CHANGING DEMOGRAPHICS OF STUDENTS AND HEALTH CARE PROFESSIONALS

The projected increase in immigration, globalization, and minority population growth has the potential to enrich the diversity of the nursing profession and to help meet the needs of an expanding culturally diverse society (Barbee & Gibson, 2001; Bessent, 1997; Bosher & Pharris, 2009; DHHS, 2000; Griffiths & Tagliareni, 1999; Grossman & Jorda,

2008; Harvath, 2008; Schumacher, Risco, & Conway, 2008; Tagliareni, 2008; Tucker-Allen & Long, 1999; Villaruel, Canales, & Torres, 2001; Wilson, 2007; Yoder, 2001). What has actually occurred is that the dramatic shift in demographics, the restructured workforce, and a less academically prepared college applicant pool have created a more diverse nursing applicant pool (Bosher & Pharris, 2009; Grossman & Jorda, 2008; Harvath, 2008; Hegge & Hallman, 2008; Kelly, 1997; Schumacher et al., 2008; Tagliareni, 2008; Tayebi, Moore-Jazayeri, & Maynard, 1998). Nursing students today represent greater diversity in age, ethnicity and race, gender, primary language, prior educational experience, family's educational background, prior work experience, and enrollment status than ever before (Jeffreys, 2004; Tagliareni, 2008).

Today's student profile characteristics can be examined to predict the potential future impact on the nursing profession (see Table 1.1). For example, recent nursing enrollment trends suggest a steady increase among some minority groups, yet no increase has been noted among Hispanic groups (Antonio, 2001; Heller, Oros, & Durney-Crowley, 2000; Ramirez, 2009; Villaruel et al., 2001). As a result, the number of Hispanic nurses is grossly disproportionate to client populations, demanding urgent and innovative recruitment efforts. Recruitment of diverse, nontraditional student populations does not assure program completion, licensure, or entry into the professional workforce. In fact, attrition is higher among nontraditional student populations (Bosher & Pharris, 2009; Braxton, 2000; Jeffreys, 2004; Seidman, 2005, 2007). Therefore, intensive recruitment efforts must be partnered with concentrated efforts aimed at enhancing academic achievement, professional integration, satisfaction, retention, graduation, and entry into the nursing professional workforce.

Unfortunately, current employment trends in nursing indicate high turnover rates, with nurses moving from workplace to workplace. High attrition rates for new nurses leaving the nursing profession are also a major concern. The nursing shortage, high acuity of patient care, diminished resources, and an aging society emphasize the need to prioritize retention of nurses in the workplace. Alleviating the nursing shortage, optimizing opportunities for career advancement, offering incentives for educational advancement, and striving to promote professional (and workplace) satisfaction are broad objectives aimed at facilitating nurse retention.

The recruitment of foreign nurses has been one strategy implemented to alleviate the nursing shortage that has contributed to the changing profile characteristics of professional nurses. Foreign nurses are a heterogeneous group, representing much diversity in profile characteristics and in prior work experience as a registered nurse. The recruitment of foreign nurses must incorporate culturally congruent strategies to ease

Table 1.1   Select Nursing Student Trends and Potential Future Impact on the
Nursing Profession

Variable	Select Nursing Student Trends	Potential Future Impact on the Nursing Profession
Age	Consistent with global and multidisciplinary trends, the enrollment of older students in nursing programs has increased over the last decade with projected increases to persist in the future.	Age at entry into the nursing profession will be older, resulting in decreased number of work years until retirement.
Ethnicity and Race	*Enrollment*: Recent nursing enrollment trends suggest a steady increase among some minority groups, however, no increase has been noted among Hispanic groups. *Retention*: Minority groups incur higher attrition rates than nonminority groups.	Currently, white, non-Hispanic nurses of European-American heritage represent approximately 90% of all registered nurses in the United States. Mismatches between the cultural diversity in society and diversity within the nursing profession will persist into the future unless strategies for recruitment and retention are more successful.
Gender	*Men*: Although the numbers of men in nursing are increasing, they remain an underrepresented minority (6%). *Women*: Support for women entering the workforce has shifted away from encouraging traditional female professions.	Men will continue to be disproportionately underrepresented in nursing. Many academically well-qualified male and female high school students with a potential interest in nursing may never enter the nursing profession.
Language	*Enrollment*: Consistent with global and national trends in higher education, nursing programs in the United States and Canada have experienced an increase in ESL populations over the past decade. *Retention*: ESL student populations have unique learning needs and incur higher attrition rates.	Although individuals with personal lived experiences in other cultures and languages can potentially meet the needs of linguistically diverse and culturally diverse client populations, they will still be disproportionately represented within the nursing profession.

(continued)

Table 1.1   Select Nursing Student Trends and Potential Future Impact on the
Nursing Profession (*continued*)

Variable	Select Nursing Student Trends	Potential Future Impact on the Nursing Profession
Prior Educational Experience	Consistent with trends in higher education worldwide, prior educational experiences are increasingly diverse with an academically less prepared applicant pool. Increases in the number of second-degree individuals have been noted. *Retention*: Academically underprepared students incur higher attrition rates.	Nurses with degrees in other fields can enrich the nursing profession by blending multidisciplinary approaches into nursing. Nurses with academically diverse experiences may broaden the overall perspective, especially with socioeconomic and educationally diverse client populations.
Family's Educational Background	Nursing programs have also seen an increase in first-generation college students, especially among student groups traditionally underrepresented in nursing. *Retention*: First-generation college students incur higher attrition rates.	First-generation college students who become nurses have the potential to enrich the diversity of the nursing profession and reach out to various socioeconomic and educationally diverse client populations.
Prior Work Experience	A restructured workforce, welfare-to-work initiatives, displaced homemakers, popularity of midlife career changes, and health care career ladder programs have expanded the nursing applicant pool, increasing its diversity in prior work experience. Many students work full- or part-time. *Retention*: Work–family–school conflicts may interfere with academic success and retention.	New graduate nurses may enter the nursing profession with a variety of prior work experiences that have the potential to enrich the nursing profession.
Enrollment Status	Almost half of all college students attend part-time. The number of part-time nursing students, especially those with multiple role responsibilities (work and family) has increased. *Retention*: Work–family–school conflicts may interfere with academic success and retention.	Part-time students will take longer to complete their education. Entry into practice will be delayed and total number of potential work years in nursing will be decreased.

the transition into the workplace setting, create multicultural workplace harmony, and promote professional satisfaction and opportunities for career advancement (Rosenkoetter & Nardi, 2007; Sherman & Eggenberger, 2008; Zizzo & Xu, 2009). Bridging the gaps between diverse groups of nurses is essential to preventing multicultural workplace conflict and promoting multicultural workplace harmony.

PREPARING CULTURALLY COMPETENT HEALTH CARE PROFESSIONALS

Goals of culturally congruent health care and multicultural workplace harmony can only be achieved by preparing health care professionals to actively engage in the process of cultural competence. Adequate preparation necessitates a diagnostic–prescriptive plan guided by a comprehensive understanding of the teaching–learning process of cultural competency development. Such a comprehensive plan must incorporate a detailed assessment and understanding of learner characteristics. Each learner characteristic provides vital information that is integral to determining special needs and strengths.

Meeting the needs of culturally diverse learners is a growing challenge in academia, the professional workplace, and within professional associations. Because all students, nurses, and other health professionals belong to one or more cultural groups before entering professional education, they bring their patterns of learned values, beliefs, and behaviors into the academic and professional setting. Values are standards that have eminent worth, meaning, and importance in one's life; values guide behavior. These cultural values are the "powerful directive forces that give order and meaning to people's thinking, decisions, and actions" (Leininger, 1995a). Cultural values guide thinking, decisions, and actions within the student and/or nurse role as well as other aspects of their lives. Students, nurses, and other health professionals also hold numerous beliefs (ideas, convictions, philosophical opinions, or tenets) that are accepted as true without requiring evidence or proof. Beliefs are often unconsciously accepted as truths (Purnell & Paulanka, 2008).

Cultural values and beliefs unconsciously and consciously guide thinking, decisions, and actions that ultimately affect the process of learning and the outcomes of learning. High levels of cultural congruence serve as a bridge to promote positive learning experiences and positive academic and/or psychological outcomes; high levels of cultural incongruence are proposed as inversely related to positive learning experiences and academic and/or psychological outcomes (Jeffreys, 2004). Cultural congruence refers to the degree of fit between the learner's values and beliefs and the values and beliefs of their surrounding environment (Constantine, Robinson, Wilton, & Caldwell, 2002; Constantine & Watt, 2002; Gloria & Kurpius, 1996). Here, the surrounding environment refers to the environment of nursing education within the nursing profession and the educational institution, workplace, or professional association setting.

Nursing is a unique culture that reflects its own cultural style. Cultural styles are the "recurring elements, expressions, and qualities that characterize a designated cultural group through their series of action-patterns, beliefs, and values" (Leininger, 1994a, p. 155). The dominant values and norms of a cultural group guide the development of cultural styles (Leininger, 1994a, p. 155). Currently (within the United States), the culture of nursing reflects many of the dominant societal values and beliefs held in the United States. Similarly, nursing education reflects many of the Western European value systems predominant in U.S. universities. Because nursing has its own set of CVB, students must become enculturated into nursing. *Enculturation* is a learning process whereby students learn to take on or live by the values, norms, and expectations of the nursing profession (Leininger, 2002a). Sufficient assistance during enculturation adjustment can minimize acculturation stress and enhance enculturation.

Another unique challenge facing nurse educators is to enculturate foreign-educated physicians and other second-career individuals who are entering nursing programs (Grossman & Jorda, 2008; Hegge & Hallman, 2008; Johnson & Johnson, 2008). Unfortunately, cultural competence as a priority professional value received delayed popularity among the nursing profession overall, with little emphasis or inclusion in nursing curricula, practice, research, theory, administration, and the literature. Consequently, today's nurse educators may be inadequately prepared to enculturate students into the new era of the nursing profession that embraces cultural diversity and supports cultural competence development. Similarly, within other health disciplines, cultural competence as a priority or even as an essential professional value received delayed attention in professional practice settings and professional curricula, thereby contributing to a multidisciplinary health care culture poorly equipped to meet the culture-specific care needs of diverse patients in a multicultural workplace environment.

Although increases in culturally diverse students have been noted in higher education and in nursing, the values and beliefs underlying nursing education have been slow to change in accordance with changing student population needs. Ethnocentric tendencies and cultural blindness have been major obstacles to the needed changes in nursing education. Ethnocentric tendencies refer to the belief that the values and beliefs traditionally held within nursing education are supreme. Consequently, traditional teaching–learning practices are upheld. Too often, cultural blindness exists in nursing education. Within the context of nursing education, *cultural blindness* is the inability to recognize the different CVB that exist among diverse student populations. Because cultural blindness does not acknowledge that differences exist, cultural imposition of dominant nursing education values and beliefs undoubtedly occur. Cultural imposition can cause cultural shock, cultural clashes, cultural pain, and cultural assault among students whose CVB are incongruent with the dominant nursing CVB (Jeffreys, 2004).

Nurse educators are challenged to explore various CVB within nursing, nursing education, higher education, and student cultures and to make culturally sensitive and appropriate decisions, actions, and innovations. Table 1.2 selectively compares and contrasts CVB of nursing education, higher education, and four other cultural groups. Based on a review of the literature, traditional views within the identified cultures were included but are in no way meant to stereotype individuals within the cultures. Readers are cautioned about making stereotypes and are reminded to explore CVB of individual learners. It is beyond the scope of this book to provide in-depth explanations about each category, yet the importance of an in-depth understanding must be recognized. The selective approach is meant to spark interest, stimulate awareness, and encourage further exploration among educators before attempting the design of culturally relevant and congruent educational strategies. This approach is critical, because the need to understand, respect, maintain, and support the different CVB of culturally diverse learners is a precursor to culturally relevant and competent education (Abrums, 2001; Bosher & Pharris, 2009; Crow, 1993; Davidhizar, Dowd, & Giger, 1998; Labun, 2002; Manifold & Rambur, 2001; Rew, 1996; Sommer, 2001; Tucker-Allen & Long, 1999; Villaruel et al., 2001; Weaver, 2001; Williams & Calvillo, 2002; Yoder, 1996; Yoder & Saylor, 2002; Yurkovich, 2001).

The teaching–learning process of cultural competence must consider the various philosophies and approaches to learning. Whether the teacher is perceived to be an authority figure, partner, coach, mentor, professional, or member of a service occupation will influence the teaching–learning process (see Table 1.2). Preferred teaching–learning styles may be active (learner-centered) or passive (teacher-centered). Although student-centered learning has long been advocated, nursing curricula have been slow to embrace this philosophy and to address the needs of diverse learner styles (Bellack, 2008). Teaching–learning strategies perceived as fun and likable by some may be perceived as aggressive (debate), competitive (gaming), threatening (Web-based, role-playing, or small group activity), boring (rote memorization), and/or irrelevant by others. Learner goals and philosophies that emphasize the "process" of learning focus on

Table 1.2   Comparison of Select Cultural Values and Beliefs

	Nursing Education	Higher Education	Chinese-American	African-American	Mexican-American	Irish-American
Orientation	Individual	Individual	Group	Group	Group	Individual
Time Perception	Present and future oriented. Punctuality valued.	Present and future oriented. Punctuality valued.	History of past important. Traditionally, lateness for appointments is expected. More recently, lateness is considered rude.	Present oriented Punctuality less important	Present oriented Relaxed punctuality	Past, present, future Flexible sense of time.
Verbal Communication	Direct, specific, and quick communication preferred. Expects individuals to indicate when something is not understood.	Depending on discipline, may have more or less elaboration and speed may not be as much of a priority as in the fast-paced health care setting common to nursing.	Moderate to low tones preferred. Loud tone associated with anger. Answers "yes" when asked if something is understood Reluctant to talk about feelings and views.	Loud tones (in comparison to other cultures) are preferred. Views and feelings are shared openly with family and trusted friends.	Personal topics may be taboo. Feelings and views only shared with trusted family and friends. "Small talk" expected to begin communication encounter.	Low contextual language where meaning is explicit rather than implicit. Personal topics are private. Thoughts and feelings shared only with close family and friends.
Nonverbal Communication	Most often consistent with dominant societal values, such as direct eye contact, handshaking, and spatial distances.	Same as nursing education	Avoid direct eye contact, especially with persons of authority and highly respected individuals.	Direct eye contact is sometimes perceived as aggressive.	Avoid direct eye contact, especially with persons of authority and highly respected individuals. Handshaking demonstrates respect.	Direct eye contact is maintained, indicating respect and trust.
Household Responsibilities	The "traditional" student did not have household or outside responsibilities. Student role is primary.	Same as nursing education. Community colleges have expanded services available to accommodate adult learner with multiple role responsibilities. Examples: weekend or evening college, day care center	Household responsibilities shared, however, specific roles expected based on gender. Male is head of family.	Household responsibilities may be divided between men and women and children. Woman is often head of family.	Household responsibilities mainly part of female role. Male dominance with male as head of family. Modesty.	Traditionally, household responsibilities part of female role; however, in recent years responsibilities shared between men and women.
Health	Professes "holistic" view of health but still strongly based on medical model with focus on symptom alleviation, use of technology, and Western medicine.	Health is not the major focus of institutions of higher education. In recent years, many colleges have eliminated or relaxed graduation requirements for courses in health, fitness, and/or physical education.	Balance between "yin and yang"	"Health is viewed as a harmony with nature."	Balance between "hot and cold."	Determined by external forces.
Nurse	"Professional". Seeking more respect from other health professionals and society.	In comparison to other disciplines, nursing had a late start in higher education. May be viewed as a vocation rather than profession.	Respected as authority figures after physicians. Nurses with advanced education are more highly respected than are nurses with less education.	Respected member of the health care team but less important than physicians.	Respected member of the health care team, however often viewed as an outsider.	Nurses are respected as members of a service-oriented field or "occupation."

Education	Within the nursing culture, disputes surrounding minimal educational requirements still persist.	Minimal education for tenure and promotion is the doctorate, although masters degree may be minimal at the community colleges.	Highly valued, especially a college education.	Highly valued, especially a college education.	Education is valued, however, access to college education has been limited historically. Families often expect females to put family first.	Education is highly valued.
Teaching and Learning	Traditional pedagogy viewed teacher as "authority" who "transmits" learning to student. Newer proponents of androgogy view teacher as partner or facilitator of learning who implements learner-centered approaches.	Same. Teaching role and load has greater emphasis at community colleges. Teaching role may be secondary to scholarly activity, publication, and research at senior colleges and research institutions.	Authority figure. True equality does not exist, therefore concept of "partner" in learning may be difficult to comprehend. High expectation within group to excel academically.	Respected authority figure. Historically, unequal opportunities for advancing education. Disproportionate numbers receive primary and secondary education in at-risk school districts, (educational disadvantaged).	Teacher is viewed as a highly respected superior. Rote learning and memorization predominates education in Mexico with little emphasis on practical application, analysis, and synthesis.	Respected professional.
Work Habits	Speed, accuracy, quality, and cost-effectiveness are valued. Completion of tasks and "keeping busy" traditionally valued.	"Keeping busy" is less valued than high quality, scholarly productivity, especially at senior colleges and research institutions.	Speed in working is not a priority. Hard work is valued.	Hard work is valued.	Work is secondary to family and other life activities. May be uncomfortable with authority persons checking work.	Hard work highly valued.
Autonomy	Competition with authority. Assertive. Autonomous decision-making within the scope of nursing practice expected.	Competitive, assertive. Academic freedom highly valued. Democratic governance, faculty-developed curricula, and professional unions/organizations valued.	Defers to person in authority, often seeking approval before making decisions. Avoids conflict and values harmony.	Self-reliance and autonomy encouraged within group. Past discrimination experiences may discourage autonomy. Females are often head of household and decision-makers.	Defers to person in authority with males as dominant decision-makers. Input of others is considered in decision-making. Autonomy for females is more difficult than for males. Avoids competition and conflict.	Autonomy and independence outside the family is encouraged while family loyalty is still maintained.
Help-Seeking Behaviors	Individual is expected to initiate help-seeking behaviors.	Same.	Stigma for seeking help for emotional disorders & stress. May be reluctant to approach for help by attempting to "save face"	Varied. May seek help within own social network before seeking outside help.	Varied. May seek help within own social network before seeking outside help.	May delay seeking help. Denial of problems is a way of coping with physical and emotional problems.
Persistence	Nursing is "hard work". Withdrawal from a nursing course is acceptable for academic and/or personal circumstances and should be decided by the individual.	Among disciplines outside of nursing, nursing may not be perceived as "hard work" or academically rigorous/challenging work for academically strong students. Views on withdrawal similar to nursing education.	Hard work is highly respected. Withdrawal decisions may be difficult and may include the family.	Withdrawal decisions may be difficult, especially if families have sacrificed greatly to assist student with educational endeavors.	Withdrawal decisions may be difficult, especially if families have sacrificed greatly to assist student with educational endeavors. Decisions may include the family. Withdrawal would be acceptable if interfering with family responsibilities.	Withdrawal decisions may be difficult because academic or personal problem must first be acknowledged.

Information obtained from: Andrews & Boyle, 1999; Campinha-Bacote, 1998a; Leininger & McFarland, 2002; Purnell & Paulanka, 2003. Adapted from Jeffreys, 2004.

the journey of "becoming" culturally competent through the integration of cognitive, practical, and affective learning. Process learners recognize that the journey itself is the "learning"; obstacles, mistakes, and hardships along the way are part of the expected developmental process that requires extra effort, sincere commitment, motivation, and persistence. Process learners realize that there is no final end product labeled "cultural competence," rather cultural competence is dynamic and ongoing. In contrast, "product" learners are focused on obtaining an end product through the mastery of content. Memorizing a multitude of "facts" about a culture becomes important rather than comprehensively understanding, applying, and appreciating the cultural context or rationale behind the "fact." There is less concern with how to learn to apply knowledge and develop skills, and even less concern with affective learning (values, attitudes, and beliefs). Product learners would be greatly disturbed, dissatisfied, and poorly motivated with an approach that views the end point for becoming culturally competent as infinite.

Perceived barriers to learning, mismatches in teacher–learner expectations, and poor learning experiences will hinder the learning process of cultural competence. For example, faculty beliefs that nonminority students are less confident in caring for culturally different clients than minority students is stereotypical and inaccurate (Jeffreys, 2000; Jeffreys & Smodlaka, 1998, 1999a, 1999b; Lim, Downie, & Nathan, 2004). Similarly, the belief that minority nurses are intrinsically equipped to care for culturally diverse clients is also inaccurate and negates the uniqueness of the many cultures that comprise the federally recognized "minority" group categories and disregards the many cultures that comprise nonminority groups. The danger is that minority students' and nurses' special educational needs with respect to providing culturally congruent care for many different groups of culturally different clients (different in culture from care provider) may be ignored. Expectations that are more, less, or different, based solely on ethnic or racial background, are grossly inadequate, because other diverse profile characteristics and their potential influence on learning must be objectively appraised.

Meeting the needs of learners representing diversity in age, ethnicity and race, gender, primary language, prior educational experience, family's educational background, prior work experience, and/or enrollment means embracing a broader, inclusive worldview that appreciates various forms of diversity. Awareness of how each profile variable can potentially influence learning is a necessary first step in understanding the multidimensional process of cultural competence development. For example, the learning needs and expectations of foreign-educated learners may be very different from what educators initially perceive, creating an obstacle for learning, achievement, and satisfaction (Billings

& Kowalski, 2008; Grossman & Jorda, 2008; Jalili-Grenier & Chase, 1997; Sherman & Eggenberger, 2008; Zizzo & Yu, 2009). Acculturation stress, adaptation, assimilation, CVB toward education, experiences with second language, and expectations can impact greatly upon learning and achievement (Bosher & Pharris, 2009; Flege & Liu, 2001; Fuertes & Westbrook, 1996; Jalili-Grenier & Chase, 1997; Kataoka-Yahiro & Abriam-Yago, 1997; Kurz, 1993; Manifold & Ramdur, 2001; Olenchak & Hebert, 2002; Smart & Smart, 1995; Upton & Lee-Thompson, 2001). Other stressors that may affect specific subgroups in nursing include: perceived cultural incongruence (Constantine et al., 2002; Maville & Huerta, 1997), perceived (or fear of) discrimination and bias (Bosher & Pharris, 2009; Kirkland, 1998), student (learner) role incongruence (Chartrand, 1990), maternal role stress (Gigliotti, 1999, 2001), perceived multiple role stress (Courage & Godbey, 1992; Gigliotti, 1999; Gigliotti, 2001; Greenhaus & Beutell, 1985; Lambert & Nugent, 1994; Loerch, Russell, & Rush, 1989), and gender role identity stress (Baker, 2001; Constantine et al., 2002; Patterson & Morris, 2002; Streubert, 1994). In addition, students who work in the health care field as unlicensed personnel, licensed practical nurses, or health care paraprofessionals may have difficulty adjusting to a new role, new worldview, and critical thinking and decision making within a nursing perspective that is guided by the professional scope of nursing practice (Jeffreys, 2004; Sweet & Fusner, 2008). Second-career students entering nursing may also bring new visions; however, second-career nursing students and graduates in accelerated programs present new challenges for professional socialization and integration (Penprase & Koczara, 2009).

New graduate nurses may experience reality shock with their new professional role, workload, and responsibilities; experienced nurses may encounter burnout. Inactive nurses returning to the workforce after a gap in work experience benefit from refresher courses and other transitional strategies to ease them into the new workplace environment (Hammer & Craig, 2008). Recently, researchers have begun to realize the need to explore the relationships between psychological distress, effort–reward imbalance, and the nursing work environment among different generations: Baby boomers, Generation X, and Generation Y (Lavoie-Tremblay et al., 2008). The generation of the Millennials challenges educators to keep pace with the social and educational technologies that these learners expect (Bellack, 2009; Zalon, 2008). For example, the net generation (1980 to 2004) expects technology, participates actively in the learning process, wants immediate response to learning, multitasks, prefers group work, and enjoys being mentored by older generations. In contrast, Generation X (1960 to 1980) are self-directed learners who are less technology proficient, can delay gratification, and seek learning with practical application.

Baby boomers (1940 to 1960) are generally less technology proficient, because technology is viewed as a new approach rather than an expected approach, are more familiar with passive learning styles, and expect a caring and connected work environment (Billings & Kowalski, 2004).

The nursing profession has the challenging opportunity to meet the unique needs of various populations of nurses, improve nurse retention, decrease the nursing shortage, and promote cultural competence. Evidence-based transitional programs, specialized orientation programs, ongoing employee workshops, refresher courses that integrate the values, skills, and knowledge needed for cultural competence in the workplace have the potential to address these needs. Unfortunately, state and certifying boards/associations have varied continuing education (CE) and competency requirements for license renewal and reentry (Yoder-Wise, 2009) and none require documentation of CE programs in cultural competence. Among other health professionals, inconsistencies in licensure renewal, certification, CE, and practice requirements also exist. For example, physicians licensed in New Jersey are now required to complete CE in cultural competence, yet this is not a universal medical requirement throughout the United States. Professional inconsistencies (in any discipline) may translate into questioning the need for the requirement, decreased motivation, resentment, and lack of commitment on the part of the professional, thereby defeating the overall goal of actively engaging the health professional in lifelong commitment to cultural competence development.

CULTURAL COMPETENCE AND CONFIDENCE

Despite the numerous complexities, changes, and challenges faced by many nursing students and nurses today, some individuals are more actively engaged in cultural competence development whereas others are not. Some individuals are more motivated to pursue cultural competence development and are more committed to the goal of culturally congruent care than others. Therefore, the evaluation of factors that may influence motivation, persistence, and commitment for cultural competency development is a necessary precursor to any educational design strategy. Confidence (self-efficacy) is one such factor that is emphasized in this book. According to Bandura (1986), the construct of self-efficacy is the individuals' perceived confidence for learning or performing specific tasks or skills necessary to achieve a particular goal. Furthermore, self-efficacy is the belief that one can perform or succeed at learning a specific task, despite obstacles and hardships, and will expend whatever energy is necessary to accomplish the task (Bandura, 1986). Consequently, confidence is inextricably linked as a major component in cultural competence development and an influencing factor in the achievement of culturally congruent care. Confidence is an integral component in the action-strategy acronym "COMPETENCE," introduced and illustrated in the next chapter. The acronym may be used by the multidisciplinary health care team to: (a) guide clinical practice with culturally diverse patients and (b) promote multicultural workplace harmony and prevent multicultural workplace conflict among culturally diverse health care workers. Later, Chapter 3 proposes a new conceptual model to understand and guide cultural competence education, research, and practice.

KEY POINT SUMMARY

- Rapid growth in worldwide migration, changes in demographic patterns, varying fertility rates, increased numbers of multiracial and multiethnic individuals, and advanced technology contribute to cultural evolution.
- Culturally congruent health care refers to health care that is customized to fit with the client's cultural values, beliefs, traditions, practices, and lifestyle.
- Health care professionals and organizations are challenged to go beyond the goal of achieving "competence" (minimum standard) toward the goal of achieving "optimal" cultural competence (standard of excellence).
- Educators everywhere are additionally challenged to learn how to lead the quest for culturally congruent health care by implementing creative, evidence-based educational activities that promote positive cultural competence learning outcomes for culturally diverse students and health care professionals aiming to reach beyond minimal competence to the achievement of optimal cultural competence.
- Two major barriers prevent a rapid effective transformation through transcultural education: (a) lack of faculty and advanced practice nurses formally prepared in transcultural nursing and in the teaching of transcultural nursing; and (b) limited research evaluating the effectiveness of teaching interventions on the development of cultural competence.
- Goals of culturally congruent health care and multicultural workplace harmony can only be achieved by preparing (teaching) health care professionals to actively engage in the (learning) process of cultural competence.

- Meeting the needs of learners representing diversity in age, ethnicity and race, gender, primary language, prior educational experience, family's educational background, prior work experience,
  and/or enrollment means embracing a broader, inclusive worldview that appreciates various forms of diversity and must consider
  the various philosophies and approaches to learning.
- Confidence (self-efficacy) is an important factor that may influence
  motivation, persistence, and commitment for cultural competency
  development.

CHAPTER 2

Dynamics of Diversity: Becoming Better Health Care Providers through Cultural Competence

Marianne R. Jeffreys, EdD, RN

Every day, nurses and other health care providers have the potential to make a positive difference in human lives by providing high-quality health care. But how do nurses and other health care providers make the greatest positive difference? How MUST nurses and health care providers in the 21st century provide quality health care amid the increasingly multicultural and global society?

The answer is twofold. First is the need to provide culturally competent, that is, culturally specific, nursing care, which is customized to fit with the patient's own cultural values, beliefs (CVB), traditions, practices, and lifestyle (Leininger, 2002c; Leininger & McFarland, 2002, 2006). Quality health care can only occur within the patient's cultural context. Second is the need to create workplaces that embrace diversity among health care professionals and that seek to promote multicultural workplace harmony and prevent multicultural workplace conflict. Both

This chapter was excerpted and adapted from Jeffreys, M.R. (2006a), Cultural competence in clinical practice. *Imprint, 53*(2), 36–41 and Jeffreys, M. R. (2008a), Dynamics of diversity: Becoming better nurses through diversity awareness. *Imprint. 55*(5), 36–41. By permission, National Student Nurses' Association.

of these endeavors begin with diversity self-awareness and diversity awareness; each is defined below. Several poignant clinical and workplace examples illustrate the significance of actively weaving cultural competence throughout all aspects of health care settings. Later, the acronym "COMPETENCE" is presented to assist health care professionals in remembering essential elements for optimal cultural competence development.

DIVERSITY AWARENESS

Diversity *self-awareness* occurs when one engages in active reflection about one's own cultural identity or identities, realizes one's own CVB, and recognizes the differences within one's own cultural group(s). Diversity *awareness* refers to an active, ongoing conscious process in which one becomes proactively aware of similarities and differences within and between various cultural groups, necessitating cultural assessment of patients and cultural sharing among health care professionals. Assessment and sharing should aim to maximize health outcomes and facilitate multicultural workplace harmony and collaboration. Diversity awareness will be most comprehensive if one recognizes the diversity of diversity and how various characteristics of diversity may influence the plan of care and/or professional collaboration. "Diversity may exist based on birthplace, citizenship status, reason for migration, migration history, food, religion, ethnicity, race, language, kinship and family networks, educational background and opportunities, employment skills and opportunities, lifestyle, gender, socioeconomic status (class), politics, past discrimination and bias experiences, health status and health risk, age, insurance coverage, and other variables that go well beyond the restrictive labels of a few ethnic and/or racial groups" (p. 5).

IS DIVERSITY AWARENESS REALLY THAT IMPORTANT FOR PATIENT CARE?

Ignoring diversity and providing culturally incongruent nursing care can adversely affect patient outcomes and jeopardize patient safety. Let's consider a nurse who has some knowledge about transcultural nursing but lacks self-confidence about performing cultural assessments and planning culturally specific care. The nurse then avoids conducting cultural assessments. Later, the nurse administers insulin and then leaves a tray of culturally forbidden foods with a diabetic patient. This nursing action is culturally incompetent and negligent. The patient will not eat the food. Even if a new tray is ordered, the time between insulin administration and eating will be delayed. Health outcomes will be adversely affected.

Additionally, cultural pain (psychological stress that occurs from cultur-ally inappropriate actions) (Leininger, 1991a; Leininger & McFarland, 2002, 2006) is emotionally stressful and also affects metabolic rate and insulin needs. This potentially fatal situation could have been prevented by conducting a cultural assessment and by accommodating the patient's CVB, and foods into the plan of care.

Equally negligent is a nurse who does not assess patients for folk medicine use. Let's imagine a patient who regularly uses herbal teas with ginseng at home and that she has brought these with her to use in the hospital. Later, the nurse administers the heart medication digoxin. Use of ginseng in conjunction with digoxin can result in drug toxicity and death. Again, this culturally incompetent and dangerous situation could have been prevented by culturally sensitive and competent nursing actions. Lack of transcultural nursing knowledge, skills, values, and confidence can result in nurses avoiding culture care assessments when planning and implementing care. The consequences can be devastating.

Overly confident nurses who think they do not need to adequately prepare, learn, or conduct routine cultural assessments can contribute to similarly devastating results. For example, making assumptions based on patient's physical appearance rather than performing an individualized cultural assessment can cause great cultural pain and set up long-lasting barriers in communication and care. Let's consider a nurse in the coro-nary intensive care unit (ICU) who provides a patient with a booklet in Spanish entitled "Mexican foods for Heart Health" and a booklet on "Free Health Service Resources for Non-U.S. Citizens" to a multiethnic bilingual (English and Spanish-speaking) patient who self-identifies as second-generation Puerto Rican and Italian-American. These nursing ac-tions are grossly inappropriate. Cultural insensitivity can cause the patient cultural pain and anguish, resulting in stress, elevated and irregular heart rate, high blood pressure, and other physiological manifestations that will adversely affect patient outcomes. When the patient is discharged home, he/she may be reluctant to return for follow-up appointments due to the culturally insensitive care received (see Exhibit 2.1 for more examples).

Exhibit 2.1   Educator-in-Action Vignette

(Note that this vignette may be adapted to new employee orientation in a health care setting, such as during a didactic classroom discussion and role play with new employee nurses [topic: culturally competent and safe medication administration]).

Students in a medical-surgical nursing course are eager to begin their new rotation on a cardiac unit. Several students are interested in pursuing advanced practice specialties as a clinical nurse specialist or as an adult nurse practitioner. Two students are interested in critical care nursing. During the preclinical conference, Professor Hart mentions that several students will administer digoxin orally to their patients. Professor Hart asks the students about nursing implications associated with digoxin administration.

Dawn says, "I know it is important to assess the apical pulse for one full minute. If the pulse is regular and at least 60 beats/minute, I will give the digoxin to my patient. The drug handbook mentioned to check serum digoxin levels first. If the digoxin level is below range or within therapeutic range, I will administer the medication."

All of the students agree that these are the most important assessments when administering digoxin.

Martine mentions that it is also important to plan ahead for discharge and begin patient teaching right away. She notes that information about the specific cardiac problem and digoxin should also be accompanied by demonstration and return demonstration of pulse-taking techniques. All of the students agree that these are important components to include in patient teaching.

Professor Hart reminds students to incorporate culture into all aspects of nursing care, including patient teaching. She comments: "A thorough health assessment must incorporate a systematic assessment of cultural values and beliefs. Please incorporate your previously learned skills about cultural assessment into your plan each week with your patients. I will be available to assist you if needed. The clinical nurse specialist (CNS) is also a good resource person in case I am busy with another student."

After the preclinical conference, Dawn quietly says to Steven, "I don't know why Professor Hart always emphasizes culture so much. Most parts of nursing care can just be done as described in our medical-surgical procedure book. Besides, how many ways can you give an oral medication? What difference does it make? I am confident that I know all I need to know about giving such a common heart drug like digoxin."

Steven replies, "I agree with you. The patients on this unit are all here for heart problems. Hearts don't have cultural values and beliefs. We should spend more time looking at rhythm strips, cardiac enzyme results, and stress test results instead of spending time with cultural assessments."

Another student, Martine, quietly thinks: "I just don't know how to approach people who are different than me. Maybe I will get a patient who is the same culture as me. I have absolutely no confidence in interviewing patients about their cultural values and beliefs. I better not try asking any questions because I might make a mistake."

Student excerpts from clinical post-conference are listed below:

Steven: My patient was a 64-year-old woman who was a religious Muslim from Egypt. When I told her that it was important to listen to her heart before giving her the heart medication, she said she did not want to take her pill and became upset. I noticed that her heart monitor showed tachycardia and arrhythmia, especially when I started to approach her with my stethoscope. Janice was assigned to the other patient in the room. Janice overheard what was going on and asked my patient if she would prefer a female nursing student to listen to her heart. My patient was agreeable. After a few minutes, Janice assessed the apical rate and administered the medication with Professor Hart observing.

Janice: Yes, I also learned that it was important to use my right hand to place the digoxin in her mouth and offer her water using my right hand. She needed my help because she had bilateral arm casts. I was sure that cultural considerations were important to assess, however, I was not totally confident that I knew enough about how I might need to accommodate drug administration procedures to her CVB. However, I was somewhat confident that I could find out this information by asking her. Before I gave her the medicine, I asked her if she had any special preferences on how I should give her the medication. She told me that she appreciated that I cared enough to ask.

Dawn: My patient was a 75-year-old recent immigrant from China who spoke some English. Her heart rate was 72 and regular. When I brought her the digoxin to take with a cold glass of water, she did not want to take the pill. At that moment, Maria, the clinical nurse specialist (CNS), entered the room. Maria explained that, consistent with traditional Chinese beliefs, my patient preferred warm beverages. When I brought my patient some hot, decaffeinated green tea, she readily took her digoxin. I guess I was overly confident about how easy it would be to administer medications without realizing cultural beliefs and customs could really make a difference. Next time, I will try to prepare better. I appreciate now how important it is to assess patients' CVB and provide culture-specific care in all aspects of care. I also appreciate the importance of collaborating with other nurses, especially the CNS who had some background knowledge about Chinese culture and my patient.

Maria also explained to me that patient teaching about digoxin started yesterday. I was surprised to hear that although there were several nurses, pharmacists, and physicians in the hospital who spoke Chinese, only one nurse (Ming) spoke the dialect understood by my patient. I thought everyone in China spoke the same language and could understand each other. I had the opportunity to speak with Ming about my patient's discharge teaching plan. Ming explained that while it was important to preserve and accommodate some of my patient's traditional values, beliefs, and health practices within the care plan, there were others that necessitated repatterning. My patient often used herbal teas at home containing ginseng; use of ginseng can result in digoxin toxicity. Before today, I did not think that detailed questions concerning herbal and dietary practices were important. Again, I was too confident that I knew everything there was to know about a particular medicine, rather than recognizing the need to individualize this to my patient's CVB, and practices. I guess I needed repatterning of my views concerning culture and safe, high-quality nursing care.

Katie: I had a similar experience. My patient would take her medication with only grapefruit juice. She told me that in Puerto Rico grapefruit juice is quite popular to promote health. After checking that there were no interactions between grapefruit juice, digoxin, and her other medications, I provided her with some juice. My patient then told me about how "hot" diseases must be treated with certain "cold" remedies. It had nothing to do with temperature. I will read about the hot and cold theory common to many Hispanic cultural groups, because I will be caring for many different patients who have many different diseases. I never realized that diseases could have different meanings and implications for patients and that these meanings could influence adherence to medication regimens.

Juanita: My patient also had digoxin ordered. He did not want to take anything by mouth because it is a religious "fasting" day. He became distressed and said he didn't want to be labeled a "difficult" patient by the staff and be ignored. Early this morning, his rhythm strips showed normal sinus rhythm with rates ranging between 74 and 86. At this time of distress about his medication, my patient's face became flushed and his pulse rate increased to 132. With my patient's permission, I contacted the hospital priest to speak with him. Afterwards, my patient was so happy because he also got to take Communion. The priest explained that it was OK to take medication orally, even on a religious fast day. My patient's pulse rate returned back to his baseline.

Martine: My patient was started on digoxin yesterday. The staff nurse asked me to reinforce patient teaching started yesterday concerning medication. I had no problem with assessing his apical pulse or getting him to take his digoxin. This was done in less than 2 minutes. I tried to look him right in the eye and then I asked him to speak up immediately if he had any questions about the medication. He turned his head away and didn't answer me right back so I left the room. I wondered what I was going to do for the rest of the day, since I had finished everything in less than 3 minutes.

However, the staff nurse sent me back to talk with the patient about discharge planning, follow-up visits, lab tests, daily self-assessment of pulse, and medication side effects. After 5 minutes, I mentally considered the nursing diagnoses: "impaired verbal communication," "noncompliance," "knowledge deficit," "ineffective coping," and "anger" for my patient. I don't think my patient liked me. I don't think he had an interest in complying with his medication regimen at home. He never looked me in the eye when I spoke to him, he used very few words to respond to me, and he kept looking at the floor during long periods of silence. When I tried to talk to him about follow-up visits at the hospital's heart-specialty clinic, he finally said that he would most likely go to the clinic on the reservation when discharged. He said he came to this hospital only because he collapsed and had a heart attack right in front of the hospital. I didn't even consider that he might live on an Indian reservation because he didn't look like an Indian—I thought he was white. At that point, I realized I probably had made many mistakes, although I really didn't understand what they were. Because I didn't have any confidence about asking questions concerning CVB, I avoided doing this. I felt really bad. On the other hand, I had been overly confident that I successfully completed all my tasks with my patient in 3 minutes. I realized that I hadn't met my patient's needs, rather I met my own needs in finishing up "tasks" using a generic approach. I told my patient I would be back soon. Then, I went to find Professor Hart.

Professor Hart and I returned to speak with my patient. This discussion revealed that he perceived the hospital environment to be threatening and "noncompliant" with his cultural feelings. No one had asked him about his cultural background, identity, values, beliefs, practices, or traditional herbal remedies. He reluctantly confided that he had been experiencing emotional stress and discomfort due to the lack of awareness, sensitivity, and understanding shown by the nurses, other health care professionals, and the organization. He termed this "lack of caring that wouldn't have occurred in the Reservation's Clinic." I realized that these culturally insensitive and incongruent incidents caused cultural pain and adversely affected my patient's well-being and health outcomes. For example, elevated heart rates and hypertension during hospitalization may have been influenced by stress caused by cultural pain. At this point, I felt so totally incompetent and questioned if I could ever become a good nurse. What should I do next? I was so confused. I was glad that Professor Hart intervened so I watch and learn how to become a culturally competent nurse.

After expressing regret and sincere concern over the factors that had caused my patient cultural pain, Professor Hart assured him that every effort would be made to provide culturally specific and congruent care. Next, Professor Hart performed a detailed and systematic cultural assessment that provided valuable information for designing a culturally specific care plan. In addition to the obvious mistakes that I made previously, I learned about several other barriers to achieving positive patient outcomes with my patient. One barrier to effective communication was my misinterpretation of my patient's periods of silence in conversation and avoidance of eye contact as indicating lack of interest. Actually, among many traditional Native American groups, silence is expected to enhance understanding and exemplifies respect for the other person. Avoidance of eye contact also indicates respect and that the person is paying close attention to what is being said. I will work very hard to prevent cultural mistakes and misinterpretations again; I realize the importance of conducting a thorough cultural assessment on all patients—it must not be avoided. Cultural competence is important!

Professor Hart encouraged questions and elaborated on the various customs and beliefs "discovered" by the students. She provided students with some additional examples using different cultural groups, reminding students to individually appraise each patient to avoid stereotypes. At the end of the discussion, Professor Hart asked students to reflect and write about the most important learning. Review of the written reflections would guide her on future assignments, teaching–learning strategies, and students' cultural competence development. Written feedback, returned to students the following week, would provide encouragement and guidance to continue on their journey for culturally congruent patient care.

Malpractice cases today may involve issues concerning cultural in-competence. Patients and family members are often winning settlements because culturally specific health care was not provided and then resulted in physical and/or emotional injury. Cases documenting the wrongful institutionalization or prolonged hospitalization of patients demonstrat-ing severe side effects of certain medications should alert nurses and physicians to screen patients' ethnic and genetic background. For ex-ample, Hispanics, Arabs, Asians, and African Americans may require lower doses of psychotropic medications (such as antidepressants) than the commonly published recommended doses (Andrews & Boyle, 2002). The growing field of ethnopharmacology documents genetic differences in how drugs are metabolized among various ethnic groups (Munoz & Hilgenberg, 2005; Purnell & Paulanka, 2008). Culturally competent nurses and physicians would also realize the importance of differenti-ating between the many subgroups within the broad ethnic/racial cat-egories to avoid stereotypical cultural assumptions and to recognize ethnic-specific pharmacogenetic differences. Pharmacogenetic differences in response to certain asthma drugs between Mexicans and Puerto Ricans with asthma is one example attesting to the need for more re-search and detailed cultural assessments (Burchard et al., 2004; Choudhry et al., 2005).

ACHIEVING CULTURALLY CONGRUENT CARE

The above case scenarios and Exhibit 2.1 illustrate the importance of culturally congruent care in meeting patient's holistic needs. According to Leininger (1991a), culturally congruent nursing care refers to "those cognitively based assistive, supportive, facilitative, or enabling acts or decisions that are tailor-made to fit with an individual's, group's, or insti-tution's CVB, and lifeways in order to provide meaningful, beneficial, and satisfying health care, or well-being services (p. 49). To "assist, support, facilitate, or enhance" culturally congruent care, Leininger (1991a) pro-posed three modes for guiding nursing decision and actions: (a) culture care preservation and/or maintenance; (b) culture care accommodation and/or negotiation; and (c) culture care repatterning and/or restructuring. The goal of culturally congruent care can only be achieved through the process of developing (learning) cultural competence.

Cultural competence is an ongoing, multidimensional learning process that integrates transcultural nursing skills in all three dimensions (cognitive, practical, and affective), involves transcultural self-efficacy

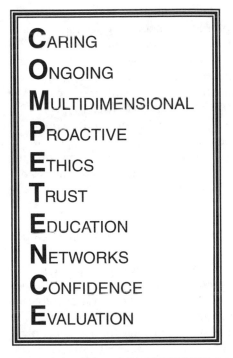

Figure 2.1   Cultural COMPETENCE Acronym for Patient Care

(confidence) as a major influencing factor, and aims to achieve culturally congruent care (Jeffreys, 2005). The acronym "COMPETENCE" is presented here to assist health care providers in remembering several essential elements for cultural competence development and achieving culturally congruent care. COMPETENCE refers to Caring, Ongoing, Multidimensional, Proactive, Ethics, Trust, Education, Networks, Confidence, and Evaluation (Figure 2.1). Each will be briefly described below:

Caring: *Demonstrate caring.*
      The essence of nursing is caring. Caring refers to actions and activities directed toward assisting, supporting, or enabling others with actual or potential needs to alleviate or improve a human condition or face death (Leininger, 1991a). Caring is essential for curing but curing is not essential for caring (Leininger, 1991a). Caring can only occur within the patients' cultural context. Patients who perceive nurses as non-caring may perceive that they have not received "care" at all. Perceptions of caring (or non-caring) can positively or negatively affect patient outcomes.

Ongoing: *Engage in ongoing cultural competence.*

Cultural competence development is ongoing. Lifelong, ongoing cultural competence development is an essential professional expectation presently and in the future. Cultural competence is not an end point or product of learning. Cultural competence is an ongoing process in which one is always attempting to "become" more culturally competent (Campinha-Bacote, 2003; Leininger & McFarland, 2002; 2006, Purnell & Paulanka, 2008). Additionally, culturally congruent care must be individually appraised, applied, and modified in an ongoing fashion throughout all aspects of patient care. Effectively weaving culture-specific care interventions throughout the care plan requires ongoing commitment and energy but will result in high quality, culturally congruent care.

Multidimensional: *Develop transcultural nursing skills in all three dimensions: cognitive, practical, and affective.*

Cultural competence in nursing is a multidimensional learning process that integrates transcultural nursing skills in all three dimensions (cognitive, practical, and affective), involves transcultural self-efficacy (confidence), and aims to achieve culturally congruent nursing care. Transcultural nursing skills are those skills necessary for assessing, planning, implementing, and evaluating culturally congruent care. Transcultural nursing skills include cognitive, practical, and affective dimensions (Jeffreys, 2000, 2005; Jeffreys & Smodlaka, 1996, 1998, 1999a, 1999b).

The cognitive learning dimension focuses on knowledge outcomes, intellectual abilities, and skills. Within the context of transcultural learning, cognitive learning skills include knowledge and comprehension about ways in which cultural factors may influence professional nursing care among patients of different cultural backgrounds and throughout various phases of the life cycle.

The practical learning dimension is similar to psychomotor learning, and focuses on motor skills or practical application of skills. Within the context of transcultural learning, practical learning skills refer to communication skills (verbal and nonverbal) needed to interview patients of different cultural backgrounds about their values and beliefs.

The affective learning dimension is concerned with attitudes, values, and beliefs and is considered most important in developing professional values and attitudes. Affective learning includes self-awareness, awareness of cultural gap (differences), acceptance, appreciation, recognition, and advocacy (Jeffreys, 2000; Jeffreys & Smodlaka, 1998). All components are essential for cultural competence development.

Proactive: *Conduct cultural assessments proactively on all patients upon initial encounter.*

Systematic cultural assessments and culture-specific care plans should be routinely initiated at the first patient contact for all patients and regularly reappraised and modified throughout nursing care interactions with patients, families, and communities. Such a proactive approach aims to actively anticipate patient needs and is preferred to a reactive approach that passively waits for patient-initiated requests, problems, misunderstandings, and cultural clashes to occur.

Ethics: *Apply ethical principles in all patient encounters.*

Culturally congruent health care is a basic human right, not a privilege (ANA, 2001, 2003, 2004, 2009; Cameron-Traub, 2002; Douglas et al., 2009; ICN, 1973; Leininger, 1991a, 1991b; UN, 1948; WHO, 2006), therefore, every human being should be entitled to culturally congruent care. The International Council of Nurses Code for Nurses (1973), the ANA Code of Ethics (2001), and the National Standards for Culturally and Linguistically Appropriate Services in Health Care (OMH, 2001) are several important documents that serve as reminders and provide guidance to health professionals. Not only are nurses and other health care providers ethically and morally obligated to provide the best culturally congruent care possible but nurses and health care providers are legally mandated to do so. Increasing numbers of lawsuits with patients claiming that culturally appropriate care was not rendered by hospitals, physicians, nurses, and other health care providers attest to the complicated legal issues that may arise from culturally incongruent care. Furthermore, patients are often winning their cases in court (Leininger & McFarland, 2002). Within the scope of professional practice, nurses and other health professionals are expected to actively seek out ways to promote culturally congruent care.

Trust: *Establish mutual trust.*

Gaining a patient's trust is a necessary first step before patients willingly share their CVB, behaviors, and practices. Until the nurse (or nursing student) has gained the patient's trust, shared information may not be entirely credible or true. Leininger (2002) advocates "moving from a mainly distrusted stranger to a trusted friend in order to obtain authentic, credible, and dependable" information (p. 91).

Education: *Participate in ongoing cultural competence education.*

All students and nurses (regardless of age, ethnicity, gender, sexual orientation, lifestyle, religion, socioeconomic status, geographic location, or race) require formalized educational experiences to meet culture care needs of diverse individuals (Andrews, 1995; Davidhizar & Giger, 2001; Jeffreys, 2000, 2002; Leininger, 1995b). At the undergraduate level, examples of formalized education to enhance cultural competence development include taking a course or series of courses in transcultural nursing or attending a transcultural nursing conference/workshop taught by qualified individuals.

Networks: *Create collaborative networks.*

Collaboration and networking with other nurses, health professionals, and organizations permit the shared pooling of necessary, specialized resources, skills, and knowledge. Within health care institutions, advanced practice nurses with a formalized educational background in general transcultural nursing skills provide on-site personal resources and referral. Advanced practice nurses with specialized education about a particular culture or cultures provide additional expertise about specific cultures. The Transcultural Nursing Society provides numerous local and global opportunities for collaboration and networking through their Web site (www.tcns.org), network of certified transcultural nurses, journal (*Journal of Transcultural Nursing*), newsletter, local chapter meetings and events, and annual conference. The Internet has made networking and dialogue with transcultural nurse experts easier than ever before.

Confidence: *Develop confidence to actively learn and perform transcultural nursing skills despite any obstacles and hardships. Avoid overly high or low confidence.*

An individual's perceived confidence (self-efficacy) for learning or performing specific tasks or skills necessary to achieve a particular goal is an important factor influencing commitment, motivation, learning, and outcome behaviors (Bandura, 1986). Individuals with low confidence for transcultural nursing skills are at risk for decreased motivation, lack of commitment, and/or avoidance of cultural considerations, when planning and implementing nursing care. Overly confident individuals are at risk for inadequate preparation in learning the transcultural nursing skills necessary to provide culturally congruent care. Individuals with strong, resilient, and realistic confidence (self-efficacy) will persist at cultural competence development despite obstacles and hardships, and will expend whatever energy is necessary (Jeffreys, 2000).

Evaluation: *Use evaluation results to improve nursing practice.*

Realistic, frequent self-appraisal of strengths, weaknesses, gaps, and barriers in the journey to develop cultural competence provides new direction for future growth and learning. Patient outcome evaluation, especially the evaluation of satisfaction and perception of culturally relevant care, provides valuable information to guide learning and nursing care decisions and actions.

DIVERSITY AWARENESS IN THE WORKPLACE

The diversity of diversity also applies to health care professionals and other coworkers—everyone belongs to one or more cultural groups. Additionally, it is important to acknowledge that diversity is dynamic or ever-changing—not static. Changes can occur within and between groups over time or individuals (and groups) can belong to different groups at different times. For example, beginning nursing students are challenged to learn the culture of nursing education and the nursing profession within the context of the cultural norms and expectations of a nursing student. Leininger (2002) refers to this as enculturation within the nursing profession. Similarly, a new graduate nurse (GN) must make the transition from a student to take on the new culture of the nursing profession as a GN (and later as a registered nurse) as well as the new organizational culture of the health care institution and the cultural nuances of a particular nursing unit. Hence, individuals—patients as well as health care professionals—belong to numerous diverse groups, each with their own unique norms, values, behaviors, and so on; yet some may be overlapping or similar.

Without appropriate diversity awareness, background knowledge, individual appraisal, and sensitivity, nurses' interactions with coworkers may adversely impact upon the workplace environment, collaboration, and patient outcomes. Consider the possible adverse effects in the following scenarios:

- Lee is a new graduate nurse who emigrated from China three years ago, prior to attending an associate degree nursing program in the United States. She graduated with a 3.5 GPA and passed the NCLEX examination in the first attempt. Her mastery of the English language in such a short time is remarkable, although she speaks with a heavy (but understandable) accent. The charge nurse assigns Lee to a Korean patient (who only speaks Korean) and says, "I am sure you will have no trouble communicating with your fellow immigrant."
- Carol is a 38-year-old white, Irish American nurse who attended a technical college for nursing five years ago as part of the state's "welfare to work initiative." She is a widowed parent of a 20-year-old, an 18-year-old, and a 3-year-old. During the weekly

multidisciplinary patient care rounds, a colleague comments about a 27-year-old single female patient with Medicaid insurance who was admitted for her third high-risk pregnancy and a history of sickle cell anemia. The colleague says, "Once someone's on public assistance, they never get off. They just get pregnant again and never want to work."

- During the weekly patient care conference, the nursing staff discusses a patient who was admitted to the hospital after a bus accident. He was traveling back to his Indian reservation when the bus collided with another vehicle. During discharge planning, one nurse says, "We usually don't get American Indian patients in this hospital. It's too bad that we don't have an Indian nurse working on our unit." Joseph, a registered nurse who self-identifies as a Black Indian (African American and Cherokee ancestry) proudly replies, "I'm Native American. We have had patients who are of Native ancestry. In fact, Mr. O'Shea in room 517 resides on one of the Mohawk reservations." The first nurse answers, "Well, I was talking about a real Indian. You and Mr. O'Shea don't look and act like real Indians." Joseph defensively replies, "What does a real Indian look like? How does a real Indian act?"

- During change of shift report, Elsa provides succinct, accurate, and pertinent details about every patient, including strategies for accommodating patient's cultural needs within the care plan. Because Elsa is reporting to Margaret, an older, more experienced nurse, Elsa has minimal direct eye contact with Margaret. Within Elsa's culture, it is considered respectful to avoid eye contact with those in authority and/or older individuals. Margaret's CVB strongly advocate direct eye contact at all times; avoidance of direct eye contact during communication is viewed as a sign of distrust. After report, Margaret tells one of her coworkers, "I just can't trust the report that Elsa gives. It is extra work to check up on everything she said."

- Juanita, a senior nursing student, says, "Because I speak Spanish fluently, many of the staff nurses and my classmates automatically think I know everything about the Puerto Rican culture and customs. Of course, I can translate information, but sometimes I feel as though some patients and families don't trust me completely because I am not Puerto Rican. It bothers me when my classmates and the staff nurses ignore my concerns. One nurse even said in front of two students 'It's all the same—Puerto Rican, Dominican, Mexican, Columbian—you all speak Spanish therefore you're all the same.' That really hurt my feelings."

PROMOTING MULTICULTURAL
WORKPLACE COMPETENCE

Legal and ethical guidelines demand that all nurses and health professionals provide culturally competent care or face consequences of negli-
gence and malpractice. Culturally competent care begins with a thorough
cultural assessment that is routinely integrated within the health assessment. Assessment, planning, implementing, and evaluating culturally
competent care requires active learning based on theoretical support, research evidence, and collaboration. Collaboration will be most effective
in an open, caring workplace environment that openly embraces a broad
view of diversity and actively engages in and encourages diversity awareness and cultural sharing among staff members.

Developing one's own cultural competence and assisting other health
professionals in their cultural competence development is a priority in
the multicultural workplace that should be emphasized in new employee
orientations, ongoing inservice educational programs, and staff meetings. Inviting guest speakers/consultants on cultural issues and cultural
competence, purchasing educational resources to enhance staff's cultural
competence, and reimbursing tuition for courses in transcultural nursing
and cultural competence (college, continuing education, and/or advanced
certificate programs) are other strategies available to foster multicultural
workplace competence (Jeffreys, 2008a). Providing high-quality, culturally competent care within a work environment that facilitates multicultural workplace harmony enhances the probability of career and workplace satisfaction—a desirable reward for any nurse. New graduates seeking employment should explore whether these opportunities are available
in prospective workplace settings.

The adapted acronym of "COMPETENCE" (Figure 2.2) can assist health care providers in remembering several essential elements for
developing multicultural workplace competence. Professional goals, societal needs, ethical considerations, and legal issues all declare the need to
prioritize cultural competence development (Jeffreys, 2002). Health care
providers can incorporate "COMPETENCE" into all aspects of their current and future professional role. The challenge remains as to whether or
not individuals will actively engage in cultural competence development
of self and others, despite real and/or perceived barriers. Overcoming
skepticism, challenging the status quo, and creating a new vision for
professional nursing that actively advocates culturally congruent care for
all patients require a strong commitment, energy, and motivation. Nurses
and other health care professionals are invited to create energetic interdisciplinary networks to develop new, innovative strategies that maximize

MULTICULTURAL WORKPLACE	
Caring	sincerely about one's own and co-workers' cultural values, and beliefs (CVB) is the first step toward developing multicultural workplace competence
Ongoing	diversity awareness and sharing of CVB among co-workers fosters a workplace climate that openly embraces diversity and encourages dialogue
Multidimensional	aspects of multicultural workplace competence include cognitive (knowledge), practical (communication skills), and affective (attitudes) dimensions
Proactive	cultural dialogue and sharing among co-workers opens up discussion, decreasing the risk of unintentional cultural mistakes, pain, and conflict
Ethics	and patient advocacy underscore the need for multicultural workplace collaboration based on research, theory, personal, and clinical experience
Trust	is an essential component for building multicultural workplace harmony that begins with self-disclosure and demonstrated respect for diverse values
Education	for developing cultural competence must include formal formats such as continuing education, college courses, and/or an advanced certificate program*
Networking	with experts in various cultures will assist one in becoming more culturally competent with patients and more culturally sensitive with co-workers
Confidence	for cultural learning and initiatives should be realistic, avoiding overconfidence and low confidence behaviors
Evaluation	appraisal of strategies implemented and learning outcomes achieved provide guidance for future innovations within multicultural workplace settings

*Jeffreys, 2008

Figure 2.2   Acronym for Multicultural Workplace Competence

cultural competence development, embrace cultural diversity, implement culturally congruent care, and optimize health.

KEY POINT SUMMARY

- In an increasingly diverse society, nurses and other health care professionals are challenged to: (a) provide culturally competent (culturally specific) care and (b) promote multicultural workplace harmony and prevent multicultural workplace conflict.
- Diversity *self-awareness* occurs when one engages in active reflection about one's own cultural identity or identities, realizes

one's own CVB, and recognizes the differences within one's own cultural group(s).

- Diversity *awareness* refers to an active, ongoing conscious process in which one becomes proactively aware of similarities and differences within and between various cultural groups, necessitating cultural assessment of patients and cultural sharing among health care professionals.
- Cultural competence is an ongoing, multidimensional learning process that integrates transcultural nursing skills in all three dimensions (cognitive, practical, and affective), involves transcultural self-efficacy (confidence) as a major influencing factor, and aims to achieve culturally congruent care.
- The acronym "COMPETENCE" assists health care providers in remembering several essential elements for cultural competence development and achieving culturally congruent patient care. COMPETENCE refers to Caring, Ongoing, Multidimensional, Proactive, Ethics, Trust, Education, Networks, Confidence, and Evaluation.
- The adapted acronym "COMPETENCE" is presented to guide health care providers in promoting multicultural workplace harmony and prevent multicultural workplace conflict.

CHAPTER 3

A Model to Guide Cultural Competence Education

Marianne R. Jeffreys, EdD, RN

Providing culturally specific and congruent care to the myriad of culturally diverse populations is a growing professional challenge. The expanding number of immigrant populations seeking health care compounded by the growing diverse nursing student population predicted in the future suggests that increasingly professional nurses will care for clients who are "culturally different." *Culturally different* clients are clients whose racial, ethnic, gender, socioeconomic, and/or religious backgrounds and/or identities are different from the health care professional or student. For educators, preparing culturally diverse nursing students to care competently for culturally different clients will be even more challenging. For health care professionals and health care institutions (HCIs), the challenge is to provide educational opportunities to enhance the cultural competency of health care professionals so that quality outcome indicators such as enhanced client satisfaction and positive health outcomes may be achieved.

Although the need to prepare students and health professionals to become culturally sensitive and competent is extremely urgent, research in the area of understanding the teaching–learning process of cultural competency has been limited. Research priorities, guided by conceptual models must shift toward strategies aimed at maximizing learner strengths, identifying learner weaknesses, and developing diagnostic-prescriptive teaching interventions. A conceptual model that depicts the multidimensional components of the teaching–learning process of cultural competency could serve as a valuable cognitive map to guide educators, researchers, and learners. Furthermore, a model that addresses factors that influence learning, motivation, persistence, and commitment for cultural competency development would offer a more comprehensive approach.

Such an approach must recognize that despite the learning opportunities presented to students, nurses, and other health professionals, some individuals persist at cultural competency development while others do not. According to Bandura (1986), learning and motivation for learning are directly influenced by self-efficacy perceptions (confidence). *Self-efficacy* is the perceived confidence for learning or performing specific tasks or skills necessary to achieve a particular goal. Moreover, self-efficacy is the belief that one can perform or succeed at learning a specific task, despite obstacles and hardships, and will expend whatever energy is necessary to accomplish the task (Bandura, 1986). Self-efficacy has been strongly linked to persistence behaviors and motivation. *Motivation* has been described as "the 'power within' that will generate actions that will result in his or her success" (Stage & Hossler, 2000, p. 173). Motivation to engage in the process of becoming culturally competent has been termed *cultural desire,* with such desire viewed as the "pivotal construct of cultural competence" (Campinha-Bacote, 2003, p. 14). As a determinant of performance, persistence, motivation, and the self-regulation of learning, self-efficacy (perceived confidence) is a major component in learning (Bandura, 1982, 1986, 1995, 1996a, 1996b, 1997; Maddux, 1995; Multon, Brown, & Lent, 1991; Pintrich & Garcia, 1994; Zimmerman, 1996). Consequently, confidence is a vital component in the process of learning cultural competence (Exhibit 2.1).

The Cultural Competence and Confidence (CCC) model (see Figure 3.1) aims to interrelate concepts that explain, describe, influence, and/or predict the phenomenon of learning (developing) cultural competence and incorporates the construct of transcultural self-efficacy (confidence) as a major influencing factor. *Transcultural self-efficacy* (TSE) is the perceived confidence for performing or learning general transcultural nursing skills among culturally different clients. *Cultural competence* is a multidimensional learning process that integrates transcultural skills in all three dimensions (cognitive, practical, and affective), involves TSE (confidence) as a major influencing factor, and aims to achieve culturally congruent care. The term *learning process* emphasizes that the cognitive, practical, and affective dimensions of TSE and transcultural skill development can change over time, as a result of formalized education and other learning experiences.

The CCC model is proposed to provide an organizing framework for understanding the multidimensional process of cultural competence and confidence by succinctly illustrating major components of the learning process (see Figure 3.1). This chapter begins by describing the initial

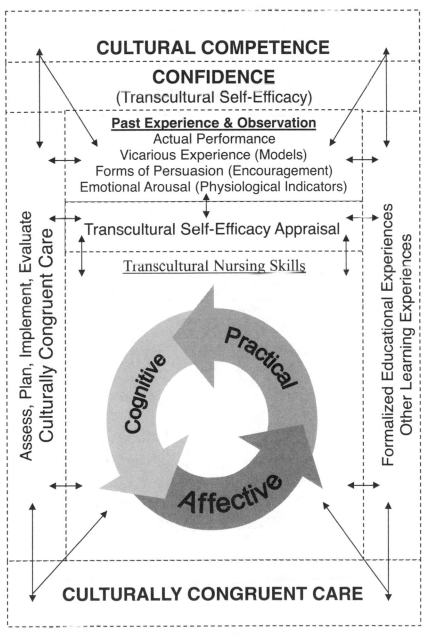

Figure 3.1 Jeffreys' Cultural Competence and Confidence (CCC) Model

conceptualization surrounding model development. Key terms and underlying assumptions will be introduced. A close-up view of TSE, cultural
competence, and culturally congruent care is depicted through the TSE
Pathway (see Figure 3.2), thereby expanding upon the major components
of the CCC model. An overview of the conceptual model and essential

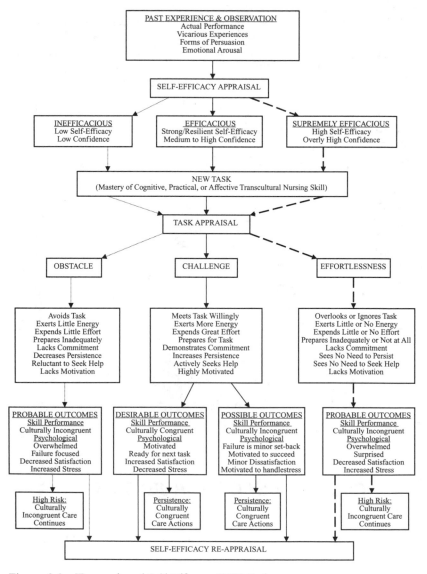

Figure 3.2 Transcultural Self-Efficacy (TSE) Pathway

background information will conclude the chapter. Lastly, the model is brought to life through a realistic "Educator-In-Action" vignette featuring cultural competence education in the health care institution (hospital setting).

BEGINNING ROOTS, OBSERVATIONS, AND INITIAL CONCEPTUALIZATION

A brief discussion of the CCC model's beginning roots from the author's observations, conceptualization, empirical support, and changes over time, demonstrating the model as developmental, tentative, dynamic, and evolving as new data become available. The model presents one perspective that will hopefully spark further inquiry into the complex yet extremely important process of developing cultural competence.

Initial ideas often evolve from multiple sources. An area of interest may be based on formal or informal observations or derived from issues in professional nursing. In the present case, both informal and formal observations led to the author's design of a series of studies and the development of the CCC model. Early on, informal observations noted that confidence, lack of confidence, or overconfidence was an intriguingly complex phenomenon that could influence learning and performance. This observation was especially noted in interactions with aquaphobics and athletes prior to the author becoming a registered nurse. Despite cognitive knowledge and psychomotor ability, learning and performance were often influenced by confidence level either directly or indirectly. Direct effects were manifested through performance outcomes; indirect effects included varying levels of avoidance behaviors, persistence, indifference, commitment, effort, satisfaction, fear, and/or stress.

Later, as an undergraduate nursing student, the author also informally observed confidence to be a factor in learning, performance, and overall success. Fellow nursing students who lacked confidence often performed poorly, despite his or her knowledge, critical thinking ability, manual dexterity, and speaking ability. Others became frustrated, simply gave up trying, and dropped out. Positive thinking peers who studied and practiced skills seemed to like nursing more and achieve better outcomes. When working as a staff nurse, the author also noted confidence to be a factor influencing professional nursing practice, career satisfaction, and career advancement. Among clients, confidence levels were also seen as variables influencing outcomes. All of these observations were informal, yet they were impressionable.

Subsequent observations as a nursing faculty member found confidence to be an important component in nursing student achievement, persistence, retention, and success. Interest in enhancing nursing student achievement became a focused area of inquiry. Review of the literature in education and psychology revealed Bandura's (1986) social cognitive theory; with self-efficacy (the perceived confidence for learning or performing specific tasks or skills necessary to achieve a particular goal) as an underlying component of the theory. Self-efficacy is task or domain specific and has been correlated with academic achievement, persistence, retention, and success; hence, self-efficacy became a targeted variable for the author's study within the context of nursing education.

During the author's doctoral dissertation study concerning first semester nontraditional associate degree student achievement and retention, individual item review of perceived self-efficacy for 60 select nursing skills suggested that students were least confident about learning specific communications skills than they were about skills in other categories (Jeffreys, 1993). Eight of the 10 communication items received responses ranking in the 30th percentile (least confident). More specifically, overall less confidence was reported for interviewing a client about "financial concerns," "religious practices and beliefs," and "ethnic food preferences." These were the only items that dealt with cultural issues in terms of socioeconomic status (class), religion, and ethnicity.

Why were students least confident about communication? Why were students less confident about items related to cultural issues? How would students have responded to items that further delineated the various dimensions of culture? According to Bandura (1986), individuals with low confidence are at greater risk for task avoidance and decreased commitment. If students are avoiding tasks or less committed to tasks associated with culture, then how can cultural assessments, culture-specific nursing care, culturally congruent care, and cultural competence be achieved? Furthermore, cultural assessments must begin with effective transcultural communication, which requires awareness, sensitivity, knowledge, and skills. Of course, "transcultural" implies the bridging of significant differences in cultural communication styles, beliefs, or practices (Kavanagh & Kennedy, 1992). If students are less confident about general communication skills, how will cultural assessments be performed (or will they be performed)? The obvious gaps and lowered confidence raised the important question, "What teaching interventions are needed to promote culturally congruent care?"

Interest in learning more about students' self-efficacy perceptions concerning specific transcultural nursing skills necessary for developing cultural competence became the author's new focused domain of inquiry. Specifically, the area of interest was to develop a composite of students' needs, values, attitudes, and skills related to transcultural nursing care and the assessment of their changes (outcomes) over time. Assessing students' needs, strengths, weaknesses, and perceptions would be the necessary precursor to the design of any teaching interventions. "Effective teaching and learning is further enhanced by frequent and ongoing evaluations of students and by adapting educational instruction based on outcome assessments" (Jeffreys & Smodlaka, 1996, p. 47). The author believed that the initial and ongoing assessment of students' self-efficacy perceptions (confidence) concerning culture care of diverse individuals would be a valuable component in transcultural nursing education. Subsequently, several studies were undertaken to explore, measure, and evaluate learners' TSE perceptions (Jeffreys, 2000; Jeffreys & Smodlaka, 1996, 1998, 1999a, 1999b). (Chapter 4 will discuss exploring, measuring, and evaluating learners through the use of the Transcultural Self-Efficacy Tool). A description of the CCC model will be presented in the following sections.

KEY TERMS

To develop a common knowledge base and avoid discrepancies in definitions, Exhibit 3.1 defines key terms important in understanding the CCC model.

Exhibit 3.1   Key Terms Associated with the Cultural Competence and Confidence Model

Transcultural self-efficacy is the perceived confidence for performing or learning transcultural nursing skills. It is the degree to which individuals perceive they have the ability to perform the specific transcultural nursing skills needed for culturally competent and congruent care (Jeffreys, 2000).

Transcultural nursing skills are those skills necessary for assessing, planning, implementing, and evaluating culturally congruent care. Transcultural nursing skills include cognitive, practical, and affective dimensions (Jeffreys, 2000).

Culturally congruent care is health care that is customized to fit with the client's cultural values, beliefs, traditions, practices, and lifestyle. Clients may include individuals, families, groups, institutions, and organizations. According to Leininger (1991a), **culturally congruent nursing care** refers to "those cognitively based assistive, supportive, facilitative, or enabling acts or decisions that are tailor-made to fit with an individual's, group's, or institution's cultural values, beliefs, and lifeways in order to provide meaningful, beneficial, and satisfying health care, or well-being services" (p. 49).

Cultural competence is a multidimensional learning process that integrates transcultural skills in all three dimensions (cognitive, practical, and

affective), involves transcultural self-efficacy (confidence) as a major influencing factor, and aims to achieve culturally congruent care. **Cultural competence
in nursing** is a multidimensional learning process that integrates transcultural
nursing skills in all three dimensions (cognitive, practical, and affective), involves transcultural self-efficacy (confidence) and aims to achieve culturally
congruent nursing care. The term "**learning process**" emphasizes that the
cognitive, practical, and affective dimensions of transcultural self-efficacy
can change over time as a result of formalized education and other learning
experiences.

The **cognitive learning dimension** is a learning dimension that focuses on
knowledge outcomes, intellectual abilities, and skills. Within the context of
transcultural learning, cognitive learning skills include knowledge and comprehension about ways in which cultural factors may influence professional
nursing care among clients of different cultural backgrounds and throughout various phases of the life cycle. **Different cultural backgrounds** refers to
clients representing various different racial, ethnic, gender, socioeconomic,
and religious groups.

The **practical learning dimension** is similar to the psychomotor learning
domain and focuses on motor skills or practical application of skills. Within
the context of transcultural learning, practical learning skills refer to communication skills (verbal and nonverbal) needed to interview clients of different
cultural backgrounds about their values and beliefs.

The **affective learning dimension** is a learning dimension concerned with
attitudes, values, and beliefs and is considered to be the most important in
developing professional values and attitudes. Affective learning includes self-
awareness, awareness of cultural gap (differences), acceptance, appreciation,
recognition, and advocacy.

PURPOSE AND GOAL OF THE MODEL

The CCC model presents an organizing framework for examining the
multidimensional factors involved in the process of learning cultural
competence in order to identify at-risk individuals, develop diagnostic-
prescriptive strategies to facilitate learning, guide innovations in teaching
and educational research, and evaluate strategy effectiveness. The main
goal of the model is to promote culturally congruent care through the
development of cultural competence. Cultural competence is influenced
by TSE, the learning of transcultural nursing skills (cognitive, practical,
and affective), formalized educational experiences, and other learning experiences. Although several models have been proposed to describe the
process of cultural competence (Campinha-Bacote, 2003; Purnell, 2008)
or the process of achieving culturally congruent care through the assessment of cultural diversity and universality (Leininger, 2002), the CCC

model focuses specifically on learning as influenced by TSE. Hence, TSE is proposed as a new construct vital to the process of cultural competence and culturally congruent care. The model is tentative and will require modification when new data become available.

ASSUMPTIONS

Based on a review of the literature and previous studies of self-efficacy (Jeffreys, 2000), several assumptions underlie the CCC model. Asterisks denote assumptions empirically tested (1 asterisk) and assumptions currently under study (2 asterisks):

1. Cultural competence is an ongoing, multidimensional learning process that integrates transcultural skills in all three dimensions (cognitive, practical, and affective), involves TSE (confidence) as a major influencing factor, and aims to achieve culturally congruent care.
2. TSE is a dynamic construct that changes over time and is influenced by formalized exposure to culture care concepts (transcultural nursing). *
3. The learning of transcultural nursing skills is influenced by self-efficacy perceptions (confidence). **
4. The performance of transcultural nursing skill competencies is directly influenced by the adequate learning of such skills and by TSE perceptions. **
5. The performance of culturally congruent nursing skills is influenced by self-efficacy perceptions and by formalized educational exposure to transcultural nursing care concepts and skills throughout the educational experience. **
6. All students and nurses (regardless of age, ethnicity, gender, sexual orientation, lifestyle, religion, socioeconomic status, geographic location, or race) require formalized educational experiences to meet culture care needs of diverse individuals. *
7. The most comprehensive learning involves the integration of cognitive, practical, and affective dimensions.
8. Learning in the cognitive, practical, and affective dimensions is paradoxically distinct yet interrelated. *
9. Learners are most confident about their attitudes (affective dimension) and least confident about their transcultural nursing knowledge (cognitive dimension). *
10. Novice learners will have lower self-efficacy perceptions than advanced learners. *

11. Inefficacious individuals are at risk for decreased motivation, lack of commitment, and/or avoidance of cultural considerations when planning and implementing nursing care.
12. Supremely efficacious (overly confident) individuals are at risk for inadequate preparation in learning the transcultural nursing skills necessary to provide culturally congruent care.
13. Early intervention with at-risk individuals will better prepare nurses to meet cultural competency. **
14. The greatest change in TSE perceptions will be detected in individuals with low self-efficacy (low confidence) initially, who have then been exposed to formalized transcultural nursing concepts and experiences.*

*Assumptions supported empirically.
**Assumptions currently under study.

AN OVERVIEW OF THE CULTURAL COMPETENCE AND CONFIDENCE (CCC) MODEL

Cultural competence in nursing is a multidimensional learning process that integrates transcultural nursing skills in all three dimensions (cognitive, practical, and affective), involves TSE (confidence), and aims to achieve culturally congruent care. Cognitive, practical, and affective dimensions of TSE can change over time as a result of formalized education and other learning experiences. Each learning dimension comprises several underlying factors or concepts. Figure 3.2 traces the proposed influences of TSE on a learner's actions, performance, and persistence for learning tasks associated with cultural competency development and culturally congruent care. TSE appraisal is a key beginning step in this process.

Self-efficacy appraisal is an individualized process influenced by four information sources: actual performances, vicarious experiences, forms of persuasion, and emotional arousal (physiological indices). Actual performances are the strongest source of efficacy information (Bandura, 1986). Successful performances can raise efficacy while unsuccessful performances lower it. Lowered self-efficacy can be psychologically stressful and dissatisfying to nursing students, nurses, and other health care professionals, further negatively impacting motivation, persistence, and cultural competency development. Individuals with low self-efficacy initially can feel devastated by failure or poor performance, and further lowered self-efficacy can cause avoidance behaviors (Bandura, 1986, 1997).

Undoubtedly, avoidance behaviors raise numerous professional, ethical, and legal issues; however, the most severe consequence is that avoidance behavior can be dangerous. For example, a student or nurse with low self-efficacy for interviewing a culturally different client about religious and ethnic values, beliefs, and practices concerning food and nutrition may avoid asking important questions. Without adequate cultural assessment, culturally incongruent care can result, causing adverse physical and emotional outcomes to the client. A nurse who reluctantly attempts to interview a culturally different client, avoids culture-specific assessments, and misinterprets client's statements and actions may fail to recognize the client's cultural pain (Jeffreys, 2005). Cultural pain refers to the "suffering, discomfort, or being greatly offended by an individual or group who shows a great lack of sensitivity toward another's cultural experience" (Leininger, 2002, p. 52). In addition to the negative emotional client outcomes, adverse physical client outcomes may occur. If a diabetic client disregards the nurse's suggested diet plan menu because of food taboos, ethnic food preferences, and/or economic constraints, the possible adverse physical health outcomes are numerous. In failing to realize why the client is not adhering to diet recommendations, an inefficacious nurse may be fearful of attempting follow-up diet teaching, lack motivation, avoid help-seeking behaviors, and become increasingly dissatisfied and anxious.

Individuals with strong (realistic) levels of self-efficacy will not be adversely affected by an occasional failure. Such individuals view an occasional failure as a temporary setback or challenge to be overcome with more effort expenditure (Bandura, 1986, 1997). In the previous case example, the realistically strong efficacious student would be motivated to seek extra assistance in the skills lab or request additional supervised opportunities in the clinical setting to ask culture-specific questions, select culturally appropriate communication style, and seek appropriate resources for culturally congruent food choices. Most likely, such a student (or nurse) would initially take the task seriously, view it with some uncertainty, and exert preparatory efforts before attempting to interview a culturally different client in the clinical setting. Preparatory efforts may include collaboration with health professionals, members of the cultural community, family, and/or client to determine the "best" or optimal culturally congruent approach.

In contrast, the supremely efficacious individual (unrealistic in self-appraisal) would view the task without uncertainty, prepare inadequately (or not at all), and potentially jeopardize patient safety if inaccurate assessments are made and appropriate assistance is not sought. Again, unsuccessful performance will lower self-efficacy; however, for the supremely efficacious individual, the goal would be that the task would now be viewed seriously and as a challenge that required adequate preparatory efforts.

Vicarious experience, or modeling, is less influential than actual performance. Models that display effort and perform tasks successfully will be more influential than models completing the task effortlessly. Self-efficacy perceptions will be further enhanced if models are similar to the individual in background and ability (Bandura, 1986; Schunk, 1987). It would be expected that novices (beginning students and new graduate nurses) have less astute skills for observing models. Because beginning students have little or no experience in the domain of nursing, such students will be at risk for selective observations that are myopic, slightly skewed, severely distorted, or limited, thereby increasing the risk for unrealistic self-appraisals. New graduates may be overwhelmed by technical tasks, fast-paced expectations to care for many acutely ill patients, the severe nursing shortage, and lack of sufficient resources. Experienced nurses or other health professionals who are novices in developing cultural competence may also need guidance in observation skills. Through the use of various structured mentoring strategies, more experienced nurses (expert nurses) and educators can enhance the power of modeling on self-efficacy appraisal and development. (Refer to Part III of this book for strategies). By assisting students and novice nurses to develop keen observation skills, educators can have a powerful influence on efficacy appraisal.

Forms of persuasion include positive verbal feedback from peers, teachers, supervisors, mentors, and significant others. Positive persuasion will only enhance efficacy if the individual's subsequent efforts turn out positively (Schunk, 1987). Therefore, positive verbal feedback should be given judiciously and honestly if it is to have any positive impact. In the TSE Pathway (see Figure 3.2), "forms of persuasion" refers to "encouragement by peers, faculty, supervisors, colleagues, mentors, or friends." Encouragement must be realistic, thus incorporating this important dimension of self-efficacy appraisal.

Physiological indices such as elevated pulse rate and sweating may indicate emotional arousal such as anxiety and/or fear. Conscious awareness of anxiety symptoms over a particular task may lower efficacy beliefs (Bandura, 1986, 1997; Schunk, 1987). For example, if a nurse repeatedly experiences anxiety symptoms such as elevated pulse rate and sweating before caring for culturally different clients (despite his or her cognitive and psychomotor ability to perform tasks), then the nurse's efficacy beliefs may be lowered, adversely affecting learning, performance, persistence, motivation, and cultural competency development. Mild anxiety associated with some uncertainty has some benefits in that individuals are more attentive to detail, recognize the need for preparatory actions, and actively seek assistance. Lack of physiological changes would accompany the expected profile of supremely efficacious individuals and adversely affect task performance.

Self-efficacy changes over time in response to new experiences and observations (Bandura, 1989; Gist & Mitchell, 1992; Saks, 1995). Cultural competence development is enhanced through carefully orchestrated education interventions, strategies to increase cultural awareness and desire, opportunities for interaction with culturally different clients, and collaboration with transcultural experts (Campinha-Bacote, 2003; Leininger, 2002a; Purnell, 2008). (See Figure 6.4). Within the CCC model, formalized educational experiences and client learning experiences that (a) carefully weave cognitive, practical, and affective transcultural nursing skills; (b) encompass assessment, planning, implementation, and evaluation; and (c) integrate self-efficacy appraisals and diagnostic-specific interventions are essential in cultural competence development and culturally congruent care. Several studies supported that culturally diverse nursing students' self-efficacy perceptions were significantly influenced by the educational and health care experiences. For example, students' course level was statistically significant in influencing perceptions in these studies examining changes in TSE perceptions (Jeffreys & Smodlaka, 1996, 1998, 1999a, 1999b; Lim et al., 2004). (See TSET Research Exhibit 6.1.) Novice (beginning) students had overall lower self-efficacy perceptions whereas advanced (more experienced) students had overall higher self-efficacy perceptions. Ethnic/racial group identity was statistically insignificant, suggesting that self-efficacy measures can be designed to capture the effect of educational experiences across culturally diverse groups; however, further empirical investigation is recommended. Bandura (1995, 1996a) pointed out that the construct of self-efficacy is of vital importance across cultures and should not be confused with Western individualism. Within hospitals and clinical agencies, changes in nurses' TSE perceptions following cultural competence educational interventions have also been reported (Dolgan, 2001; Platter, 2005; Velez, 2005).

Carefully designed self-efficacy measures (survey tools) can be used to appraise the initial self-efficacy levels for particular tasks and skills prior to designing educational interventions. Review of survey data to identify inefficacious and supremely efficacious individuals will allow for early intervention and assistance in enhancing realistic self-efficacy appraisal. Because Bandura (1982, 1989, 1996a) recommended situation- or task-specific tools to measure self-efficacy and proposed other guidelines in self-efficacy tool development, educators and researchers should selectively choose a reliable and valid self-efficacy tool specifically matching their research needs. Often, this means that a new tool must be developed. The instrument design process is complex and time-consuming; however, specific steps should be followed to enhance the validity and reliability of findings (Jeffreys & Smodlaka, 1996; Waltz, Strickland, & Lenz, 2005). Chapter 4 comprehensively describes an empirically tested tool, the Transcultural Self-Efficacy Tool (TSET) for measurement and evaluation of TSE. Chapter 4 also introduces the new Cultural Competence Clinical Evaluation Tool (CCCET) and Clinical Setting Assessment Tool-Diversity and Disparity (CSAT-DD) designed to measure and evaluate several previously untested assumptions of the CCC model. (See Chapter 4 for details). Ongoing comparative studies of TSET, CCCET, and CSAT-DD data across various settings will expand the depth of empirical support for the CCC model.

Exhibit 3.2   Educator-In-Action Vignette

Jeannette, a clinical nurse educator at a hospital, is puzzled by some of the comments written on the anonymous evaluation forms following a hospital-sponsored cultural competence development workshop. Jeannette tells Trudy, another clinical nurse educator, "I just don't understand these comments. This nurse scored 96% on the post-workshop multiple choice test. This nurse knew almost all the answers. We went over so many details about the culture and even provided handouts delineating the major facts." Jeannette proceeds to share the nurse's written comments with Trudy. (See below).

Nurse: "I know that culture-specific nursing interventions can make a difference in client outcomes. I am aware that some of my patients have cultural values and beliefs that are different from my own. I want to become a more culturally competent nurse so I read journal articles about culture whenever they are published in *RN* magazine. Sometimes the articles give great ideas about how to communicate appropriately with culturally different clients and even provide some understandable assessment tools. The hospital workshop on 'Meeting the Needs of Russian Immigrants' provided me with new knowledge about one of the many cultural groups that we encounter regularly at our hospital. Unfortunately, I just don't feel very confident about my abilities as a culturally competent nurse so I don't really try to develop culture-specific care plans or directly ask clients about their CVB. I feel as though I am prying. Besides, I might make a mistake. If culturally different clients ask me for something that isn't too extraordinary or against the usual hospital policy, I do try to accommodate them unless things get too busy."

Trudy replies, "The nurse's comments suggest that she or he has some cultural knowledge, cultural desire, self-awareness, conscious awareness of cultural diversity, conscious awareness of cultural incompetence, exposure to cultural assessment skills and tools, and many interactions with culturally different clients, yet lacks confidence. Cultural competence and culturally congruent care outcomes are strongly linked to confidence. Specifically, transcultural self-efficacy is the perceived confidence for performing or learning transcultural nursing skills. It is the degree to which individuals perceive they have the ability to perform the specific transcultural nursing skills needed for culturally competent and congruent care."

Trudy proceeds to share the CCC model and the TSE Pathway with Jeannette, discussing the major and minor components in each. Jeannette then recognizes that cultural competence is a multidimensional learning process that integrates transcultural skills in all three dimensions (cognitive, practical, and affective) and involves TSE (confidence) as a major influencing factor.

Based on the model, Jeannette and Trudy plan to develop future learner-centered educational experiences that (a) carefully weave cognitive, practical, and affective transcultural nursing skills; (b) encompass assessment, planning, implementation, and evaluation; and (c) integrate self-efficacy appraisals and diagnostic-specific interventions.

KEY POINT SUMMARY

- The CCC model interrelates concepts that explain, describe, influence, and/or predict the phenomenon of learning (developing) cultural competence and incorporates the construct of TSE (confidence) as a major influencing factor.
- TSE is the perceived confidence for performing or learning transcultural nursing skills.
- Within the CCC model, formalized educational experiences and client learning experiences that (a) carefully weave cognitive, practical, and affective transcultural nursing skills; (b) encompass assessment, planning, implementation, and evaluation; and (c) integrate self-efficacy appraisals and diagnostic-specific interventions are essential in cultural competence development and culturally congruent care.
- Self-efficacy appraisal is an individualized process influenced by four information sources: actual performances, vicarious experiences, forms of persuasion, and emotional arousal (physiological indices).
- The TSE Pathway traces the proposed influences of TSE on a learner's actions, performance, and persistence for learning tasks associated with cultural competence development and culturally congruent care.

PART II

Tools for Assessment and Evaluation

Educators and researchers are continually challenged to measure changes following educational interventions. Part II addresses this challenge by introducing several quantitative questionnaires and assessment tools and discussing implementation and data interpretation strategies in a detailed, user-friendly approach easily adapted by novice and advanced researchers. Chapter 4 begins by introducing a quantitative tool (questionnaire) that measures and evaluates learners' confidence—the Transcultural Self-Efficacy Tool (TSET).

The TSET, which the author has previously used in grant-funded projects and studies, has prompted requests for use or study from numerous graduate students, faculty, employee educators, and health care professionals in various disciplines from around the world. Their requests informed the first edition of this book with its detailed discussion about the TSET and the conceptual model underlying it; and they also inform this second edition. An exponential increase in such requests (and completed studies) has made it quite clear that the TSET offers tools that speak to current conditions and issues in education and practice. As such, the major components, features, and psychometric properties (reliability and validity) of the 83-item questionnaire are presented, using a systematic and reader-friendly approach. Tables summarize vital instrument information.

The chapter also discusses the Cultural Competence Clinical Evaluation Tool (CCCET), a new tool adapted from the TSET that contains three subscales measuring different dimensions of clinical cultural competence behaviors: (a) the extent of culturally specific care (Subscale 1);

(b) cultural assessment (Subscale 2); and (c) culturally sensitive and professionally appropriate attitudes, values, or beliefs including awareness, acceptance, recognition, appreciation, and advocacy necessary for providing culturally sensitive professional nursing care (Subscale 3) as rated by the student or employee and the teacher or agency evaluator. The Clinical Setting Assessment Tool: Diversity and Disparity (CSAT-DD), a user-friendly tool to collect data about the clinical practicum/agency site, specifically focusing on descriptions of diverse client populations (Part I) and 28 high-priority clinical problems, is introduced. Additional assessment measures, applied uses, evaluation strategies, and the "Educator-In-Action" vignette conclude the chapter, offering multiple options and ideas for educators and researchers.

Chapter 5 offers resources for establishing prioritized, diagnostic-prescriptive, evidence-based cultural competence education. For example, inefficacious (low confidence) individuals are at risk for decreased motivation, lack of commitment, and/or avoidance of cultural considerations when planning and implementing nursing care. In addition, supremely efficacious (overly confident) individuals are at risk for inadequate preparation in learning the transcultural nursing skills necessary to provide culturally congruent care. Implications for educators are presented. Pragmatic suggestions for avoiding pitfalls in educational research design and data interpretation are also offered. The "Educator-In-Action" vignette provides a clear example of how educators may easily integrate this guided approach within their own teaching practice.

CHAPTER 4

Transcultural Self-Efficacy Tool (TSET), Cultural Competence Clinical Evaluation Tool (CCCET), and Clinical Setting Assessment Tool–Diversity and Disparity (CSAT-DD)

Marianne R. Jeffreys, EdD, RN

- What are student's needs, values, attitudes, and skills concerning transcultural nursing?
- Which transcultural nursing skills do students perceive with more confidence?
- Which transcultural nursing skills do students perceive with less confidence?
- What are the differences in transcultural self-efficacy perceptions between novice and advanced groups?
- What are the changes in transcultural self-efficacy perceptions following formalized educational experiences and/or other learning experiences?
- What demographic factors influence transcultural self-efficacy perceptions?

These questions prompted the design of the Transcultural Self-Efficacy Tool (TSET). The beginning part of the chapter will discuss the exploration, measurement, and evaluation of confidence through the use of the TSET (Jeffreys Toolkit 2010, Item 1). Major components, features, and psychometric properties (reliability and validity) of the TSET will be highlighted. To address the issue of TSE predicting cultural competence behaviors in clinical, a brief discussion of a current multiphase study will follow. The purpose of the study is to examine the influence of cultural competence education on undergraduate and graduate nursing students' transcultural self-efficacy perceptions, extent of culturally specific care provided for culturally diverse clients, frequency of cultural assessment, and the development of culturally sensitive and professionally appropriate attitudes, values, or beliefs (Jeffreys & Dogan, 2007). The study also involves the adaptation of the TSET into the Cultural Competence Clinical Evaluation Tool (CCCET) discussed in forthcoming sections within this chapter. Finally, The Clinical Setting Assessment Tool: Diversity and Disparity (CSAT-DD), a user-friendly tool to collect data about the clinical practicum/agency site, specifically focusing on descriptions of diverse client populations (Part I) and clinical problems targeting the 28 focus areas of the Healthy People 2010 document (Part II) will be introduced. Additional assessment measures, applied uses, and evaluation strategies will conclude the chapter.

TRANSCULTURAL SELF-EFFICACY TOOL DESCRIPTION

Major Components and Features

The TSET was originally designed to measure and evaluate students' confidence for performing general transcultural nursing skills among diverse populations. A generalist approach, focusing on general transcultural nursing skills, was considered most appropriate for learners without previous formal education and background in transcultural nursing, especially those who would care for clients of many different cultural backgrounds. The generalist approach emphasizes broad transcultural nursing principles, concepts, theories, and research study findings to care for clients of many different cultures (Leininger, 1989). In contrast, a specialist approach is most appropriate for learners who have mastered general transcultural nursing skills developed through formalized educational and interactive experiences. A specialist approach aims to prepare an individual as a "specialist" in one or more select cultural groups, requiring a series of specialized transcultural courses and concentrated fieldwork (Leininger, 1989; Leininger & McFarland, 2002, 2006).

To address the question, How can transcultural self-efficacy (TSE) perceptions be explored, measured, and evaluated validly among novice and advanced students? a literature review was conducted, focusing on transcultural nursing, cultural issues, self-efficacy, learning theories, and instrumentation. The majority of self-efficacy tools described in the nursing literature pertained to client education. One self-efficacy scale, the Cultural Self-Efficacy Scale (Bernal & Froman, 1987), was designed to measure cultural self-efficacy perceptions of community health nurses within three specific client populations (black, Latino, and Southeast Asian). No self-efficacy tool had been specifically designed that would measure student's perceived self-efficacy for performing general transcultural nursing skills among clients of different cultures. Furthermore, no questionnaire had been designed for culturally diverse nursing students who must learn to care for many different groups of culturally diverse clients.

Therefore, the design of a new instrument was necessary. The author's decision to create a new instrument was further substantiated by self-efficacy theory that supports the design of detailed questionnaires (focused on specific tasks or skills) within the desired domain of inquiry (Bandura, 1982, 1989, 1997). The process of designing a new instrument included item development, item sequence, subscale sequence, expert content review, expert psychometric review, revised draft, pretest, minor revisions, and a second pretest (Jeffreys & Smodlaka, 1996).

Based on the literature and the results of a two-phase evaluation study (Jeffreys & Smodlaka, 1996), the 83-item TSET (Jeffreys, 1994) contains three subscales presented in the following sequence: Cognitive (25 items), Practical (28 items), and Affective (30 items). Separate subscales were created for two main reasons: (a) the most comprehensive learning includes coordinated learning in the cognitive, practical (psychomotor), and affective domains; and (b) self-efficacy theory purports that different dimensions within a specific domain of inquiry require separate subscales for accurate measurement and evaluation (Bandura, 1982, 1989). The Cognitive Subscale asks respondents to rate their confidence about their knowledge concerning the ways cultural factors may influence nursing care. The Practical Subscale asks respondents to rate their confidence for interviewing clients of different cultural backgrounds to learn about their values and beliefs; 28 culture-related interview topics are presented as items. Attitudes, values, and beliefs are addressed in the Affective Subscale.

Consistent with self-efficacy measurement tool guidelines (Bandura, 1977, 1982, 1989), items are close-ended and positively phrased; a 10-point rating scale from 1 (not confident) to 10 (totally confident) is used. Approximate completion time is 20 minutes. Table 4.1 depicts the major

Table 4.1 Transcultural Self-Efficacy Tool (TSET): Major Components, Features, and Rationale

TSET Description	Rationale
General Content Areas (Subscales) 1. Cognitive 2. Practical 3. Affective	Taxonomy of educational objectives (different dimensions of learning)[1] Self-efficacy theory (different dimensions within a specific domain require separate subscales)[2]
Number of Items = 83 25–30 items on each subscale Cognitive (25 items) Practical (28 items) Affective (30 items)	Instrument length may affect reliability and validity[3] Select the least number of unique items to capture construct while avoiding redundancy[3]
General Item Content 1. Specific to culture care issues or transcultural nursing 2. Appropriate for entry-level nursing students	Target purpose[4] Original target audience[4] Entry level is the most basic level, therefore items will have broader application and future use
Individual Item Content 1. Addresses only one issue 2. Clear and succinct 3. Avoids redundancy between items	Stimulate valid and reliable responses from the targeted population[3]
Item Structure 1. Close-ended 2. Positively phrased	Consistent with self-efficacy theory and scales[2]
Rating Scale 10-point rating scale from 1 (not confident) to 10 (totally confident)	Bandura's use of 10-point scales[2] More discriminating than the 6-point rating scale[4]
Item Sequence 1. Clustering items sequentially as they occur (Example: pregnancy, birth, etc.) 2. Least stressful to more stressful or complex	Psychometric guidelines[3] Taxonomy for affective objectives[1] Self-efficacy theory and scales[2,5]
Emphasis on Individual Efficacy Appraisal 1. Personalized items and directions using second pronoun 2. Highlighting and underlining important words	Psychometric guidelines[3] Increase reliability and validity of responses[3]
Subscale Sequence 1. Cognitive 2. Practical 3. Affective	Prevents anchoring effect as supported by pretesting various forms of TSET subscale sequence[4]

[1] Bloom (1956); Harrow (1972); Krathwohl, Bloom, & Masia (1964)
[2] Bandura (1977, 1982, 1986, 1989)   [3] Sudman & Bradburn (1991)
[4] Jeffreys & Smodlaka (1996)   [5] Cervone & Peake (1990).

components and features with the underlying rationale for each component and feature.

Psychometric Properties: Validity

A series of four studies were initially conducted to estimate the psychometric properties of the TSET. Psychometric properties broadly refer to the results obtained from specific statistical tests for estimating instrument validity and reliability. Results provide estimates for the validity and the reliability of the instrument. Details about the initial validity and reliability tests and their results will be outlined in the following sections. Subsequent validity and reliability estimates from subsequent studies will be integrated throughout the narrative text and/or in the "TSET Research Exhibits."

Validity is concerned with the degree to which an instrument measures what it is supposed to measure. For the TSET, a general question was asked: Does the TSET accurately measure what it is supposed to measure? In order to answer this broad question, three more specific questions were asked, differentiating between content validity, construct validity, and criterion-related validity.

Content Validity

Content validity is concerned with whether the instrument and its items are representative of the desired content area and is best assessed by content experts (Waltz, Strickland, & Lenz, 2005; Polit & Beck, 2004). For the TSET, the question posed was: Is the TSET and its items representative of the desired content area? The identified content area targeted the transcultural nursing skills necessary for the transcultural nurse generalist who may be caring for clients of many different cultural backgrounds. Additionally, items needed to represent this content domain and be readable and appropriate for novice undergraduate nursing students. Information about the intended purpose, desired content area, and self-efficacy theory was distributed to the content experts. Content validity was established by six doctoral prepared nurses certified in transcultural nursing (Jeffreys & Smodlaka, 1996).

Construct Validity

Assessment of construct validity evaluates the degree to which a tool measures the construct being studied. Construct validation attempts to validate the tool's underlying theoretical concepts and proposed relationships between the concepts (Munro, 2005; Polit & Beck, 2004; Rattray & Jones, 2007). An instrument whose performance is consistent with the underlying conceptual expectations demonstrates adequate construct validity (Carmines & Zeller, 1979). To answer the question, To what degree does the TSET measure transcultural self-efficacy? a contrasted group approach and a factor analysis were conducted.

Contrasted Group Approach

Two initial studies used the contrasted group approach for estimating construct validity and addressed the question, Are mean scores on the TSET significantly different between two contrasted groups (novice students and advanced students)? Consistent findings from the initial longitudinal study and cross-sectional study supported that the TSET detected differences in transcultural self-efficacy perceptions within groups and between groups on all of the subscales (Jeffreys, 2000; Jeffreys & Smodlaka, 1999a, 1999b). Several underlying theoretical assumptions were supported in these studies, namely:

- Transcultural self-efficacy is a dynamic construct that changes over time and is influenced by formalized exposure to culture care concepts (transcultural nursing).
- Learners are most confident about their attitudes (affective dimension) and least confident about their transcultural nursing knowledge (cognitive dimension)
- Novice learners will have lower self-efficacy perceptions than advanced learners.
- The greatest change in transcultural self-efficacy perceptions will be detected in individuals with low self-efficacy (low confidence) initially, who have then been exposed to formalized transcultural nursing concepts and experiences.

Subsequent studies using contrasting groups of learners in the academic setting (students) and clinical agency setting (nurses) also demonstrated significant differences pre- and post-cultural competence educational intervention, thus lending continued support for the TSET's construct validity (Dolgan, 2001; Lim et al., 2004; MacQuarrie, 2004; Toney, 2004; Velez, 2005). See other studies in TSET Research Exhibits 6.1, 6.2, 6.3, 6.4, 6.5, 10.1, and 10.2.

Factor Analysis: Initial Approach

Next, factor analyses evaluated the degree to which individual items clustered around one or more conceptual dimension. Items that cluster together (to become a "factor") should make sense conceptually, thus supporting the underlying conceptual framework and attesting to the construct validity of the instrument. The factor analysis studies (Jeffreys &

Dogan, 2009; Jeffreys & Smodlaka, 1998) broadly explored "What is the factor composition of the TSET?"

Several different statistical procedures may be employed in factor analysis. Each procedure contains certain errors or assumptions; therefore all factor analysis options were appraised. Review of statistical theory and collaboration with a psychometric expert guided the decision-making process. The process employed in the initial factor analysis study is presented first, followed by the subsequent study utilizing statistical procedures and techniques not yet developed in 1995. The first step of factor analysis begins with a matrix of correlation coefficients between items (Comrey, 1973; Munro, 2005). Items should contribute uniquely and satisfactorily to the instrument, avoiding any redundancy between items. Generally, items that correlate below 0.30 are not sufficiently related and therefore do not contribute to the construct's measurement; items that correlate above 0.70 are considered redundant and unnecessary (Ferketich, 1991). The question, Do all items on the TSET contribute uniquely and sufficiently to the TSE construct? was evaluated via an inter-item correlation matrix. All items correlated between 0.30 and 0.70, therefore, it was assumed that all TSET items contributed uniquely and sufficiently to the TSE construct (Jeffreys, 2000; Jeffreys & Smodlaka, 1998).

The next issue pertained to the assessment of intercorrelations between the three subscales. Within self-efficacy theory, separate subscales should be designed to measure the distinct dimensions within a domain of inquiry. In the assessment of self-efficacy, intercorrelations between subscales corroborate that each subscale measures different dimensions within the domain (Bandura, 1989). To answer the question, Are the Cognitive, Practical, and Affective Subscales correlated with each other? subscale scores were computed. Intercorrelations between subscales were statistically significant and ranged from 0.53 (Cognitive and Affective) to 0.62 (Cognitive and Practical) and 0.68 (Practical and Affective). These results helped validate the following assumptions in the underlying framework:

- Learning in the cognitive, practical, and affective dimensions is paradoxically distinct yet interrelated.
- Learners are most confident about their attitudes (affective dimension) and least confident about their transcultural nursing knowledge (cognitive dimension).

Factor analysis studies are sometimes used for determining parsimony through item deletion, meaning that items that do not load on a factor are deleted to make the instrument shorter. Using conventional procedures for factor analysis as reported in the literature prior to 1995 (Gilley & Uhlig, 1993; Kim & Mueller, 1978; Nunnally & Bernstein, 1994), a principal component analysis with the varimax rotation yielded a nine-factor structure for the study sample (Jeffreys, 2000; Jeffreys & Smodlaka, 1998). With factor loadings set at 0.50, 70 items loaded on the 9 factors; none of the 70 items loaded significantly on any other factor. "All nine factors had eigenvalues greater than 1.00, accounted for 62% of the total variance, and contained at least three items whose difference in loading on the other factors was greater than 0.30" (Jeffreys & Smodlaka, 1998, p. 223). The question, Should any items be dropped? was considered. Because dropping items after just one factor analysis study should be viewed cautiously (Comrey, 1973) and because the inter-item correlation matrix indicated that each item contributed uniquely and significantly to the TSE construct, no items were dropped.

Factors derived from an analysis provide one interpretation of the data and are useful for understanding relationships within a specific domain; however, the interpretation should be confirmed with other types of evidence (Comrey, 1973). Additionally, construct validation should focus on the degree to which an instrument is consistent with the related literature and underlying conceptual framework, (Carmines & Zeller, 1979), therefore, this was also examined. For the TSET, supporting evidence included several key theoretical issues. First, the factors related to the literature in transcultural nursing and the underlying conceptual framework. Items that clustered together made sense conceptually and were accordingly labeled: recognition, kinship and social factors, professional nursing care, cultural background and identity, life cycle transitional phenomena, awareness of cultural gap, communication, self-awareness, and appreciation (Jeffreys, 2000; Jeffreys & Smodlaka, 1998). Second, items that clustered together were from the same subscale, clustering exclusively on the Cognitive, Practical, or Affective Subscale. Subscale exclusivity most likely implies that within each broad educational category, as captured in the three TSET subscales, there are several underlying theoretical dimensions that contribute to the TSE construct (Jeffreys & Smodlaka, 1998). Third, students were most confident about Affective Subscale factors and least confident about Cognitive Subscale factors. Fourth, changes in mean scores on each of the nine factors occurred in the expected direction for novice and advanced students (means were higher for advanced students on all of the factors).

Results from this phase of the initial factor analysis study helped validate the following assumptions:

- Learning in the cognitive, practical, and affective dimensions is paradoxically distinct yet interrelated.

- Learners are most confident about their attitudes (affective dimension) and least confident about their transcultural nursing knowledge (cognitive dimension)
- Novice learners will have lower self-efficacy perceptions than advanced learners.

Factor analysis: Latest techniques and comparative findings. Since the initial factor analysis study, new statistical techniques have been developed that permit more sophisticated analyses. Using a sample of 272 culturally diverse associate degree nursing students, Jeffreys and Dogan (2009) explored the factorial composition of the TSET by conducting a Common Exploratory Factor Analysis (CEFA). The reader is encouraged to note that CEFA is different from Principal Component Analysis (PCA); the rationale for conducting another factor analysis study using new statistical techniques will be described briefly.

"Both Exploratory Factor Analysis (EFA) and Principal Component Analysis (PCA) are multivariate statistical techniques widely used in social and behavioral sciences (Ledesma & Valero-Mora, 2007). PCA is a more popular method for factor extraction, because it is the default method provided in many popular statistical software packages. As Costello and Osborne (2005) point out, however, PCA is not a true method of factor analysis "'and there is disagreement among statistical theorists about when it should be used, if at all' (p. 2)" (Jeffreys & Dogan, 2010).

Jeffreys and Dogan (2010) also implemented two other similarly underused (if not ignored) methods in analyzing survey data. First, the most recent data imputation techniques were used in dealing with missing data. Second, the standard errors of factor loadings were used in determining the factor structure of the TSET. Specifically, standard errors for factor loadings were computed and utilized in deciding if a given item loads significantly on a factor and whether the difference between the factor loadings of two or more items on the same factor are statistically significant. (Details about these procedures and the technical differences between the PCA and CEFA may be found in Jeffreys & Dogan, 2010).

The CEFA comprising 69 of the 83 items yielded 4 factors: "Knowledge and Understanding," "Interview," "Awareness, Acceptance, and Appreciation," and "Recognition" with internal consistency ranging from 0.94 to 0.98. Notably, all of the items within a factor came from a single subscale of the TSET. Consistent with the item-exclusive factor loadings on subscales demonstrated in the previous factor analysis study (Jeffreys & Smodlaka, 1998), what this most probably implies is that within each broad educational learning domain, as captured by the three TSET subscales, there are several underlying theoretical dimensions that contribute to the construct of transcultural self-efficacy. Furthermore, the internal consistency of each of the factors was quite high, ranging from 0.94 to 0.98, attesting to the coherence of the underlying conceptual structure; reliability of the total instrument was 0.99 (Jeffreys & Dogan, 2010). Unlike the previous study in which 70 items yielded 9 factors consisting of items that loaded exclusively within the originally conceptualized subscale (Jeffreys & Smodlaka, 1998), the number of factors came closer to the initial conceptualization of subscales. However, validation of a construct must focus on the degree to which an instrument is consistent with the underlying theoretical framework and related literature. If the performance of an instrument is consistent with the theoretically proposed expectations, then it is concluded that the instrument is construct valid (Carmines & Zeller, 1979).

The factorial composition of the TSET continues to be consistent with the underlying theoretical framework and the related literature in nursing, education, and psychology (self-efficacy). Notably, Factor 1 incorporated all 25 items on the Cognitive Subscale with factor loadings ranging from 0.63 to 0.80 and all items correlating positively with the total score (0.68 to 0.83). The Cognitive Subscale targeted the cognitive learning domain conceptualized by Bloom et al. (Bloom, Englehart, Furst, Hill, & Krathwohl, 1956), focusing on the first two levels of "knowledge and understanding." Using the more valid and newer CEFA approach yielded a coherent factor structure within the cognitive learning domain whereby all items loaded exclusively and significantly on this subscale, demonstrating high internal consistency (Crohnbach's alpha = 0.97). The previous PCA statistical approach (Jeffreys & Smodlaka, 1998) separated items in the Cognitive Subscale into two factors: Professional Nursing Care (nine items) and Lifecycle Transitional Phenomena (eight items). The content validity experts previously validated that the 25 items (developed from the transcultural literature) within the Cognitive Subscale were appropriate and relevant for this learning domain within the full context of transcultural self-efficacy. The 2009 CEFA analyses (Jeffreys & Dogan, 2010) supported the ratings by the content validity experts, thereby lending greater validity to the TSET.

Educational experts support that sufficient background knowledge and understanding is needed in order to apply information practically. As conceptualized in the TSET and the CCC model, interviewing clients about cultural values and beliefs is essential for the completion of a comprehensive health history, development of a culture-specific/culturally competent and congruent care plan, and provision of culturally congruent care. Using the CEFA approach, Factor 2 (Interview) contained 22 of the 28 items on the Practical Subscale with factor loadings ranging from 0.67 to 0.86, all items correlating positively with the total score (correlation coefficients ranged from 0.77 to 0.89), and demonstrated high reliability (Cronbach's alpha = 0.98). The labeling of Factor 2 as "Interview" was considered appropriate for the underlying conceptual framework that purports that the teaching and learning of cultural competence must carefully weave together cognitive, practical, and affective learning. Although Factor 2 excluded six of the items dealing with asking clients about verbal and nonverbal communication, space and touch, time perception, language preference, and English comprehension, all of the other essential expert-rated interview topics loaded exclusively on this one factor. One possible explanation for the item exclusion may be that the respondents assumed that in order to conduct an interview, assessment of English comprehension, etc. would be obviously essential. Previously (Jeffreys & Smodlaka, 1998), these six items loaded separately on Factor 7, labeled "Communication."

Transcultural experts and educational leaders continually attest to the importance of affective learning domain on integrating foundational and key professional values within a professional education (Andrews, 1995; Leininger & McFarland, 2002, 2006; Neumann & Forsyth, 2008). Although the 1998 study (Jeffreys & Smodlaka) yielded four separate factors consisting of items loading exclusively on the Affective Subscale, the most recent CEFA study analyses generated two factors labeled "Awareness, Acceptance, and Appreciation" (Factor 3) and "Recognition" (Factor 4) (Jeffreys & Dogan, 2010). Factor 3 addressed: (a) all three items dealing with awareness of own cultural group and biases, (b) awareness of insensitive and prejudicial treatment among different cultural backgrounds; (c) all three items concerned with accepting differences and similarities between cultural groups and client's refusal of treatment based on beliefs; and (d) all five items associated with appreciation. The factor loadings for this factor ranged from 0.51 to 0.87, all items correlated positively with the total score (correlation coefficients ranged from 0.61 to 0.85), and the factor was highly reliable (Cronbach's alpha = 0.94).

Factor 4 (Recognition) contained 10 of the 11 items that addressed recognition in the affective dimension. Respondents were asked to recognize, among clients of different cultural backgrounds, the impact of select elements (political factors, values, roles, socioeconomic factors) on health care practices, the need to foster cultural care through nursing strategies (preservation/maintenance, accommodation/negotiation, repatterning/restructuring), importance of home remedies and folk medicine, and the need to prevent cultural imposition and ethnocentric views. Excluded from the factor was the item about inadequacies in the U.S. health care system. The factor loadings for this factor ranged from 0.55 to 0.80. Cronbach's alpha for the set of items loading on this factor was 0.94. All items correlated positively with total score; the correlation coefficients ranged from 0.68 to 0.83.

Originally conceptualized as one dimension tapping on affective learning, the latest analyses (Jeffreys & Dogan, 2010) may suggest that within the respondents' perspective, recognition (Factor 4) involved a different type or level of affective learning. Several transcultural experts have identified "awareness" as the essential, first, or key element required for cultural competence development (Andrews & Boyle, 2008; Campinha-Bacote, 2003; Giger & Davidhizar, 2008; Leininger & McFarland, 2002, 2006; Purnell & Paulanka, 2008; Spector, 2008). This awareness includes self-awareness as well as awareness of various aspects of culturally different clients. Recognition may include a different level of assessment that blends together knowledge, practical skills, and awareness. But, notably, all of these components are considered essential in the development of cultural competence and in the provision of culturally congruent nursing care. Perhaps focus groups with similar and/or different learner/health care provider professional populations will lend greater insight into the perceived differences between "awareness, acceptance, and appreciation" and "recognition."

Consistent with the 1998 study (Jeffreys & Smodlaka), virtually all Affective Subscale items under the heading "Recognition" clustered together. In the CEFA study (Jeffreys & Dogan, 2010), only the item about recognizing inadequacies in the U.S. health care system was excluded. This item was added to the TSET upon the suggestion of several of the content validity experts. Previously, all items clustered together under "Recognition." Since the development of the TSET in 1994 (Jeffreys, 1994), changes within the U.S. health care system have been ongoing; some of these changes may be reflected in the respondents' views of this item. Additionally, the 2009 study sample included students within one associate degree program (n = 272). Generally, associate degree nursing students do not receive as much background course work grounded in the complexities of the U.S. health care system. Researchers in other countries have also requested changing this item to mention their respective country and/or deleting this item. Because one purpose of factorial analyses may be to refine instrument items and create more parsimonious instruments that capture a valid measure/assessment of the targeted construct, consideration of deleting this item following repeated CEFA studies using different health care professional populations is warranted.

Factor Analysis: Conclusive Summary

Conclusively, the latest CEFA study (Jeffreys & Dogan, 2010) continues to support that the TSET assesses the multidimensional nature of transcultural self-efficacy while also differentiating between three types of learning: cognitive, practical, and affective. Additionally, each TSET item continues to contribute to the reliability of the underlying constructs, as evidenced by the positive and high item to total score correlations. Furthermore, the TSET continues to demonstrate high levels of internal consistency and had a coherent factor structure supportive of the underlying conceptual framework (CCC model). The benefits of this support allow the researcher/educator to move beyond mere assessment to the design, implementation, and evaluation of diagnostic-prescriptive teaching strategies for cultural competence education.

Criterion-Related Validity

Another important consideration pertains to the assessment of criterion-related validity. Criterion-related validity examines the degree to which the subject's performance on the measurement tool and the subject's actual behavior are related (LoBiondo-Wood & Haber, 1998; Polit & Beck, 2004). In other words, criterion-related validity addresses "How is performance on a measurement tool and actual behavior related?" and may be assessed using different approaches. For the TSET, predictive validity was examined. Predictive validity examines the degree of correlation between the measure of the concept and a future measure of the same concept. An underlying theoretical assumption was that transcultural self-efficacy (TSE) is a dynamic construct that changes over time and is influenced by formalized exposure to culture care concepts (transcultural nursing). The question, Does the TSET measure changes in TSE after formalized exposure to transcultural nursing? was most directly addressed in a longitudinal study. Results indicated statistically significant differences in TSE perceptions between the first and fourth clinical semester (Jeffreys & Smodlaka, 1999a). The greatest changes were detected in students with lower self-efficacy initially, who had then been exposed to a two-year educational experience that integrated transcultural nursing concepts, issues, and skills within theory and clinical work. In a cross-sectional study, TSE scores also demonstrated changes in the expected (predicted) direction. Demographic variables (age, gender, income, ethnicity, and racial group identity) did not influence TSE perceptions or the types of changes in TSE perceptions (Jeffreys & Smodlaka, 1999b). The results supported the following underlying assumptions:

- Transcultural self-efficacy is a dynamic construct that changes over time and is influenced by formalized exposure to culture care concepts (transcultural nursing).
- Learners are most confident about their attitudes (affective dimension) and least confident about their transcultural nursing knowledge (cognitive dimension)
- All students and nurses (regardless of age, ethnicity, gender, sexual orientation, lifestyle, religion, socioeconomic status, geographic

location, or race) require formalized educational experiences to meet culture care needs of diverse individuals.

- Novice learners will have lower self-efficacy perceptions than advanced learners.
- The greatest change in transcultural self-efficacy perceptions will be detected in individuals with low self-efficacy (low confidence) initially, who have then been exposed to formalized transcultural nursing concepts and experiences.

Predictive validity is also concerned with the degree to which an individual's performance on the questionnaire correlates with a predetermined outcome behavior. The desired outcome behavior is a high level of cultural competent behaviors resulting in culturally congruent care; however the evaluation of cultural competency in the clinical setting is complex. The potential for changed behaviors with known observations, confounded by the limited availability of qualified observers and valid measurement strategies, presents challenges for directly estimating predictions of TSE on actual behavior. According to Bandura's theory (1986), resilient (strong) self-efficacy perceptions result in higher levels of goal commitment, motivation, persistence, learning, and skill performance. Commitment and motivation are essential components in achieving cultural competency (Campinha-Bacote, 1999, 2003; Chang, 1995), therefore, it can only be assumed that transcultural self-efficacy perceptions will directly influence cultural competency through commitment and motivation. Other studies indicated that self-efficacy is a mediator of commitment and motivation, thereby affecting outcome behaviors (Bandura, 1996a, 1996b, 1997; Bandura & Schunk, 1981; Lent, Lopez, & Bieschke, 1993; Mone, Baker, & Jeffries, 1995; Saks, 1995).

To address this issue of TSE predicting cultural competence behaviors in clinical, a multiphase study is currently under way. The purpose of the study is to examine the influence of cultural competence education on undergraduate and graduate nursing students' transcultural self-efficacy perceptions, extent of culturally specific care provided for culturally diverse clients, frequency of cultural assessment, and the development of culturally sensitive and professionally appropriate attitudes, values, or beliefs (Jeffreys & Dogan, 2007). The study also involves the adaptation of the TSET into the CCCET discussed in forthcoming sections within this chapter.

Other Validity Findings

Harper's Delphi study involving 35 expert international nurse researchers determined that of six other cultural questionnaires reported in the nursing literature, the TSET measures the most attributes of cultural competence identified by the expert panel (Harper, 2008). All of the cultural competence instruments evaluated, except the TSET, contained less than half of the items identified by the expert panel as important to achieving cultural competence. The TSET contained 52 items or 66% of the items from the Delphi rounds. In a systematic review of 45 instruments measuring cultural competence, Gozu et al. (2007) reported that most instruments are poorly constructed, lacking acceptable psychometric properties; however, they noted that the TSET had more detailed psychometric testing and consistently demonstrated high validity and reliability. In addition to acknowledging the high validity and reliability of the TSET, Krentzman and Townsend's review also noted its use with diverse respondents (Krentzman & Townsend, 2008). Capell et al.'s (2007) review of cultural competence instruments also noted the consistently high validity and reliability of the TSET, yet recommended further testing of all instruments for social desirability and to determine if they correlate with culturally competent behaviors or enhanced client outcomes. (See Chapter 5 for social desirability response bias and the TSET.)

Psychometric Properties: Reliability

An instrument cannot be valid without demonstrated reliability. Reliability refers to the degree of accuracy and consistency in measurement. Reliability examines the extent to which an instrument provides the same results on repeated uses (LoBiondo-Wood and Haber, 1998; Polit & Beck, 2004).

Usually, reliability tests are performed each time the instrument is used, because instrument reliability is population-specific rather than an inherent instrument property (Nunnally & Bernstein, 1994). With the TSET, the broad question concerning reliability asked, To what extent does the TSET provide the same results on repeated uses with different samples? In order to answer this question, two more specific questions were asked, differentiating between internal consistency and stability.

Internal Consistency

Internal consistency is concerned with the degree to which questionnaire items correlate with each other and reflect the same concept. High levels of internal consistency in the total instrument and within its subscales permit tallying of items for the purpose of scoring and data analysis (LoBiondo-Wood & Haber, 1998; Nunnally & Bernstein, 1994). The question, To what degree are items on the TSET internally consistent? could also be phrased to ask, To what degree do TSET items correlate with each other

Table 4.2   Summary of TSET Reliability Tests and
Results (Jeffreys, 2000)

Type Assessed	Method	Results
Internal Consistency	Cronbach's alpha	.92 to .98
	Split-half	.76 to .92
Stability	Test-retest	.63 to .75

and reflect the same construct? Another important question, Is the internal consistency of the TSET adequate? necessitated comprehension of methodological guidelines concerning minimal adequacy results. Reliability tests are reported as reliability coefficients. Perfectly correlated items would be demonstrated by a coefficient of 1.00. Generally, a reliability coefficient of 0.70 is considered acceptable for new instruments. In contrast, a minimum reliability coefficient of 0.80 is considered adequate for well-established instruments (Nunnally & Bernstein, 1994).

These questions led to two approaches for reliability testing: Cronbach's alpha (coefficient alpha) and split-half reliability. Cronbach's alpha is the preferred measure of internal consistency because all items are compared with each other and with the total questionnaire. In split-half reliability, one half of the instrument or subscale is compared with the other half. This approach is less accurate and often yields lower results (Nunnally & Bernstein, 1994). Consistent with this methodological assumption, split-half reliability results on the total TSET and its subscales were lower, ranging from 0.76 to 0.92. Cronbach's alpha was calculated across several studies, each time yielding coefficient alpha ranging from 0.92 to 0.98 on the total TSET instrument and its subscales (Jeffreys, 2000). Additionally, alpha coefficients ranged from 0.87 to 0.95 when testing for the internal consistency of items within each of the identified nine factors (Jeffreys, 2000; Jeffreys & Smodlaka, 1998). The initial results indicated that the TSET had high estimates of reliability (internal consistency) and supported the use of subscale scoring to measure the various dimensions of TSE perceptions (see Table 4.2). Subsequent TSET use by other researchers demonstrated overall high levels of reliability and internal consistency (see TSET Research Exhibits 6.1, 6.3, 6.4, and 6.5 for some examples).

Stability

Stability aims to measure whether the measurement of the construct is stable and addresses To what degree will the same results be obtained on repeated instrument administrations? One desired use of the TSET was to detect TSE perceptual changes over time; therefore it was essential to use the test-retest method for assessing stability. Consistent with recommended protocols for test-retest methodology (Carmines & Zeller, 1979; Nunnally & Bernstein, 1994), a two-week interval between TSET administration was selected. Specifically, the test-retest method explored the questions, To what degree will the same results be obtained on two administrations of the TSET following a two-week interval? To what degree is the TSET stable? and, Is the stability of the TSET adequate?

Because test-retest reliability is considered the least conclusive measure of reliability, it was anticipated that results would be lower than with the split-half or Cronbach's alpha methods. Test-retest correlation coefficients for the total TSET ranged from 0.63 to 0.75, suggesting moderate stability. However, it should be noted that lower values may actually signify that the trait changes over time, independent of the instrument's stability (Carmines & Zeller, 1979). It is possible to surmise students' exposure to multidimensional learning experiences via assignments, classroom, and clinical settings over two weeks could make a slight positive difference. Table 4.1 summarizes TSET reliability results in the initial instrument studies (Jeffreys & Smodlaka, 1996, 1998, 1999a, 1999b). (See TSET Research Exhibits Chapter 6 & 10 for other examples.)

Scoring

As mentioned previously, the high levels of internal consistency within the whole TSET instrument and within each subscale supported the use of scores for data analyses. Bandura (1986) recommended assessing both the strength and magnitude (level) of self-efficacy. A review of literature by Lee and Bobko (1994) identified five different ways of operationalizing self-efficacy based on Bandura's recommendations. Consistent with many other self-efficacy instruments (Bandura, 1989; Berry, West, & Dennehey, 1989; Brown, Lent, & Larkin, 1989; Cervone, 1989; Hackett, 1985; Lent, Brown, & Larkin, 1986, 1987; Shell, Murphy, & Bruning, 1989), scoring of the TSET initially included subscale calculations of self-efficacy strength (SEST) and self-efficacy level (SEL). SEST refers to the average strength of self-efficacy perceptions within a particular dimension (subscale) of the construct. On the TSET, SEST scores are calculated by totaling subscale item responses and dividing by the number of subscale items, resulting in the mean score (Table 4.3). SEST scores are used most often in self-efficacy studies (Lee & Bobko, 1994). One must be aware that because SEST scores present the average score, low or high item responses may be hidden within the average (mean). SEST scores can be used to detect changes over time, compare with a demographic variable, or compare within the group.

Table 4.3   Self-Efficacy Strength (SEST) Score Calculation: Subscale Mean

	Cognitive Subscale	Practical Subscale	Affective Subscale
Formula			
$\dfrac{\text{Item Response Sum}}{\text{\# of Subscale Items}}$	$\dfrac{\text{Add Item Responses}}{25}$	$\dfrac{\text{Add Item Responses}}{28}$	$\dfrac{\text{Add Item Responses}}{30}$
Application	$\dfrac{140}{25}$	$\dfrac{220}{28}$	$\dfrac{210}{30}$
	SEST = 5.6	SEST = 7.9	SEST = 7.0

SEL refers to the number of items perceived at a specified minimum level of confidence. In studies with phobics and low academic achievers, SEL has been used to identify individuals with "low efficacy" and then track SEL changes following treatment interventions. Individuals with less than 20% confidence are inefficacious and are at high risk for avoidance behaviors and severe stress (Bandura, 1977, 1982; Bandura & Schunk, 1981). Although this benchmark has been used with phobics and academic low achievers, this benchmark has been adjusted in samples where greater self-efficacy perceptions have been anticipated. For example, Bandura and Schunk (1981) raised the benchmark to 40%, reflecting a "moderate degree of assurance" (p. 594). Some self-efficacy studies have not included the evaluation of self-efficacy level (Lee & Bobko, 1994). Other researchers have noted redundancy between the two measures and have chosen to only report one measure (score) of self-efficacy (Cervone, 1989).

On the TSET, SEL initially referred to the number of subscale items students perceived with more than 20% confidence; however, the 20% benchmark may need to be raised in samples where greater self-efficacy perceptions are observed, desirable, and/or expected. In order for SEL scores to be meaningful, they must discriminate within the sample. If the benchmark is too low for the sample, then most (or even all) of the sample will have the same SEL score. For example, in several studies, the 20% SEL benchmark resulted in few students (Jeffreys & Smodlaka, 1999a, 1999b; Lim, Downie, & Nathan, 2004) and few nurses (Toney, 2004) who did not meet the 20% benchmark. Future studies may wish to raise the benchmark standards, especially if the overall goal is to enhance cultural competence and provide high levels of culturally congruent care to culturally diverse patients. The question remains, What is an appropriate benchmark for professional nurses (and for students studying to become professional nurses)? Statistical methods (standard-setting research) could be employed to mirror the "standards" or "benchmarks" procedures used in large-scale assessments; however, access to large nationwide samples pose an overwhelming obstacle for this approach. The 20% (or even 40%) benchmark does not seem to be discriminating among nursing students or nurses, an optimistic sign suggesting that, overall, nursing students and nurses interacting with and caring for culturally diverse clients meet this low benchmark. The 20% or 40% benchmark was initially selected based on Bandura's work with phobics and academically low-achieving children who usually did not meet these benchmarks prior to therapeutic intervention. Based on study results of various researchers using the TSET, the 20% or 40% benchmark and SEL calculation no longer seems appropriate. The next step would be standard-setting research to determine the appropriate benchmark for student and registered nurse groups. In lieu of standard-setting research, researchers using the TSET are redirected back to other researchers' recommendations who elected to eliminate SEL calculations based on redundancy and/or indiscriminate findings with SEST scores (Cervone, 1989; Lee & Bobko, 1994).

Grouping samples into low, medium, and high-efficacy groups based on SEST, SEL, and/or some other criterion permits further comparative analyses and the identification of at-risk individuals (inefficacious or supremely efficacious). Inefficacious individuals are at risk for avoiding tasks; supremely efficacious (overly confident) individuals are at risk because of inadequate preparation and/or viewing the task as unimportant (Bandura, 1982). Several different methods may be used for group categorization and comparison; several sample methods are proposed; however, future studies are needed to assess validation. (Jeffreys Toolkit 2010, Item 1 instructions). The study purpose and sample may guide method selection for group categorization. For example, coding may occur in the following manner: (a) low (students who select a 1 or 2 response on 80% or more of the subscale items); (b) high (students who select a 9 or 10 response on 80% or more of the subscale items; and (c) medium (students who select a 3 through 8 response on 80% or more of the subscale items or who do not fall into the low or high group) (Jeffreys & Smodlaka, 1999a, 1999b; Lim et al., 2004; Toney, 2004). Alternatively (in samples with few 1 or 2 responses/subscale), respondents with any 1 or 2 responses may be categorized as low SEL, if adhering to the proposed 20% confidence benchmark indicating "low" or "at-risk." The definition of the "high" group could be "respondents who selected 9 and 10 responses for all subscale items." Here, the medium group would constitute respondents who did not fall into the other two groups. In other samples (especially where low self-efficacy perceptions can be anticipated to be less prevalent), still other techniques may be employed for grouping. For example, the 20% benchmark for SEL could be raised to 40% (Bandura & Schunk, 1981). Another approach involves percentages or standard deviations to compute low, middle, and high groups. For example, the medium group can be defined as plus or minus one standard deviation from the subscale mean. Respondents below this criterion would be labeled "low"; respondents above this criterion would constitute the "high" group. Further research is needed to appraise various approaches.

In summary, SEST scores are most often used in self-efficacy studies (Lee & Bobko, 1994). Calculation of SEST scores for each of the TSET subscales is routinely recommended whenever the TSET is used. TSET SEL scores are an additional, supplemental approach for analyzing data; however, standard-setting research to determine actual benchmark levels is now recommended. Different methods can be employed to group individuals into low-efficacy, medium-efficacy, and high-efficacy groups for the purpose of identifying at-risk individuals and tracking changes. Again, standard-setting research, using very large samples, will provide empirical evidence for the grouping approach selected. In lieu of a very large sample, low-medium-high groupings can still be used and data appraised recognizing limitations posed.

Evaluating Transcultural Self-Efficacy Perceptions

Although the TSET was specifically designed to measure and evaluate undergraduate nursing students' confidence for performing general transcultural nursing skills among diverse populations, nurse researchers have requested the TSET for use with graduate students and/or for use with nurses working in various clinical agencies. Researchers in other health professions worldwide have requested the TSET for review and possible use, adaptation, and/or translation. Because the TSET does not selectively target specific cultural groups, rather it broadly asks respondents to consider general principles related to culturally different clients, it has broader application among culturally diverse health care professionals who provide care for many diverse culturally different clients. The generalist approach (as emphasized in the TSET) was considered most appropriate for learners without previous formal education and background in transcultural nursing and/or the transcultural nurse generalist who will provide care for clients of many different cultural backgrounds.

One underlying assumption of the TSET is that all students and nurses (regardless of age, ethnicity, gender, sexual orientation, lifestyle, religion, socioeconomic status, geographic location, or race) require formalized educational experiences to meet culture care needs of diverse individuals. (The same assumption applies across other health professional disciplines). Unfortunately, the numbers of nurses and other health professionals who have received formal education experiences in transcultural topics and cultural competence are few (AAMC, 2005; ADA, 2005, 2007; Andrews, 1995; APA, 1994; APTA, 2008; Gerstein et al., 2009; Harper, 2008; Leininger, 1995b; Leininger & McFarland, 2002; Lubinski & Matteliano, 2008; NASW, 2001, 2007, 2009; Nochajski

& Matteliano, 2008; Panzarella & Matteliano, 2008; Ponterotto et al., 2010; Suh, 2004; Wilson & Houghtaling, 2001). Only relatively recently have accrediting agencies, professional organizations, journals, textbooks, and films, included culture and culturally congruent care as an essential dimension in achieving quality health outcomes. Therefore, it was reasonable to assume that an instrument that is readable and appropriate for novice undergraduate students is also appropriate for other populations.

Usability may be applicable to populations who have had little or no formalized education experiences in transcultural nursing and cultural competence and/or those without opportunities for field application/ interaction with culturally different clients and/or nurses/health professionals. Usability may also extend to populations who have had formal and/or informal exposure to transcultural nursing, culturally different clients, and culturally different health care professional colleagues. For example, Toney (2004) used the TSET to measure TSE among community health nurses who frequently encounter culturally diverse clients in their clinical practice.

Cultural competence of health care providers is a worldwide concern and the TSET has the potential to assist educators evaluate cultural competence education initiatives. Within the discipline of medicine, the TSET has been adapted for use with physicians in Australia (Shadbolt, 2004). Another new version of the TSET, appropriate for multidisciplinary health care providers is being piloted through a grant-funded study at a large HCI (see TSET Research Exhibit 10.1). Use of the TSET translated into other languages will expand the depth of knowledge concerning cultural competence education, identify universal differences and similarities, and provide further empirical support for the TSET's validity and reliability across cultures and languages. Ultimately, it is the study purpose, design, research questions/hypotheses, and sample that must guide a researcher's decision to use the TSET. Future research with the TSET among similar and different populations will expand knowledge concerning TSE and the TSET.

Evaluation of TSE perceptions may be used for a variety of purposes targeting the individual and/or groups (See Exhibit 4.1).

Exhibit 4.1   Educator-In-Action Vignette

Professor Quest becomes interested in exploring, measuring, and evaluating undergraduate students' baseline self-efficacy perceptions prior to the design and implementation of educational innovations (EI) or interventions to develop cultural competence. He plans to systematically reevaluate self-efficacy perceptions following the implementation of EI. Following a literature review, Professor Quest contemplates the use of the TSET to explore baseline TSE perceptions, conduct follow-up measures of TSE after EI are introduced into the curriculum, and evaluate changes within the three dimensions of learning. He is also interested in evaluating culturally competent actions in the clinical setting.

He decides to pilot the TSET with a small group of approximately 30 first-semester students. After obtaining permission to use the TSET (Jeffreys 2010 Toolkit Item 19; See Preface, page xix), Professor Quest prepares a "Pilot Test Worksheet" (Table 4.4) to guide evaluation of the TSET for use with his prospective larger study.

Based on the pilot test results, he determines priority areas for EI, searches the literature for evidence-based EI, and designs or adapts cultural competence EI. Professor Quest uses the Cultural Competence Documentation Log (Jeffreys 2010 Toolkit Item 20) as a template to document and organize his EI, measurement, and evaluation plans. He expands upon the template to develop a research plan (Table 4.5) that corresponds with his research problem statement and questions (see below). Early collaboration with a statistician assists Professor Quest in the decision-making process and plan for statistical analysis.

Problem Statement

What is the influence of cultural competence education on nursing students' transcultural self-efficacy perceptions, extent of culturally specific care provided for culturally diverse clients, frequency of cultural assessment, and the development of culturally sensitive and professionally appropriate attitudes, values, or beliefs?

Research Questions

1. Which transcultural nursing skills do students perceive with more confidence?
2. Which transcultural nursing skills do students perceive with less confidence?
3. What are the changes in TSE perceptions following formalized educational experiences and/or other learning experiences?
4. To what extent is culture-specific care provided by students during the clinical practicum?
5. Which cultural assessments are implemented more frequently with culturally diverse clients during the clinical practicum?
6. Which cultural assessments are implemented less frequently with culturally diverse clients during the clinical practicum?
7. To what extent do culturally sensitive and professionally appropriate attitudes, values, or beliefs change during the clinical practicum?
8. What is the diversity of clients in the clinical area?
9. What is the diversity of health problems in the clinical area?
10. What are the demographic characteristics of students?

Table 4.4   Pilot Test Data Worksheet

	Cognitive	Practical	Affective	Total TSET
Completion Time				X
Item Responses				
Range	X	X	X	
Mode	X	X	X	
Median	X	X	X	
Frequency (each item option)	X	X	X	
Subscale Mean (SEST)	X	X	X	
Reliability Tests				
Crohnbach alpha	X	X	X	X
Split-half	X	X	X	X
Validity Tests				
Construct (Hypothesis-testing approach): Students will be least confident about their knowledge and most confident about their attitudes, values, and beliefs	Are SEST scores the lowest?	Are SEST scores neither the highest nor lowest?	Are SEST scores the highest?	

The purposes are to:

1. Develop a composite/baseline of learners' needs, values, attitudes, and skills concerning transcultural nursing (or health care).
2. Identify general transcultural skills perceived with more confidence (or those as less difficult or stressful).
3. Identify general transcultural skills perceived with less confidence (or those as more difficult or stressful).
4. Identify differences within groups.
5. Identify differences between groups.
6. Identify at-risk individuals (low confidence or overly confident).
7. Evaluate the effectiveness of specific teaching interventions.
8. Assess changes in transcultural self-efficacy perceptions over time.

Although self-report instruments present certain limitations, the construct of self-efficacy can only be evaluated by self-appraisal and self-report (Bandura, 1996a, 1996b; 1997). Choice of a valid and reliable instrument will help decrease the limitations associated with measurement error and increase the confidence with which researchers interpret data. Using the TSET, several different approaches can be implemented to yield

Table 4.5 Research Plan: Questions, Data Collection, Educational Innovation, Data Analyses

Research Questions*	Pretest Data Collection	Educational Innovations (EI)**	Posttest Data Collection	Data Analyses
1. Which transcultural nursing skills do students perceive with more confidence? 2. Which transcultural nursing skills do students perceive with less confidence?	Personal Coding Page TSET Give before EI As above			Calculate item means Rank order means from highest to lowest Rank order means from lowest to highest
3. What are the changes in TSE perceptions following formalized educational experiences and/or other learning experiences?	As above		Personal Coding Page TSET	Calculate subscale SEST scores and compare pretest scores with posttest scores Check for statistically significant changes (t-test) Group into low, medium, high groups and compare pretest and posttest for each subscale
4. To what extent is culture-specific care provided by students during the clinical practicum?			Personal Coding Page CCET-SV CCET-TV Give after EI	Calculate frequency and % Rank order Compare SV and TV

Question	Instrument	Analysis
5. Which cultural assessments are implemented more frequently with culturally diverse clients during the clinical practicum?	As above	As above Rank order from highest to lowest
6. Which cultural assessments are implemented less frequently with culturally diverse clients during the clinical practicum?	As above	Rank order from lowest to highest
7. To what extent do culturally sensitive and professionally appropriate attitudes, values, or beliefs change during the clinical practicum?	As above	Calculate frequency and % Rank order Compare SV and TV
8. What is the diversity of clients in the clinical area?	CSAT-DD Clinical instructor completes at end of semester after EI	Calculate frequency and %
9. What is the diversity of health problems in the clinical area?	As above	As above
10. What are the demographic characteristics of students?	DDS Attach after TSET Give before EI	As above

*Questions can easily be adapted for undergraduate and graduate students in nursing and other health professions, nurses, and other health care professionals (providers) employed in HCI.
** See Chapters 6–13 for examples of educational innovations (EI).

valuable information necessary to guide future research, education, and practice. The selected approach will be determined by the study purpose, design, research questions/hypotheses, sample, and researcher. Ongoing instrument evaluation must be an integral component in every study. Comparison of SEST scores, SEL scores, groups (low, medium, high), individual item responses, and factor mean scores can be used to answer research questions/hypotheses. Collection of appropriate and relevant demographic data will be valuable in interpreting findings and may be useful for descriptive or inferential statistical analyses. (Jeffreys Toolkit 2010, Items 8 and 9 present examples of demographic data potentially relevant for collection with the TSET). Researchers' examination of the results in relation to the proposed underlying assumptions of the CCC model can further substantiate the proposed theoretical assumptions. For example, among various study samples, respondents are most confident about their affective skills and least confident about their knowledge (Lim et al., 2004; Toney, 2004; Wilson & Houghtaling, 2001). (See TSET Research Exhibits in Chapter 6 and 10). Strategies for interpreting transcultural self-efficacy perceptions will be discussed in Chapter 5.

CULTURAL COMPETENCE CLINICAL EVALUATION TOOL

Major Components and Features

The CCCET is a new tool adapted from the TSET (Jeffreys, 1994, 2000, 2006; Jeffreys & Smodlaka, 1996, 1998, 1999a, 1999b). Specifically, the TSET's existing items were maintained; however, the rating scale and directions were adapted to permit the students'/learners' self-evaluation of clinical cultural competence and teachers'/agency evaluator's evaluation of clinical cultural competence. Statistical consultation focused on issues concerning instructions, relationship of item to rating scale and directions, optical scanning capability, and proposed data analyses. The CCCET contains three subscales measuring different dimensions of clinical cultural competence behaviors: (a) the extent of culturally specific care (Subscale 1); (b) cultural assessment (Subscale 2); and (c) culturally sensitive and professionally appropriate attitudes, values, or beliefs including awareness, acceptance, recognition, appreciation, advocacy necessary for providing culturally sensitive professional nursing care (Subscale 3). Consistent with the TSET, a 10-point rating scale is used as indicated below:

- Subscale 1 (Provision of culture-specific care): "Not at all" (1) to "totally" (10)
- Subscale 2 (Cultural Assessment): "Never" (1) to "always" (10)

- Subscale 3 (Cultural sensitivity): "Not at all" (1) to "to a great extent" (10)

In addition, respondents had the option of selecting A ([clinical] area not available) or B (diverse clients not available). For example, if nurses or students were not in the maternity/labor and delivery/postpartum unit, selection of choice "A" (area not available) would be appropriate for items related to birth and pregnancy. The intended use of the CCCET was to determine baseline information, identify areas of strengths, weaknesses, and gaps, and to evaluate change following educational intervention and/or increased exposure to culturally diverse clients and/or increased exposure to the clinical topic/area not previously available. Students and teachers independently complete the CCCET at the end of the clinical experience; approximate completion time is 20 minutes (Jeffreys Toolkit 2010, Items 3 and 4). Following the design and preliminary psychometric evaluation of the CCCET-Student Version (SV) and CCCET-Teacher Version (TV) with undergraduate and graduate nursing students, an employee version (CCCET-EV) and Agency Evaluator version (CCCET-AEV) were created for use in clinical agencies. (Jeffreys Toolkit 2010, Items 5 and 6) Questionnaire items remained the same; however, several words were changed in the directions to accommodate the change in population and setting.

Psychometric Properties: Validity

A series of three studies was planned to estimate the psychometric properties of the CCCET-SV and CCCET-TV.

Content Validity

Three content validity experts (doctoral prepared nurses internationally recognized as experts in transcultural nursing) reviewed both versions of the CCCET. The Content Validity Index (CVI) was 0.91 for both the teacher and the student versions of the instrument, indicating that the experts found the items highly relevant and representative of the domain. Experts' comments were appraised by the nurse researcher and statistician. No items required modification.

Concurrent Validity

The CCCET-SV and CCCET-TV was piloted with both undergraduate and graduate nursing students. For the undergraduates, the CCCET was piloted with three semesters of second semester associate degree nursing students (n = 161) enrolled in a 15-week medical-surgical clinical course. Because the intended purpose was to evaluate cultural competence in the clinical setting, the particular undergraduate medical-surgical course was selected for the pilot because the course: (a) contains the most credit hours and clinical experiences of any other course in the associate degree curriculum; and (b) is the first course that requires successful completion of the nursing fundamentals course in which students participate in multidimensional course activities incorporating transcultural nursing. Students independently completed the CCCET at the end of the clinical practicum. To allow matching of CCCET-TV and CCCET-SV, clinical instructors completed the CCCET-TV for each student at the end of the second clinical course, placing the completed CCCET-TV and student's CCCET-SV in an envelope prior to sealing and returning to the researcher. Preliminary data analyses are currently underway.

For the graduate student pilot, the CCCET has been administered to graduate nursing students enrolled in either one of the two clinical courses in the clinical nurse specialist (CNS) adult health or geriatric curriculum. The CCCET is completed at the end of the semester by students and teachers/preceptors. To allow matching of CCCET-TV and CCCET-SV, clinical instructors/preceptors complete the CCCET-TV for each student at the end of the second clinical course, placing the completed CCCET-TV and student's CCCET-SV in an envelope prior to sealing and returning to the researcher. Preliminary data analyses are currently underway.

Psychometric Properties: Reliability

After verifying that there were no significant differences between the three semesters of undergraduate nursing students, data was collapsed for aggregate analyses. Using a sample of 161 students, reliability (Crohnbach's alpha) for the total CCCET-SV (0.99) and each of the subscales was quite high, ranging from 0.97 to 0.98. Reliability (Crohnbach's alpha) for the teacher version was also high at 0.95 for the total CCCET-TV and moderate to high for each of the subscales (0.85–0.98). It must be mentioned that due to a large number of A (area not available) and B (diverse clients not available) responses, the actual number of valid cases entered into the reliability analysis was comparatively low. The importance of A and B responses, from a curricular standpoint must not be minimized because these responses provide valuable information that can appraise current clinical experiences and offer insights needed to guide curricular change.

Scoring

The mean and standard deviation of items and subscales, along with frequency distribution, is the chosen method of data analysis. Outcomes of these analyses will help answer the following questions and guide curricular/program change (See Exhibit 4.1):

1. To what extent is culture-specific care provided in the clinical setting?
2. Which cultural assessments are implemented most frequently with culturally diverse clients?
3. Which cultural assessments are implemented least frequently with culturally diverse clients?
4. To what extent did culturally sensitive and professionally appropriate attitudes, values, or beliefs change?
5. What is the influence of select demographic variables on the dependent variables?
6. How similar or different are ratings between student or employee and teacher/preceptor or agency evaluator?
7. What areas/topics of clinical practice are available?
8. What areas/topics of clinical practice are unavailable?
9. To what extent are culturally diverse clients available in the clinical site?
10. What is the influence of transcultural self-efficacy perceptions on cultural competence (behaviors and attitudes) in the clinical setting?
11. What is the influence of teaching intervention(s) on cultural competence (behaviors and attitudes) in the clinical setting?

CLINICAL SETTING ASSESSMENT TOOL – DIVERSITY AND DISPARITY

Major Components and Features

The CSAT-DD is a user-friendly tool to collect data about the clinical practicum/agency site, specifically focusing on descriptions of diverse client populations (Part I) and clinical problems targeting the twenty-eight focus areas of the Healthy People 2010 document (Part II). (Jeffreys Toolkit 2010, Item 7). The first page gathers information about the type of agency (e. g., private, public, etc.) and whether the instructor/preceptor/agency evaluator completed a college level course and/or continuing education (CE) units in transcultural nursing or cultural competence in health care. The 15 items in Part I gather information about the demographic makeup of the client population (age, ethnicity, languages spoken, religion, etc.) as well as identifying the most prevalent characteristics represented. Part II (28 items) identifies the five most frequent focus areas evident in the clinical setting. This tool is intended for descriptive use but could be used to examine the relationship between select variables on the CSAT-DD and other items or scores on the TSET and/or CCCET. Information can be used to evaluate amount and type of exposure of student/learner/nurse to culturally diverse clients and Healthy People 2010 focus areas.

OTHER ASSESSMENT TOOLS

Several other user-friendly assessment tools are described in Chapters 6, 10, and 13. The assessment tools, found in the Jeffreys Toolkit 2010 (Items 10–17), can be used alone or in conjunction with other toolkit items. The assessment tools are:

- Self-Assessment Tool-Academic (SAT-A)
- Self-Assessment Tool-Health Care Institutions (SAT-HCI)
- Self-Assessment Tool-Professional Associations (SAT-PA)
- Active Promoter Assessment Tool-Academic (APAT-A)
- Active Promoter Assessment Tool-Health Care Institutions/ Professional Associations (APAT-HCIPA)
- Systematic Inquiry: Academic (SI-A)
- Systematic Inquiry: Health Care Institutions (SI-HCI)
- Systematic Inquiry: Professional Associations (SI-PA)
- Demographic Data Sheet-Undergraduate (DDS-U)
- Demographic Data Sheet-Nurses (DDS-N)

KEY POINT SUMMARY

- Based on the literature and the results of a two-phase evaluation study, the 83-item TSET was designed to measure and evaluate students' confidence for performing general transcultural nursing skills among diverse populations.
- The process of designing the TSET included item development, item sequence, subscale sequence, expert content review, expert psychometric review, revised draft, pretest, minor revisions, and a second pretest.
- The TSET contains three subscales presented in the following sequence: Cognitive (25 items), Practical (28 items), and Affective (30 items).
- Validity tests addressed content validity, criterion-related validity, and construct validity.

- Research findings supported that the TSET detected differences in transcultural self-efficacy perceptions within groups and between groups.
- Reliability tests for internal consistency and stability indicated adequate reliability.
- The TSET has been used with nursing students, nurses, physicians (physician version), and multidisciplinary health care providers (health care provider version).
- The CCCET contains three subscales measuring different dimensions of clinical cultural competence behaviors: (a) the extent of culturally specific care (Subscale 1); (b) cultural assessment (Subscale 2); and (c) culturally sensitive and professionally appropriate attitudes, values, or beliefs (Subscale 3).
- The CSAT-DD is a user-friendly tool to collect data about the clinical practicum/agency site, specifically focusing on descriptions of diverse client populations (Part I) and clinical problems (Part II).

CHAPTER 5

A Guide for Interpreting Learners' Transcultural Self-Efficacy Perceptions, Identifying At-Risk Individuals, and Avoiding Pitfalls

Marianne R. Jeffreys, EdD, RN

Empirical support for self-efficacy as a predictor of cultural competence is more difficult to establish than conceptually acknowledging that self-efficacy plays a vital role in cultural competence development and culturally congruent care actions. Theoretical background information must be carefully considered when interpreting findings and demonstrating empirical support. For example, the Cultural Competence and Confidence (CCC) model (see Figure 3.1) illustrates the proposed connections between the foundational concepts. Chapter 3 details major components underlying the conceptual model, incorporating the main theoretical tenets of Bandura's self-efficacy theory (Bandura, 1982, 1986, 1989, 1997). Finally, Figure 3.2 depicted the directional pathways involved in TSE, cultural competence development, and culturally congruent care actions, further expanding upon theoretical background information.

Because the evaluation of self-efficacy relies on respondents' self-perceptions, there will always be some error associated with self-report measures; however, the only way that self-efficacy can be measured is with a self-report measurement tool. Despite the limitations that self-report measurement tools present, efforts can be made to increase the usability and interpretation of results by using a valid measurement tool and by customizing various steps and components of the research process to appropriately complement each other. Avoiding pitfalls in the initial research design will improve the interpretation of findings. Similarly, avoiding pitfalls in the interpretation of findings will enhance the study's validity and future usability and generalizability.

Making sense of transcultural self-efficacy (TSE) perceptions is a key component in this interpretive process. This chapter guides educators in the interpretation of TSE perceptions and in avoiding pitfalls in research design and interpretation. The identification of at-risk individuals through the interpretation of findings is highlighted.

INTERPRETATION

Making sense of TSE perceptions must be grounded in self-efficacy theory. A quick overview of essential theoretical elements will aid in interpretation. One must know what to look for, what data findings suggest, and how to subsequently formulate valid empirical conclusions. Several main theoretical features emphasizing connections to data interpretation are presented.

A key concept in Bandura's (1986) social cognitive theory is that learning and motivation for learning is directly influenced by self-efficacy perceptions, which are domain- and task-specific. Individuals with strong self-efficacy perceptions in a specific domain think, feel, and act differently from those who are inefficacious or those who are overly confident. Therefore, when interpreting findings, one will look for ways to differentiate between individuals who demonstrate strong (resilient) self-efficacy, low self-efficacy (inefficacious), or supremely high self-efficacy (overconfidence). For example, TSE perceptions as measured by the Transcultural Self-Efficacy Tool (TSET) can be differentiated by Self-Efficacy Strength (SEST) subscale scores, comparison of factor mean scores, and/or grouping into low, medium, and high groups based on the selected grouping methodology. See Chapter 4 for details on the TSET.

Strong (resilient) self-efficacy enhances sociocognitive functioning in several ways: (a) new or difficult tasks are viewed as challenges that are accepted willingly; (b) great preparatory efforts are exhibited; (c) strong goal commitment and persistence behaviors are enhanced; (d) failures and setbacks are attributed to insufficient effort; and (e) more energy is expended to overcome failures, hardships, setbacks, and potential stressors in an effort to achieve goals (Bandura, 1986). A strong (resilient) self-efficacy to withstand failures combined with some uncertainty (task perceived as a challenge rather than self-doubts about capability) will encourage preparatory efforts and thus enhance performance outcomes (Bandura, 1982, 1989). It is presumed that such individuals are highly motivated and actively seek help to maximize their transcultural nursing skills and cultural competence development. Based on the proposed pathways (see Figure 3.2), resilient individuals would be the most likely to persist in cultural competence development and the most likely to achieve culturally congruent care actions.

At-Risk Individuals

In contrast, the inefficacious individual (one with low confidence levels) is at risk for lowered persistence, motivation, and goal commitment. He or she may give up when obstacles or hardships are encountered. Such individuals may easily become discouraged if they do not quickly grasp new concepts, skills, or knowledge. That is, they may view transcultural learning tasks as overwhelming and insurmountable obstacles, threats, and hardships to be avoided. Consequently, decreased effort may be engaged, and lowered persistence with transcultural nursing skills may ensue. Low self-efficacy can affect cultural competence development directly, if individuals give up without even trying and then avoid cultural assessments, or indirectly, through poor nursing outcomes and/or through negative psychological outcomes. Poor nursing outcomes (achievement of negative client health outcomes) may be caused by culturally incongruent care. Such individuals become increasingly overwhelmed, focused on failure, dissatisfied, and stressed (see Figure 3.2).

Interpretation of data to identify inefficacious individuals is therefore crucial. In addition, individuals with low self-efficacy benefit the most with diagnostic-specific interventions designed to enhance self-efficacy and other academic and psychological outcomes (Brown, Lent, & Larkin, 1989; Jeffeys & Smodlaka, 1999a; Lent, Brown, & Larkin, 1987; Zimmerman, 1995). Early identification of inefficacious students followed by diagnostic-prescriptive interventions can help students maximize strengths, minimize weakness, and facilitate success (Jeffreys, 1993, 2000, 2001, 2002, 2004; Jeffreys & Smodlaka, 1998, 1999a, 1999b). Because inefficacious individuals often lose motivation and are reluctant to actively seek assistance, the educator plays a key role in initiating actions with inefficacious individuals. (The broad term *educator* is used to describe any qualified individual in the position to provide transcultural educational interventions. Examples include qualified nursing faculty, clinical educators, preceptors, nurse managers, mentors, certified transcultural nurses, nurses with advanced certification in cultural competence, and nursing organizational leaders). Although self-efficacy appraisal is task-specific, repeated failures and negative psychological outcomes decrease self-efficacy for learning and performing the necessary tasks for becoming a culturally competent registered nurse, thereby lowering persistence and commitment behaviors overall.

Other at-risk individuals are those who are supremely efficacious (overly confident). Supremely efficacious individuals may be totally unaware of their weaknesses, underestimate the task or its importance, overlook the task, overestimate their abilities, and overrate their strengths (Bandura, 1982). Consequently, overly confident individuals may not see the need for adequate preparation, restructuring of priorities, or time management to accommodate transcultural tasks. Therefore, such individuals may not be adequately prepared. Cultural competency development is affected indirectly through poor skill outcomes and negative psychological outcomes. Poor, weak, or unsuccessful performances can lead to feeling overwhelmed, surprised or shocked, dissatisfied, and stressed. Unfortunately, some supremely efficacious individuals may not even be aware that culturally incongruent care actions have impacted adversely on a client's emotional and physical health outcomes.

Because supremely efficacious individuals often lack motivation for the task and see no need to seek assistance, the educator plays a key role in initiating actions with overly confident individuals. Early identification of supremely efficacious individuals can help individuals realistically appraise one's strengths and weaknesses and recognize the need for adequate preparation for the achievement of successful outcomes. Because students, (especially beginning students) may not know what to expect in nursing, students may need much guidance in ongoing self-appraisal. Realistic self-efficacy appraisal allows one to seek action to enhance strengths and remedy weaknesses. Unfortunately, supremely efficacious individuals may not be restricted to beginning students, but may encompass nurses and other health care professionals at various career stages.

Curricular and Program Appraisal

Although the identification of at-risk individuals followed by teaching interventions is one proposed purpose of interpreting self-efficacy perceptions, interpretation may also be done to guide curricular and program innovations. (Program refers to hospital/agency employee orientation programs, inservice education, and continuing education). For example, if first semester baccalaureate nursing students complete the TSET and consistently report lower confidence for five particular items on the Cognitive Subscale, this flags that these empirical findings should be further explored. Soliciting qualitative comments may add richness to the data and allow greater insight. Examining the first semester nursing course in relation to these items/topics may uncover an educational gap, suggesting supplementary educational strategies to enhance transcultural nursing skills specifically to these topics. Administration of the Cultural Competence Clinical Evaluation Tool (CCCET) may further identify areas of strengths, weaknesses, and provide evidence of the opportunities available to interact with culturally diverse clients within a particular area of practice. Yet, if it makes sense that first semester students would have lower confidence for a cluster of items, then this helps validate the measurement tool and lends greater support for overall study results. For example, if students report lower confidence for topics not covered in the current course or in any previous courses, it makes conceptual sense that students would have lower confidence. However, if students just completed a course focused on maternal and child health yet reported lower confidence for TSET Cognitive Subscale items "pregnancy," "birth," and "growth and development," there would be cause for concern. The same example could apply for new nurse orientation to the maternity unit. Exploring underlying course, curricular, and program objectives and desired outcomes would be necessary. Using a longitudinal study design will permit the examination of within-group changes over time, providing data on the impact of subsequent courses and other educational experiences throughout the curriculum or program.

AVOIDING PITFALLS

As with all data interpretation, but especially with data involving self-report measurement tools and the measurement of constructs that are difficult to measure, data interpretation must be viewed cautiously. Interpretation must be realistic. An overconfident or inefficacious approach in data interpretation should be avoided, because both approaches can interfere with the best interpretation that will have the most practical significance and usability. Consciously recognizing study limitations and avoiding overgeneralization of results will help keep overconfidence in check. Acknowledging the positive findings rather than negating all results because of slight imperfections in study design or other limitations is another consideration. Recognizing that statistically insignificant results can have practical significance and recognizing that statistically significant results do not always yield meaningful findings or practical significance are equally important. The following sections discuss strategies for avoiding pitfalls in research design and interpretation.

Recognize Limitations Related to Measurement Level

Self-efficacy measurement tools are reported to provide data at the ordinal or interval level of measurement. Ordinal measurement shows relative rankings whereby the intervals between numbers on the scale are not necessarily equal. At the interval level of measurement, distances between the numbers are equal. In both ordinal and interval measurement there is no absolute zero point. Generally, interval-level data permit more sophisticated statistical analyses, (parametric statistics versus nonparametric statistics); however, within the social sciences there is much controversy about classification of the level of measurement and the appropriateness of selected statistical analyses (Knapp, 1990, 1993; LoBiondo-Wood & Haber, 1998). Individual consideration and the acknowledgment of study limitations are the recommended actions (Knapp, 1990, 1993).

Typically, self-efficacy studies have reported mean and standard deviations (Bandura, 1989; Lee & Bobko, 1994). The mean is a measure of central tendency and the standard deviation is a measure of variability associated with interval-level data; however, when reported with ordinal-level data, limitations in interpretation must be acknowledged. When interpreting data, one must be aware that individuals who select a "3" response on a 10-point self-efficacy rating scale are not necessarily half as confident as individuals who select a "6" response. What can be interpreted is that the former individuals are less confident than the latter group as measured by that particular rating scale. Similarly, an individual with a mean subscale score of 7.0 is not exactly "twice" as confident as an individual scoring a mean of 3.5 (see Exhibit 5.1).

Exhibit 5.1   Educator-In-Action Vignette

Without adequate preparation and thoughtful consideration before and during research design, implementation, and data analysis, the interpretation of findings can be inaccurate and have devastating consequences. Consider the possible adverse effects of the following incorrect interpretations. Contrast the potential effects of the alternative, improved interpretation.

Situation A

Using the TSET pretest and posttest results from a sample of 15 senior baccalaureate nursing students who enrolled in a transcultural nursing course elective, t-test results indicate statistically insignificant changes in TSE on all subscales.

Professor Quick states, "These results prove that the transcultural nursing course elective is not significant in developing cultural competence. We should cancel this course and reallocate funds toward the medical-surgical clinical courses."

Professor Best states, "It is not surprising that statistically significant results did not occur with such a small, self-selected convenience sample. The transcultural nursing course should be a required prerequisite or corequisite course to the clinical courses to enhance cultural competence development and permit application. A larger, more representative and diverse (not self-selected) sample will decrease the probability of a Type II error."

Situation B

The following TSET scores are obtained:

	Sample Mean (n = 87)	Standard Deviation	Case 1	Case 2	Case 3	Case 4
Cognitive	5.43	2.21	5.86	9.22	3.07	6.54
Practical	6.34	1.96	6.97	9.34	4.27	6.97
Affective	7.56	1.74	8.04	9.87	5.71	7.66

Professor Quick states, "Cognitive Subscale scores show that Case 2 is more than three times as knowledgeable about culture-specific care as Case 3. It would be a good idea to match Case 2 and 3 together because Case 2 would be a good role model. Cognitive Subscale scores are lowest overall so it will be more important to emphasize knowledge (content) about specific cultures. Affective Subscale scores are highest so this dimension of learning should not be a priority. The curriculum should be modified based on these results."

Professor Best states, "Consistent with the underlying conceptual framework of the CCC model, the data suggest that students in this sample are least confident about their knowledge and most confident about their attitudes, values, and beliefs. Learning that purposely integrates cognitive, practical, and affective dimensions optimizes learning outcomes; therefore, educational interventions should continue to emphasize and integrate all three components. Besides, affective learning is viewed as the most powerful in influencing professional development and cognitive learning.

Scores for Case 2 suggest that he or she may be overly confident, whereas scores for Case 3 suggest that he or she may be inefficacious. According to the CCC model and the TSE Pathway, both Case 2 and Case 3 could be identified as 'at-risk' for providing culturally incongruent care; however, limitations due to measurement prevent absolute categorization or exact comparisons of scores between individuals. Follow-up assessment and intervention with the identified at-risk individuals is appropriate and indicated. We should not generalize these first-time results and change the curriculum, but rather continue to collect data and compare results.

The best approach may be to adhere to the conventional analyses used in self-efficacy studies (interval level), interpret findings cautiously by acknowledging study limitations, repeat studies and compare results, and observe other outcome measures to substantiate findings. Because it is impossible to measure self-efficacy at such an exact level that distinguishes self-efficacy perceptions equally between individuals and between questionnaire response choices, researchers must go beyond this limitation to appreciate and value the findings generated in self-efficacy studies. Striving to control for other possible extraneous variables through a well-planned research design will enhance the validity and generalizability of findings (Ferguson, 2004).

Pretest Before Educational Intervention

When evaluating the effectiveness or impact of a specific educational intervention, the comparison of baseline data with outcome data strengthens the study. Using a pretest and posttest approach with a longitudinal sample will enhance the interpretability of findings. Administration of a self-efficacy measurement tool (e.g., the TSET) prior to the initiation of any specific transcultural teaching intervention, followed by a posttest administration immediately after the intervention, will permit the most control and decrease the risk of extraneous variables affecting results. Without a pretest, the researcher/educator cannot be sure that the educational intervention caused any change in the targeted population. Because it will be difficult to evaluate changes in cultural competency in the clinical area (see Chapter 3), it will be increasingly important to evaluate changes in TSE. According to Bandura (1986, 1997), changes in transcultural self-efficacy through the use of pretest and posttest become more important to measure, especially when other performance outcome indicators may be difficult to evaluate. The underlying premise is that self-efficacy is a mediator and predictor of outcome performance behaviors and outcomes (Bandura, 1996a, 1996b, 1997; Bandura & Schunk, 1981; Lent, Lopez, & Bieschke, 1993; Mone, Baker, & Jeffries, 1995; Saks, 1995).

Observe for Curricular/Program Consistency

Consistency in educational experiences between time of pretest and posttest is especially important when evaluating the impact of a curriculum or workshop series using an integrated approach to cultural competence development. The premise underlying a series of educational experiences (such as in a curriculum or clinical agency workshop series) is that each educational experience will build upon previous learning. Learning experiences carefully coordinated to complement each other by weaving together learning in the cognitive, practical, and affective domains are most desirable. Active learning experiences designed to build on previous learning adds to depth and synthesis. Learners who are passive tourists, spectators, or mentally inattentive will not be actively engaged in the process of becoming culturally competent.

To accomplish the learning of cultural competence at higher depth and synthesis, careful thought and consideration must take into account the feasibility of offering sequenced, high-quality, learner-centered experiences. Sequencing courses, requiring pre-requisites and corequisites that make sense conceptually, and avoiding class waivers simply for pure convenience will optimize the learning experience and help control for extraneous variables. Ideally, educators who wish to measure the impact of transcultural nursing integrated throughout a curriculum (series of courses or educational experiences) should administer a pretest to all students similarly on their first class session of the first foundational transcultural nursing course and before exposure to transcultural educational interventions. Within the HCI, providing a foundation for cultural competence development during the initial employee orientation program (EOP) should be followed by a carefully planned sequence of employee inservice programs and unit-based educational initiatives (see Chapters 10, 11, 12).

In academia, if some students are waived from taking the first foundational transcultural course to take several other courses first because of scheduling or other non-educational requests, the evaluation of TSE will be confounded by curricular inconsistency and by the weakening of transcultural concepts throughout. One desired outcome supporting sequencing of courses is that all students will have had the same exposure to transcultural concepts, skills, and theory. More enlightened learners within a class can reach higher (optimal) levels of cultural competence development by sharing insights with each other at a higher level of synthesis. Learners without a common foundational experience will not have this advantage. Course expectations with mixed learner groups will have different, less effective educational outcomes because learning must be adjusted to accommodate learners without the prerequisite knowledge, skills, and values (see Figure 6.4).

Determine Sufficient Sample Size

Determining sufficient sample size is a necessary precursor to enhance success in any study. Sample size will be determined by study purpose, literature review, conceptual framework, design, hypotheses/research questions, sampling technique, data collection, instruments, and data analyses. Although various sampling techniques may be employed, the advantages and disadvantages of different sampling techniques are not discussed here; rather, the focus is on sample size. However, it must be mentioned that most self-efficacy studies (and nursing studies) utilize nonprobability samples (convenience, purposive, quota).

First, all steps of the research process must be carefully considered before attempting to determine sample size. (The word "determine" is used rather than "calculate" because factors other than a mathematical formula must be considered). Second, feasibility of attaining desired sample size must be appraised. Third, aiming for more than the minimum number in the sample is advisable because unforeseen circumstances may reduce the usable data (e.g., incomplete questionnaires and/or lack of identifiers for matching questionnaires).

The most common pitfall concerning sample size is that sample size is too small to provide robust data. Certain statistical analyses cannot even be performed via computerized statistical software packages unless a minimum number of cases are present. Occasionally, the statistical tests with small samples may be processed; however, statistical significance will never be achieved. The danger is that even if there is a change in the anticipated direction, it may not be detected in small sample sizes. Cohen's (1977) power analysis is a statistical procedure used to determine three levels of effect size for the desired power based on the probability of a Type II error. (A Type II error refers to the acceptance of a null hypothesis when it should have been rejected). Statistical consultation and power analysis prior to the study implementation is valuable; however, other factors must be considered. Other considerations in sample size determination, particularly relevant for possible proposed purposes in TSE studies, are listed:

- Longitudinal studies require larger samples because mortality (dropouts) may occur.
- Longer time intervals between longitudinal data collection times require larger samples.
- Sample means will be affected by extreme scores especially in small samples.
- Factor analysis studies require large samples.
- Comparisons based on select demographic variables require sufficient respondents representing each demographic variable.

Collect Sufficient Demographic Data

The collection of sufficient demographic data will be valuable for four main reasons. First, demographic data will help determine whether the actual sample is truly representative of the targeted sample. Second, demographic data can be used to compare and contrast transcultural self-efficacy perceptions between samples, permitting the expansion of scientific knowledge. Third, demographic data can be used to examine within-group differences based on demographic factors. Fourth, demographic data can help substantiate the underlying assumptions and directional conceptual relationships proposed in the CCC model and TSE Pathway.

Significant differences in TSE perceptions based on demographic variables can be desirable if differences are consistent with the underlying theoretical framework. For example, the CCC model purports that novice learners will have lower self-efficacy perceptions than advanced learners. Demographic data distinguishing between novices and advanced learners must therefore be collected and analyzed. In contrast, lack of statistically significant differences in TSE perceptions based on such variables as race, ethnicity, language, religion, or socioeconomic status supports the underlying theoretical assumption that all learners (despite race, ethnicity, etc.) benefit from transcultural nursing educational experiences to provide culturally congruent care for culturally different clients (Jeffreys & Smodlaka, 1998, 1999a, 1999b; Lim et al., 2004).

Deciding what type of demographic data should be collected will depend upon the purpose and nature of the research investigation. It behooves the researcher/educator to critically appraise what demographic data could prove valuable prior to finalizing the study design and long before collecting data. (Jeffreys 2010 Toolkit Items 8 and 9 provide some examples). One general guideline is that sociodemographic questions should be placed last (Sudman & Bradburn, 1991). Some additional guidelines are listed below:

- Demographic data that is never collected are lost forever. (Plan ahead.)
- Too many questions are overwhelming. (Ponder pertinence.)
- Unclear questions are confusing. (Make categories and questions clear.)
- Unnecessary personal questions are offensive. (Ask only what is necessary.)
- Avoid haphazard sequencing of questions. (Present the least non-threatening questions first followed by more sensitive or personal questions [Sudman & Bradburn, 1991].)
- Data collected inconsistently have limited validity and usefulness. (Collect consistently.)
- The collection of invalid data is wasteful. (Collect carefully.)

Obtain Institutional Review Board Approval

Educators and/or researchers should be familiar with their institution's procedure and guidelines concerning Institutional Review Board (IRB) approval. Generally, teaching interventions and strategies for evaluating the effectiveness of teaching interventions do not require IRB approval if such teaching and outcome evaluations are typical expectations of the academic process and if findings will not be disseminated publicly. Initially, educators may not intend to publish, display, or present information, therefore, they do not seek IRB approval before beginning their assessments, interventions, and outcome evaluation. Unfortunately, this limits the usability of findings beyond the immediate institutional setting. The revitalization of nursing education must begin with educators taking active responsibility for using evidence-based teaching interventions and sharing their knowledge with others through the dissemination of educational research (Diekelmann, 2002; Diekelmann & Ironside, 2002; Drevdahl, Stackman, Purdy, & Louie, 2002; Jeffreys, 2004; National League for Nursing, 2002a, 2002b; Riley, Beal, Levi, & McCausland, 2002; Storch & Gamroth, 2002; Tanner, 2002; Young & Diekelmann, 2002). Because IRB approval must be obtained before a study is initiated and because every educational intervention has the potential to make a difference (positive or negative) in the process of cultural competence development, nurse educators must seriously consider the benefits and take the extra step in obtaining IRB approval.

Minimize Social Desirability Response Bias

Social desirability response bias refers to the tendency of some respondents to provide the "socially expected" response rather than true feelings (LoBiondo-Wood & Haber, 1998; Polit & Beck, 2005; Waltz, Strickland, & Lenz, 2005). Within the nursing profession, it could be assumed that cultural competence is a professional expectation; therefore, some researchers may be concerned about using self-report measurement tools to assess cultural competence. Bandura (1982) suggests that self-efficacy appraisals tend to be more conservative, especially when judgments are reported publicly, identification of respondents is possible, or direct observations of performance behaviors will occur. In other words, it may be "socially desirable" to present more conservative views of oneself. "Because there is no way to tell whether the respondent is telling the truth or responding in a socially desirable way, the researcher usually is forced to assume that the respondent is telling the truth" (LoBiondo-Wood & Haber, 1998, p. 318).

Although researchers must acknowledge that social desirability response bias may always exist in self-report instruments, several strategies may greatly reduce the effect of social desirability response bias on the results. To minimize social desirability response bias on the TSET, the author composed a letter of consent, informing respondents of the nature of the study, its educational benefits to nursing students, confidentiality, and voluntary participation (Jeffreys & Smodlaka, 1996). Several studies revealed that TSE perceptions were similar, whether or not respondents replied anonymously. Anonymous data and matched data using student identity numbers resulted in respondents selecting responses ranging from 1 (not confident) to 10 (totally confident) (Jeffreys & Smodlaka, 1996, 1998, 1999a, 1999b). Taking extra measures to assure student confidentiality and publicizing these measures can also minimize social desirability response bias. For example, asking respondents to wait to begin questionnaire completion until the data collector and instructor leave the room, appealing to respondents to complete questionnaires quietly and independently of each other, requesting students to place questionnaires in a sealed envelope, using a personal coding cover page for anonymity, and matching questionnaires (Jeffreys Toolkit 2010, Item 18) and reinforcing steps mentioned in the consent form can reassure respondents. The latter steps speak to the need for consistency in data collection.

Control Data Collection Procedures

Multiple data collectors and/or multiple data collection sites can complicate data collection consistency; however, steps can be taken to control data collection procedures. Collaboration with a liaison from each data collection site via written and telephone or personal correspondence should emphasize the need for consistent data collection procedures and clearly delineate the procedure steps. An information packet should contain a cover letter describing the nature of the study, instructions for instrument administration and return, and the instrument (and optical scanning sheets if needed). Numbered steps and written statements for data collectors to read to respondents at specific intervals enhance consistency in data collection. A group setting with a designated time for instrument completion is the preferred method for collecting TSET and CCCET data. Self-efficacy appraisal involves a complex thinking process that should be focused, undisturbed, uninterrupted, and precise. Eliminating distracters or other extraneous factors during instrument completion is vital for maximizing the validity of study results. If questionnaires are mailed to individuals, there is less control (consistency) in the data collection process. Asynchronous online questionnaire completion also has less control than synchronous online completion. An accompanying letter should request individuals to first set aside a specified amount of undisturbed time toward instrument completion.

Watch for History as a Threat to Internal Validity

In addition to the independent variable, an event outside a study may occur that could influence the dependent variable. This threat to internal validity is referred to as history. Although researchers should be cognizant of various threats to internal validity (maturation, testing, instrumentation, mortality, and selection bias), only history will be highlighted here in relation to TSE and cultural competence development. Historical events could potentially influence perceptions positively or negatively. During longitudinal studies designed for the purpose of assessing the effectiveness of specific educational experiences for cultural competence development, researchers must closely watch for the possibility of outside influences. In a study involving one-time data collection, history as a threat to internal validity has a different impact. Noting any significant historical events immediately before data collection will be important, especially if comparison between samples at different points in time and/or geographic locations will be conducted. Watching for extraneous events and considering possible implications is an ongoing process. Several examples are provided:

- The JCAHO introduces "cultural competence" as a requirement for accreditation.
- A registered nurse licensing examination features new test items that target cultural competence.
- A health center receives grant funding to provide emergency care to new refugees from a foreign country.
- Following a local outbreak of tuberculosis, an emergency room is overcrowded with uninsured illegal immigrants seeking health care.
- A heroic act by a member of an ethnic and religious minority group is well publicized locally in a predominantly white Protestant community.
- Several racial riots break out on campus, seriously injuring several nursing students.
- Worldwide terrorist acts lead to war.
- National financial incentives emphasize the development of culture-specific health care.

Test Technology

A trial test run with the technology required to scan questionnaires, process data, and analyze data will prevent potential pitfalls interfering with data use and interpretation. The technology trial test may require the expertise of computer experts, statisticians, psychometricians, and/or research assistants; therefore, early collaboration (before data collection) is essential. Various software programs are available for creating questionnaires; however, some programs may be more compatible with existing technological resources than others. It would be quite unfortunate if completed questionnaires cannot be scanned due to a technological problem. For example, the TSET formatted using Remark software must be scanned using Remark software; data can then easily be transferred into the SPSS program for data analysis. In contrast, the TSET typed format uses separate optical scanning forms. The completed optical scanning forms are then scanned using compatible software and an optical scanning machine. A computer expert may need to create a program for "reading" the scanning forms.

Without exploring the existing technological capabilities and/or limitations, a researcher may be stuck with data that cannot be easily processed. Checking the conditions of site licensing guidelines and/or the need for licensing renewals is another consideration. Computer technology and optical scanning equipment can ease the accuracy and speed at which questionnaires are processed. Testing technology ahead of time will avoid serious pitfalls.

KEY POINT SUMMARY

- Differentiating between individuals who demonstrate strong (resilient) self-efficacy, low self-efficacy (inefficacious), or supremely high self-efficacy (overconfidence) is integral to the interpretive process.
- It is presumed that individuals with resilient self-efficacy are highly motivated and actively seek help to maximize their transcultural nursing skills and cultural competence development.
- Low self-efficacy can affect cultural competence development directly, if individuals give up without even trying and then avoid cultural assessments or indirectly through poor nursing outcomes and/or through negative psychological outcomes.
- Supremely efficacious individuals may be totally unaware of their weaknesses, underestimate the task or its importance, overlook the task, overestimate their abilities, and overrate their strengths.

Overly confident individuals may not see the need for adequate preparation, restructuring of priorities, or time management to accommodate transcultural tasks.

- Strategies for avoiding pitfalls in TSE research design and interpretation include:
  - Recognize limitations related to measurement level.
  - Pretest before educational intervention.
  - Observe for curricular/program consistency.
  - Determine sufficient sample size.
  - Collect sufficient demographic data.
  - Obtain IRB approval.
  - Minimize social desirability response bias.
  - Control data collection procedures.
  - Watch for history as a threat to internal validity.
  - Test technology.

PART III

Educational Activities for Easy Application

Part III offers a wide selection of educational activities that can easily be applied by educators everywhere. Three chapters (6, 10, and 13) provide a general overview and menu of activities and strategies for use in three respective areas: academic setting, health care institution, and professional associations. Chapter discussions, corresponding diagrams, and toolkit items explore the steps essential for optimal cultural competence development:

- Self-assessment
- Active promotion
- Systematic inquiry
- Decisive action
- Innovation
- Measurement
- Evaluation

Five chapters (7, 8, 9, 11, and 12) creatively link strategies together via detailed case exemplars that spotlight various populations and settings.

Chapter 6 introduces readers to strategies for uncovering, discovering, and exploring educational opportunities toward cultural competency, beginning with faculty, and extending to student, self-assessment. The corresponding toolkit item provides excellent resources for easy use. Inquiry, action, and innovation at the curriculum level involve the philosophy, conceptual framework, program objectives and outcomes, courses, course components, and horizontal and vertical threads. At the course level, inquiry, action, and innovation involve the course outline, instructional media, learning activities, course components, and clinical settings. Detailed examples include the teaching of cultural competence through innovative use of textbooks, reading assignments, videos, computer-assisted instruction, virtual learning platforms, Web page, nursing skills laboratory, clinical settings, immersion experiences, service-learning, written assignments, presentations, examinations, and supplementary resources. These resources involve the library, enrichment programs, nursing student club, nursing student resource center (or Nursing Neighborhood), bulletin boards, honor society chapter, local organization, and guest speakers. Action-focused strategies for educational innovation and ideas for evaluating educational interventions are described, concluding with a descriptive "Educator-In-Action" vignette. Several TSET Research Exhibits demonstrate the evaluation of various educational interventions implemented by researchers and institutions throughout the United States at undergraduate and graduate levels.

Chapter 7 spotlights the *Cultural Discovery* approach for integrating general transcultural nursing concepts and skills within a first semester course. Designed to provide meaningful experiences and stimulate critical thinking among nontraditional, culturally diverse students who must learn to care for many clients of diverse cultural backgrounds, the strategy is easily adaptable to various academic levels as well as health care institutions. *Cultural Discovery* includes several components in conjunction with the Leininger Acculturation Health Care Assessment Enabler for Cultural Patterns in Traditional and Nontraditional Lifeways, specifically: background reading assignments, classroom activity component, collaborative library introductory program, videotape program, interview, literature review, reflection, and written paper assignment. Implemented over an 8-week period, *Cultural Discovery* assisted beginning nursing students to systematically conduct a basic general cultural assessment, identify some similarities and differences among individuals within cultural groups, distinguish between varying dimensions of acculturation, and discover the importance of culturally congruent nursing care. *Cultural Discovery* is easily adaptable to health care institutions (HCI). Using the COMPETENCE acronym and framework described in Chapter 2, a multidimensional integrated 15-step adapted HCI approach is presented. The adapted strategy proposes multiple, flexible, yet interactive and scaffolded teaching–learning strategies that recognize the time constraints of working nurses amidst different shifts, coupled with varying levels of motivation.

Chapter 8 describes a multidimensional strategy for teaching and learning cultural competence in graduate nursing education with a specific focus on the innovative field trip experience (IFTE). First, a brief overview of the literature in nursing and higher education provides the essential background information underlying strategy development, implementation, and evaluation, including a discussion of how the Cultural Competence and Confidence (CCC) model guided development. Next, a brief overview of the transcultural nursing core course within the Clinical Nurse Specialist (CNS) curriculum is highlighted. Four case exemplars, supplemented by detailed tables and figures, demonstrate easy application. Case exemplars include: Asian Indian women and prenatal care; Amish culture and immunization beliefs and practices; Orthodox Jewish community and end-of-life care; and African American Women and Arthritic Pain Management Using Complementary and Alternative Medicine (CAM). A discussion of cognitive, practical, and affective learning outcomes and implications for nurse educators conclude the chapter.

Chapter 9 describes the process of developing a culturally congruent approach to faculty advisement and helpfulness, which includes self-assessment, literature review, consultation and collaboration, student assessment, analysis, plan, communication, and interaction. Culturally congruent and culturally incongruent faculty actions, student perspectives, and their influence on academic, psychological, and retention outcomes are examined. The illustrated Nursing Undergraduate Retention and Success (NURS) model (Jeffreys, 2004) enriches the chapter with its road map for examining the multidimensional factors that affect undergraduate nursing student retention and success, including students' cultural values and beliefs.

Chapter 10 presents strategies for systematic inquiry into already existing facets of the HCI, along with suggested activities for developing new initiatives, actions, educational innovation, and evaluation. An illustrated self-assessment strategy (with the corresponding toolkit item) for direct application within HCIs, a sample questionnaire to guide prioritization, and a sample list for determining target populations are essential tools to guide cultural competence education and justify resource allocation. Numerous educational activities are integrated throughout the chapter, highlighting key areas such as institutional mission and philosophy, new employee orientation, newsletter and publications, inservice education, staff meetings, patient care conferences, walking rounds and report, special events, continuing education, and networking. The "Educator-In-Action" vignette demonstrates several strategies thoughtfully integrated to maximize the vast resources of culturally diverse health professionals within an HCI servicing different groups of patients.

Chapter 11 describes a process of visibly integrating cultural competence throughout an existing employee orientation program (EOP). A well-planned EOP should: (a) substantively emphasize cultural competence throughout most content areas; (b) provide strategies and incentives for nurses to implement culture-specific care directly on their assigned unit or setting; and (c) intrinsically motivate nurses to actively engage in the ongoing quest for developing cultural competence in self and in others. Illustrative case exemplars, supplemented by detailed figures, are threaded throughout the chapter, demonstrating easy application for a variety of unit-based or site-based settings, including school health nursing. Evaluation of EOP components, including formative and summative evaluation strategies, concludes the chapter.

The ongoing accessible opportunities for cultural competence education at the HCI and other employee settings offer tremendous possibilities for optimal cultural competence. Chapter 12 describes an 11-step process for designing, implementing, and evaluating an employee inservice (EI) program, with a user-friendly diagram depicting the steps. Two case exemplars (perioperative nursing and bone marrow transplant [BMT] unit) demonstrate how this process can be adapted by other staff/employee nurse educators interested in developing diagnostic-prescriptive employee inservice programs for nurses and other licensed and unlicensed health care personnel. The EI exemplars were designed for nurses already working in a health care institution; however, the case exemplars have applicability for other health care personnel as well as other patient populations and settings. Additionally, the exemplars illustrate how the inservice can be implemented as a component of a larger, full-day inservice program or as a separate, shorter, unit-based inservice. Evaluation of EI components, including formative and summative evaluation strategies, concludes the chapter.

Professional associations possess a potentially powerful and extensive ability to network with diverse groups of professionals beyond a single health care institution or academic setting, highlighting their influence on promoting, disseminating, and advancing cultural competence education. Chapter 13 presents strategies for identifying educational opportunities within professional associations for promoting cultural competence education; recognizing and overcoming barriers and challenges; and developing action-focused strategies for educational innovation. An illustrated strategy (with corresponding toolkit item) provides resources for direct application within these associations, with numerous educational activities. A thought-provoking table compares and contrasts educational topics and titles, challenging associations to go "beyond topic and title to search for substantive evidence of cultural competence." The

"Educator-In-Action" vignette presents a realistic scenario that illustrates several ongoing challenges facing professional associations.

Chapter 14 suggests important implications for educators everywhere. Educators are challenged to commit to a focused and transformational change that will not only advance the science and art of cultural competence education, but will also result in culturally congruent care, ultimately benefiting health care consumers worldwide. The urgent expansion of educational research on the teaching and learning of optimal cultural competence is emphasized, and areas for further inquiry, research, and goal setting are proposed. Extensive references are provided at the end of the book.

CHAPTER 6

Academic Settings: General Overview, Inquiry, Action, and Innovation

Marianne R. Jeffreys, EdD, RN

Any educational setting can provide numerous opportunities for promoting cultural competence; however, the academic setting can make the greatest impact here. This is true primarily because the main function of the academic setting is "education" and for the student "learning," which can be maximized through a well-planned, coordinated approach (see Figure 6.1). Leininger (2002) proposed four approaches for effectively integrating transcultural nursing within the academic setting: (a) transcultural concepts, skills, and principles integrated within an existing curriculum; (b) select culture care modules incorporated within a curriculum; (c) a series of coordinated, substantive transcultural nursing courses with field experiences; and (d) a major degree program or track in transcultural nursing (graduate level).

In this chapter, emphasis is given to the first approach because it has the broadest and most immediate application across academic settings and degree programs. In addition, an integrated approach has the potential to positively affect the greatest number of "future" nurses. Without an initial, formalized exposure to transcultural nursing, how will nursing students even know of its existence, realize its significance, and develop the beginning knowledge, skills, values, and confidence necessary for learning and performing culturally congruent nursing care? Furthermore, how will students be aware of the vast possibilities for ongoing learning

Academic Settings

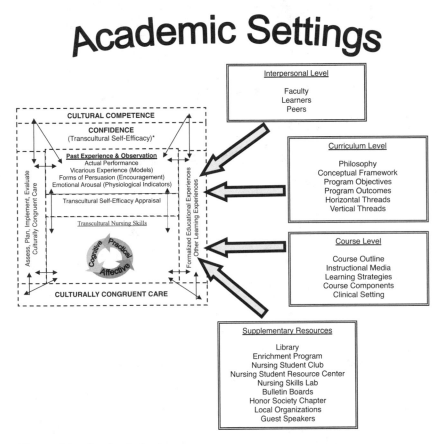

Figure 6.1   Academic Settings

in cultural competence development or advanced degree options? Early, stimulated interest in transcultural nursing may later prompt pursuit of a specialized degree program or track in transcultural nursing.

As lifelong, ongoing cultural competence development is an essential professional expectation, it is extremely urgent that initial education emphasizes cultural competence. Entry-level education offers the greatest possibilities, particularly the first nursing "fundamentals" course, because it provides the foundation for all future nursing courses and nursing practice. Optimally, a required prerequisite or corequisite transcultural nursing course will further enhance the possibility for a stronger foundation for cultural competence development; however, an additional course may not be feasible, especially with the time and credit constraints of associate degree nursing programs. Numerically, entry-level education has the potential to make enormous strides in cultural competence development because enrollment in such programs is greater than any other degree programs. This educational and professional goal can only occur with well-qualified, committed nursing faculty and through the use of culturally congruent teaching–learning strategies that address students' diverse cultural values and beliefs (CVB).

Nurse educators are empowered to make a tremendous difference by introducing, fostering, and nurturing cultural competence development. Each individual faculty member is empowered to make a positive difference; however, the greatest impact will be achieved through a coordinated, holistic group effort that thoughtfully weaves together nursing course components, nursing curriculum, and supplementary resources. Certain factors within the academic setting may support cultural competence development, yet other factors may restrict its development. This chapter aims to: (a) uncover, discover, and explore educational opportunities (within academia) for promoting cultural competency; (b) describe action-focused strategies for educational innovation; and (c) present ideas for evaluation (and reevaluation) of educational innovation implementation. Figures, tables, "Innovation in Cultural Competence" insert exhibits, and the "Educator-In-Action" vignette provide supplementary information to expand upon narrative text features. Major emphasis is placed on individual instructor appraisal and course-level appraisal.

FACULTY SELF-ASSESSMENT

Promoting cultural competency in academia requires considerable, sincere effort that begins with self-assessment, in which the nurse educator systematically appraises the various dimensions that can impact upon the educational process and on the achievement of educational outcomes (Jeffreys, 2004). A systematic assessment can be initiated using the cultural dimensions listed in Table 1.2, and illustrated in Figure 6.2. (A user-friendly Self-Assessment Tool-Academic [SAT-A] is available in the Cultural Competence Education Resource Toolkit [Jeffreys, 2010]). The SAT-A may be used individually and/or in groups. (See instructions in Preface, page xix). The realization that there are multidimensional variables influencing student–faculty interaction is overwhelming; yet, these variables are essential to evaluate before developing a culturally congruent educational approach. Sometimes nurse educators may be "unconsciously incompetent" in their educational approach with culturally diverse (different) students. According to Purnell (2008), an educator is unconsciously incompetent when she or he is not aware of cultural differences or when, unknowingly, carrying out actions that are not culturally congruent. Behaviors such as cultural blindness, cultural imposition, and

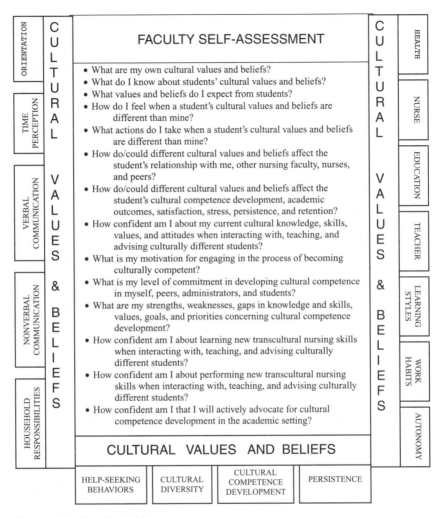

Figure 6.2 Faculty Self-Assessment

culturally incongruent actions can cause cultural pain to others (Leininger & McFarland, 2002). Consciously attempting to implement culturally congruent behaviors and avoiding incompetence is a key component in facilitating cultural competence development among culturally diverse learners.

First, self-awareness of one's own CVB is essential. Although the nursing faculty member may be immersed within the "culture" of nursing education and be familiar with long-held nursing education CVB, it is important to be aware of the unconscious and conscious CVB that exist in nursing education and in one's own values and belief systems. Faculty must be aware that their own CVB, held long before entering into the nursing culture, may influence values, beliefs, practices, behaviors, and actions consciously and unconsciously. For example, a nursing faculty member whose traditional cultural values favor direct eye contact for all communication and who views lack of eye contact suspiciously will need to be consciously aware of his or her underlying values and beliefs and aim to consciously avoid distrusting students based solely on this nonverbal cue (Jeffreys, 2004).

Second, awareness of one's knowledge about different CVB, especially the CVB that most directly affect the teaching–learning process and cultural competence development, must be explored (see Figure 6.2). Although Table 1.2 presents a snapshot approach of selected CVB that may impact upon the educational experience, it does allow for a quick comparison of different CVB. One benefit of this approach is that it evokes the awareness that there may be other CVB in various cultures of which the nurse educator is unaware. The realization that one is not and cannot be "culturally competent" all of the time is often a powerful awakening. Becoming conscious of one's incompetence is often a humbling experience but often sparks a desire for obtaining cultural knowledge. Awareness of differences and similarities between values and beliefs espoused in higher education, nursing education, and individual student CVB can also lend new insight into why conflicts, misunderstandings, and alternate priorities predominate. Such raised awareness can help determine whether specific factors are supportive or restrictive toward the goal of developing cultural competence among culturally diverse students who can guide culture-specific educational interventions. Added within this mix of diversity are academically underprepared students, foreign-trained physicians entering nursing programs, and second-career individuals (Botstein, 2008; Grossman & Jorda, 2008; Harvath, 2008; Hegge & Hallman, 2008; Kirst, 2008; Pressler & Kenner, 2009).

Embedded in this self-assessment is the appraisal of one's understanding about the multidimensional factors influencing nursing student learning, achievement, retention, success, and cultural competence development. Educational views, policy, learning styles, and values about education differ across cultures (Callister, Khalaf, & Keller, 2000; Crow, 1993; Flinn, 2004; Keane, 1993; Lattanzi & Purnell, 2006; Purnell & Paulanka, 2008; Nurmi & Aunola, 2001; Rew, 1996; Stigler & Hiebert, 1998; Stolder et al., 2007; Winters & Owens, 1993; Yoder, 2001) and impact upon learning, achievement, and persistence (Labun, 2002; Nurmi & Aunola, 2001; Ransdell, 2001a, 2001b; Ransdell, Hawkins, & Adams, 2001a, 2001b; Yoder, 1996). Unless nurse educators conduct a systematic appraisal of all of the multidimensional components, a full understanding will not truly be achieved. Nurse educators should reflect on the last time a thorough, updated review of the literature on cultural competence, the teaching–learning process, and diverse students was conducted. Appraisal of one's desire for updated knowledge and commitment should be critically determined. Evaluating one's knowledge about student expectations and perceptions should be appraised. Lack of knowledge or limited knowledge in this area identifies areas for further self-development; however, one must have the desire to obtain knowledge and be committed to the pursuit of such an endeavor or knowledge quest. Finally, self-assessment should conclude with a listing of strengths, weaknesses, gaps in knowledge, goals, commitment, and priorities.

The nurse educator must assess one's cultural desire or motivation for engaging in the process of becoming culturally competent. Within this construct of cultural desire is the concept of caring for others (Campinha-Bacote, 2003). Cultural knowledge is the process of searching and obtaining a thorough educational foundation about various CVB in an attempt to comprehend and empathize with others' perspectives. Along with awareness, cultural desire and cultural knowledge are essential steps toward becoming culturally competent (Campinha-Bacote, 2003). Thoroughly reflecting on the feelings experienced and actions taken when students' CVB are different from one's own CVB can further one's insight. Because the process of cultural competence is ongoing, the nurse educator should examine one's commitment toward achieving this goal. True commitment necessitates time, energy, persistence, extra effort to overcome obstacles, and willingness to learn from mistakes.

Comprehensive understanding, skill, and desire are essential but not enough to effectively make a positive difference in cultural competence development. The author believes that resilient transcultural self-efficacy (TSE) (confidence) is the integral component necessary in the process of cultural competence development (of self and in others). TSE is the mediating factor that enhances persistence in cultural competence development despite obstacles, hardships, or stressors. Resilient TSE perceptions embrace lifelong learning in the quest to become *more* culturally competent and in the quest to assist others (learners) to become more culturally competent. Educators with resilient TSE perceptions persist in their endeavors to be active transcultural advocates or promoters of cultural competence in all dimensions of the educational setting and professional practice.

Faculty self-assessment as "active promoter of cultural competence development" is a necessary precursor for successful strategy development. Table 6.1 provides a guide for appraising values, beliefs, and actions and for determining whether or not one is an active role model in cultural competence development. It is proposed that the "actions taken to promote cultural competence development" is what makes one an

Table 6.1   Nurse Educator's Self-Assessment: Active Promoter of Cultural
Competence Development

Promoter	Values, Beliefs, and Actions	Promoter
Yes	Views cultural competence as important in own life *and shares beliefs with students**	No
Yes	Views cultural competence as important in students' education, professional development, and future practice *and shares view with students*	No
Yes	Views own nurse educator role to include active involvement in promoting cultural competence development among students *and shares view with students*	No
Yes	Routinely updates own knowledge and skills to enhance cultural competence *and shares relevant information with students*	No
Yes	Attends professional events concerning cultural competence development *and shares positive and relevant experiences with students*	No
Yes	Views professional event participation concerning cultural competence development as important in students' education and/or professional development, and future practice *and shares view with students*	No
Yes	*Offers incentives to encourage student participation in professional events*	No
Yes	Maintains professional partnerships focused on cultural competence development *and shares positive and relevant experiences with students*	No
Yes	Maintains membership(s) in professional organizations whose primary mission is cultural competence development *and shares positive and relevant experiences with students*	No
Yes	Views student memberships in nursing organizations/associations (whose primary mission is cultural competence development) as important in students' education and/or professional development, and future practice *and shares view with students*	No
Yes	*Offers incentives to encourage student participation in memberships in nursing organizations/ associations committed to cultural competence development*	No
Yes	Recognizes actual and potential barriers hindering student's development of cultural competence *and initiates strategies to remove barriers*	No
Yes	*Implements strategies to encourage student development of cultural competence*	No
Yes	*Evaluates strategies implemented to encourage student development of cultural competence*	No

*Active promotor/facilitator actions are indicated by italics active role model. Table 6.1 can also provide a guide for organizational self-assessment to determine if schools of nursing, educational institutions, and organizations are "active promoters" or if there are factors restricting cultural competence development. (A user-friendly Active Promoter Assessment Tool-Academic [APAT-A] is available in the Cultural Competence Education Resource Toolkit [Jeffreys, 2010]. The APAT-A may be used individually and/or in groups. (See instructions in Preface, page xix).

Participation in cultural competence conferences, workshops, events, meetings, and relevant professional memberships exemplify a professional commitment to lifelong learning and cultural competence development that can be motivating and uplifting to students. Professional nurses serve as role models through their commitment to learning and the nursing profession. Because students have most exposure to the nursing profession through faculty guidance, nurse educators exert powerful influence on students. If faculty do not value cultural competence activities for their own professional development, then it is hard to imagine that they would have a positive impact on encouraging students' active development. Similarly, if nurse educators are actively involved in cultural competence activities, yet do not actively publicize their views, involvement, participation, and contribution, positive professional role modeling will not be evident to students. Vicarious learning through role modeling and forms of persuasion (encouragement) are powerful influences on self-efficacy appraisal, motivation, and persistence behaviors (Bandura, 1986).

After self-assessment, nurse educators who have not optimally shared positive views, values, beliefs, and experiences with students should make a concerted effort to do so. It is, however, not enough to profess values and beliefs to students; nurse educators must be sincerely committed and take positive actions in order to "make a difference" and enhance cultural competence development. To do this, nurse educators must recognize actual and potential barriers hindering student's cultural competence development, propose innovative solutions, take action, initiate strategies, evaluate educational innovations, and create new innovations based on evaluative data.

EVALUATION IN THE ACADEMIC SETTING

As students, educators, administrators, and health care consumers become more astute collectively in recognizing that culturally congruent health care is a right – not a privilege – it becomes increasingly urgent to closely examine how visible (or invisible) cultural competency development is actively present in the academic setting. At the undergraduate and graduate setting, examination at the curricular, program, school, and course level requires courage, commitment, time, energy, and a systematic plan. A systematic evaluative inquiry can be guided by two additional questions: (1) To what degree is cultural competence an integral component?; and (2) How do all the cultural components fit together? (Figure 6.3). A thorough evaluation (Jeffreys Toolkit 2010, Item 15) serves as a valuable precursor to informed decisions, responsible actions, and new diagnostic-prescriptive educational innovations toward the overall goal of achieving optimal cultural competence. The following sections address key features for inquiry, action, and innovation within the academic setting.

Curriculum

Systematic curriculum evaluation via quantitative and qualitative methods helps identify program strengths, weaknesses, inconsistencies, and gaps. Jeffreys Toolkit (2010) Item 15 (Systematic Inquiry: Academic (SI-A) offers a user-friendly quantitative and qualitative approach for systematic appraisal decisions, corresponding actions, notations/reflections, prioritization, and future planning. Reflective self-appraisal on an individual level and a program level is necessary for enhancing the scholarship of teaching (Brady et al., 2008; Drevdahl, Stackman, Purdy, & Louie, 2002; Emerson & Records, 2008; Harvath, 2008; Pressler & Kenner, 2009; Reeves, 2001; Young & Diekelmann, 2002). Concept-mapping that focuses on cultural competence as a concept helps trace the concept throughout the curriculum. On close scrutiny, curricular threads of culture and cultural competency should be equally and substantially evident throughout the program's philosophy, conceptual framework, program objectives, program outcomes, courses, and all course components. Examination of curricular threads must differentiate between horizontal and vertical threads. For example, horizontal threads are interested in the "process" of learning; therefore, horizontal threads must be introduced early, integrated purposely, and intricately woven throughout the curriculum to create a durable fabric that provides long-lasting learning and desirable outcomes.

In contrast, vertical threads are "content" oriented; they build from simple foundational content to more complex content. For example, moving from nursing care of the individual to family and then community demonstrates movement from simple dimensions to more complex dimensions. Applying "content" to care of the individual, care of the family, and care of the community should consider culture-specific measures within the plan of care. For example, the "content" of breast cancer screening should address culturally congruent measures to optimize

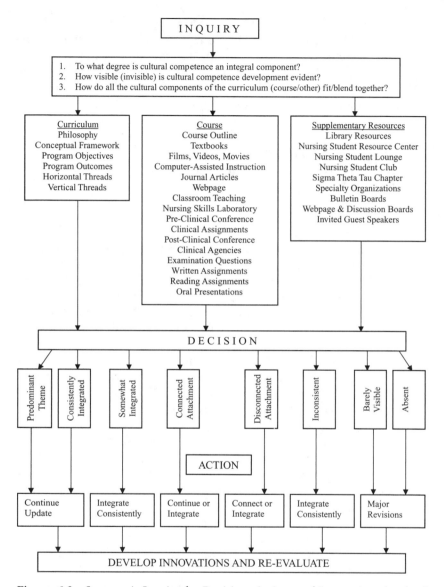

Figure 6.3   Systematic Inquiry for Decision, Action, and Innovation: Academic Setting

screening by reaching out to culturally diverse individuals, families, and communities. Curricular vertical and horizontal threads should be complementary, consistent, and appropriate for each educational level. Appropriate selection and sequencing of courses should be justified with a clear rationale. Foundational prerequisite courses, corequisite courses, and subsequent courses must fit together and build upon each other.

Although less discussed in the nursing literature, strategy-mapping throughout the curriculum is another important evaluative method. Strategy-mapping traces various student-centered learning approaches, thereby assessing another necessary curricular dimension. Because diverse learners have diverse learning needs, strengths, values, and beliefs, weaving different multidimensional active learning activities throughout the course and curriculum will be most beneficial (Bellack, 2009; Brookfield, 1986; Campbell-Heider et al., 2006; Flinn, 2004; Gaffney, 2000; Hughes & Hood, 2007; Hunter, 2008; Kelly, 1997; Kennedy, Fisher, Fontaine, & Martin-Holland, 2008; Williams & Calvillo, 2002; Yoder, 2001) (see Table 6.2). Student's CVB will influence how various strategies are valued, interpreted, and used; therefore, nurse educators should take this into consideration while planning, implementing, and evaluating activities. Students need to understand and appreciate the conditions under which specific learning strategies may be more or less effective, rather than assuming that certain ones are best (Pintrich & Garcia, 1994). Explaining the value of different teaching–learning activities may be indicated to optimally facilitate learning among culturally diverse and academically diverse learners.

Specific activities have advantages and disadvantages. Pairing students eliminates the potential for an audience and enhances the potential for in-depth quality student interactions that can foster cognitive and affective growth (Christiaens & Baldwin, 2002). Groups, however, provide greater opportunities for diverse thinking. Outcome benefits can be maximized with clear directions, group rules, well-matched group composition, effective leadership, immediate feedback and guidance, reflection, and adequate time allocation (Huff, 1997). Storytelling with reflection is another effective strategy, especially among culturally diverse learners (Forneris & Campbell, 2009; Koenig & Zorn, 2002). For many students, gaming, debates, and role play provide an effective mechanism for active, fun learning that results in cognitive, psychomotor, and/or affective outcomes (Candela, Michael, & Mitchell, 2003; Cowen & Tesh, 2002; Kramer, 1995; Jeffreys, 1991; Pimple, Schmidt, & Tidwell, 2003); yet, individual competitiveness may be contrary to some students' CVB. The Internet (Web-based courses) provides opportunities for interactive learning in pairs, small groups, and large groups via individual e-mail, group e-mails, course chat rooms, course discussion boards, and wiki (Bolan, 2003; Christianson, Tiene, & Luft, 2002; Ciesielka, 2008; Dorrian & Wache, 2008; Harden, 2003; Koeckeritz, Malkiewicz, & Henderson, 2002; MacIntosh, MacKay, Mallet-Boucher, & Wiggins, 2002; O'Neill, Fisher, & Newbold, 2009; Rash, 2008; Sternberger, 2002; Wink, 2009). Most recently, webcasting permits audio and visual presentations via the Internet, including live class participation via personal computers (DiMaria-Ghalili, Ostrow, & Rodney, 2005; O'Neill et al., 2009;

Table 6.2   Acronym for Meeting the Needs of Diverse Learners

DEVELOPMENTAL	A developmental approach is recommended whereby a comprehensive, broad introduction to cultural competence and transcultural nursing provides a foundation for subsequent cultural competence education. Subsequent teaching–learning strategies purposefully weave together and build upon prior formalized and informal learning in order to foster optimal cultural competence development. The developmental approach integrates cognitive, practical, and affective learning at increasingly higher levels throughout the educational process.
IMMEDIATE	Immediate relevance and direct application into the clinical or work setting is consistent with adult learning theory that recognizes the uniqueness of adult learner populations.
VARIETY	A wide variety of learner-centered teaching–learning activities partnered with a wide variety of case study examples representing a wide variety of cultural groups and clinical needs is recommended for the wide variety of academically and culturally diverse health care professionals and students requiring ongoing cultural competence education.
EVIDENCE-BASED	Empirically supported teaching–learning strategies should begin the repertoire of teaching–learning strategies implemented and evaluated in academic, health care, and professional association settings. Adaptation of existing strategies and the design of new teaching–learning strategies should be routinely appraised for the achievement of successful outcomes. Both formative and summative evaluations, routinely conducted, will add to the repertoire of evidence-based teaching–learning strategies most effective in cultural competence education. Evaluating what strategies work best for various sub-groups of diverse learner will be instrumental in meeting the needs of diverse learners and enhancing optimal cultural competence education.
RESOURCES	Pooling together appropriate human, financial, scholarly, and space/equipment resources will maximize opportunities for a positive learning experience and enhance optimal cultural competence development. Without sufficient resources, cultural competence education will be adversely affected.
SELECTIVE	Selective case scenarios and learning experiences should be guided by pre-determined priority needs of learners or key targeted patient groups (clinical setting) or students (academic or continuing education setting).
EXPERIENTIAL	Guided and mentored experiential learning experiences, preceded by key preparatory learning activities, provide a tremendous opportunity for developing optimal cultural competence. Actual performance of transcultural nursing skills or culturally specific actions is most influential in transcultural self-efficacy appraisal and the further development of cultural competence knowledge, skills attitudes, and confidence.

Ostrow & DiMaria-Ghalili, 2005; Pressler & Kenner, 2009). Other new technology, such as pod-casting, permits various options that can enhance learning, especially among nontraditional learners with ESL, dyslexia, and/or multiple role responsibilities (Forbes & Hickey, 2008; Pressler & Kenner, 2009). Virtual learning platforms offer students a unique opportunity to transfer and apply knowledge and skills within a wide range of culturally diverse virtual patients (Edwards et al., 2007). The virtual learning platform creates a "safe" learning environment whereby students get exposed to cultures and situations that they may not ever experience and/or have limited experience within the school's clinical agencies (see Exhibit 6.1). Students must be computer-literate, confident, and motivated if computer-based strategies are to be effective. Nurse educators have many learner-centered student interactive strategies from which to choose; however, the educator must be adequately prepared, knowledgeable of student variables, committed, and caring, if strategies are to be successful (Jeffreys, 2004).

Exhibit 6.1   Innovations in Cultural Competence Development: Virtual Learning Platform

Title: Monarch General Hospital: Enhancing BSN Student Interaction with Culturally Diverse Virtual Patients

Authors: Phyllis Barham, RN, MS, Richardean Benjamin, CNS, MPH, PhD, Phyllis Eaton, CNS, PhD, Kay Palmer, MSN, CRRN, Carolyn Rutledge, CFNP, PhD, and Lynn Wiles, RN, PhD
© Old Dominion University School of Nursing, Norfolk, VA

Abstract

The Old Dominion University Bachelor of Science in Nursing curriculum uses an innovative program assigning students to culturally diverse videotaped patients situated in Monarch General Hospital (MGH). MGH, a faculty-developed, computer-generated virtual learning platform, provides students with any-time/any-place interactive and repetitive practice options via the Web. A lexicon-based program allows students to interact with videotaped patients, whose health issues are impacted by culture, thus emphasizing the importance of addressing culture during health encounters. These assignments provide all students with exposure to important cultural issues often encountered in practice. Patient cases cross the life span and are used in courses throughout the undergraduate curriculum. In addition to interviewing the culturally diverse virtual patients, students are presented additional information about the cultures represented when the patients themselves present videotaped information about their culture and through the provision of other cultural informational links in the MGH library.

Inconsistent and/or insufficient integration of cultural competence curricular threads, learning activities, strategies, opportunities, and incentives throughout the nursing curriculum restricts cultural competence development and is confusing to students. Curricular inconsistency is incongruent with the creation of a true community of culturally diverse nursing learners – essential for culturally inclusive professional socialization, development, and growth. Curricular inconsistency is also counterproductive to earlier cultural competence promoting efforts; inconsistency confounds students and compounds educational outcomes. In contrast, consistent vertical and horizontal threads, purposely woven throughout the curriculum, are a program strength that can only support student learning and success.

Curricular mapping and a detailed critique of the philosophy, conceptual framework, program objectives, program outcomes, and curricular threads is an ambitious endeavor, requiring much courage, humility, honesty, and dedication. It is often a humbling experience to realize that one's curriculum necessitates an intensive overhaul or detailed tune-up in cultural competence (or any other area as well). Concept-mapping and strategy-mapping provide methods for tracing curricular threads and learning activities, identifying gaps, and detecting overlapping areas. More recently, electronic-based strategies have facilitated the ease of ongoing and collaborative curriculum evaluation (Miller, Koyanagi, & Morgan, 2005). Inquiries must extend beyond the immediate nursing program to examine the possibility of seamless articulation into more advanced nursing programs (that build upon foundational cultural competence learning) at the same school, neighboring and/or affiliating schools, and/or nursing programs nationally recognized as leaders in cultural competence development.

Certain factors will enhance the ability to conduct an intensive curriculum critique. These include psychological factors, practical factors, and expertise factors. Ideally, all conditions should be favorable for a critique to be most successful and valid. Psychological factors include: intrinsic motivation, extrinsic motivation, commitment, willingness to make changes, open-mindedness, satisfaction, minimal stress, workplace harmony, positive group dynamics, and perceived positive reinforcement. Practical factors include time, workload, financial resources, administrative support, secretarial support, technical resources, facilities, and energy. Expertise factors include the level of expertise (educational preparation and actual task experience) in evaluation, curriculum development and evaluation, curriculum process via group interaction, concept-mapping, cultural competence development, teaching and learning cultural competence, teaching and learning process, adult learners, culturally diverse students, and learner characteristics.

Unfortunately, there is a critical shortage of nursing faculty that is projected to increase in the future (Adams, Murdock, Valiga, McGinnis, & Wolfertz, 2002; Jarrett et al., 2008; NLN, 2002a, 2002b; Rizzolo, 2002; Rosenkoetter & Nardi, 2007; Stevenson, 2003; Schumacher, Risco, & Conway, 2008). Furthermore, the number of faculty formally prepared in the teaching and learning of nursing and in the curriculum development is tragically declining. For example, the number of graduates specifically prepared in nursing education via master's programs with education tracks has declined to only 116 graduates in 2000 (Rizzolo, 2002). Although advanced (post-master's) certificate programs in nursing education have increased, the usual three to five required courses generally do not include a separate course (or a substantive course) in teaching culturally diverse students and cultural competence education throughout the curriculum. The prevalence of part-time adjunct faculty within nursing programs (frequently teaching in the clinical setting) often means that proportionately the number of faculty within a school of nursing with a full-time focus on curriculum development and evaluation is slim. In addition, the number of faculty formally prepared with courses in transcultural nursing is grossly inadequate (Andrews, 1995; Jeffreys, 2002; Leininger, 1995b). Combining the desired faculty attributes to include preparation in both areas, result in even lower numbers. Faculty experienced in curriculum and cultural competency will need to lead and mentor others in this evaluative process.

Establishing cultural competence curriculum evaluation as a research agenda within a school of nursing fosters accountability across the curriculum, promotes team faculty action, and yields valuable data to guide future curricular innovations. Discovering whether cultural competence education throughout the curriculum results in the desired changes requires measurement with a valid and reliable tool. TSET Research Exhibits 6.1 and 6.2 illustrate how the TSET can be used to evaluate transcultural nursing threads and cultural competence threads integrated within undergraduate and graduate curricula.

TSET Research Exhibit 6.1   Evaluating the Effectiveness of Cultural Competence Threads throughout a Baccalaureate Curriculum

Perceived Cultural Competency of Nursing Students
Patricia Burrell, PhD, APRN, APMHCNS-BC, CNE
Professor of Nursing
Hawaii Pacific University
Kaneohe, HI

Abstract

Transcultural nursing leads health care in preparing culturally appropriate practitioners. Students expand their knowledge about the culture
of nursing, their own cultures, and the culture of others.

The Hawaii Pacific University, School of Nursing received a 3-year
grant from the U.S. Department of Health and Human Services Administration (HRSA) to assist in developing culturally competent practitioners. We established a research agenda to measure the effectiveness of the Transcultural Nursing threads throughout the curriculum.
We asked, "What is the self-efficacy of an ethnically and culturally
diverse student body in their utilization of basic transcultural nursing
skills?"

249 students have completed the incoming and exiting surveys.

Jeffreys' Transcultural Self-Efficacy Tool (TSET) (2006), an 83-item
questionnaire was used to collect data on the students' confidence in
using basic transcultural nursing skills.

In the affective area, their attitudes and beliefs about culture and nursing, 3.5% of the incoming group scored low, 60.23% scored medium,
and 36.23% scored high. In the graduating group, 0.02% scored low,
3.25% scored medium, and 96.75% scored high.

It appears that the majority of the students perceived themselves as
having high self-efficacy in all areas when entering the clinical aspect of
the nursing program. Upon graduation, it appears as if their own beliefs
and values and attitudes toward culture and nursing increased.

Research Report

Purpose: To measure the effectiveness of transcultural nursing threads
throughout the curriculum.

Research Question: What is the self-efficacy of an ethnically and culturally diverse student body in their utilization of basic transcultural
nursing skills?

Study Design: Prospective

Sample:

Size: 249
Type of learner: BSN students
Demographics: African American, Caucasian, Chinese, Filipino, Japanese, Korean, Mexican, Mixed-Race, Micronesian, Samoan, Spanish

TSET Data Collection

Pretest: Data were collected prior to the first clinical nursing course
Posttest: Data were collected at NCLEX prep before graduation and after completing the 2.5 years of clinical nursing courses.

Educational interventions/teaching–learning strategies: Cultural competency threads throughout the curriculum

TSET Reliability (Crohnbach's alpha)
    Total TSET: 0.810
    Cognitive Subscale: 0.987
    Practical Subscale: 0.991
    Affective Subscale: 0.397

Data Analysis

SEL Scores were used for grouping into High, Medium, and Low:

Low: Select 1 or 2 responses on 80% or more items
High: Select 9 or 10 responses on 80% or more items
Medium: Select 3 through 8 responses on 80% items or does not fall into low or high

Subscale	High	Medium	Low
Cognitive			
Pretest	22.83%	71.01%	6.31%
Posttest	13.89%	15.47%	73.54%
Practical			
Pretest	20.68%	69.42%	3.90%
Posttest	50.51%	47.60%	1.89%
Affective			
Pretest	36.23%	60.23%	3.5%
Posttest	96.75%	3.25%	0.02%

Advocacy (Responses to TSET items 82 and 83)

Advocacy (Item 82 and 83)	High	Medium	Low
Pretest	57.34%	42.22%	0.44%
Posttest	72.72%	24.9%	2.38%

Discussion: Overall, increases in TSE perceptions from pretest (beginning of nursing clinical courses) to posttest (end of nursing program) occurred on all subscales following the integration of transcultural nursing throughout the BSN curriculum. Additional analyses targeting the two items dealing with cultural advocacy demonstrated an increase in self-efficacy as advocates for culturally congruent care.

Curricular Implications
    1. Results will be used to guide future curricular innovations
    2. Continue collecting data using TSET

Dissemination of Results:

3rd Hong Kong Nursing Forum, University of Hong Kong, June 2009
Hawaii Pacific University. Scholarship Day, Kaneohe, Hawaii, January, 2008.
TCN 34th conference, Minneapolis, Minnesota, September, 2008
Nurse Educators Conference, Hong Kong Polytechnic University, Kowloon, Hong Kong, SAR, November, 2007.
Australasian Nurse Educators Conference, Wellington, New Zealand, October, 2007.

TSET Research Exhibit 6.2   Evaluating Enhancement of Cultural Competence throughout a DNP Program

Enhancement of Cultural Competence and Evidence-Based Practice Knowledge for Faculty and Doctor of Nursing Practice Students in the Pace University, Lienhard School of Nursing, Department of Graduate Studies, New York, NY
Primary Investigator: Joanne K. Singleton, PhD, RN, FNP-BC, FNAP
Co-Investigator: Rona F. Levin, PhD, RN

Abstract

Two common and critical threads across all LSN programs are evidence-based practice (EBP) and cultural competence and sensitivity. In the

DNP curriculum, knowledge and skills in cultural competence and evidence-based practice must be enhanced to ensure the design, implementation, and ongoing evaluation of care aimed at improving outcomes for all, and in particular for vulnerable groups. Our methods include curriculum enhancement in cultural competence and EBP. The goal is to improve transcultural self-efficacy and EBP in DNP students and faculty.

Transcultural self-efficacy is defined as "perceived confidence for performing or learning transcultural nursing skills...needed for culturally competent and congruent care" (Jeffreys, 2006, p. 31). The development of cultural competence is a multidimensional process that integrates cognitive, practical, and affective learning. One's own perception of confidence, or self-efficacy, to learn or perform specific tasks or skills influences learning and motivation to learn (Bandua, 1986). Learning cultural competence in nursing integrates cognitive, practical, and affective transcultural nursing skills, involves confidence in trascultural self-efficacy, and is directed toward providing culturally congruent care. Transcultural self-efficacy and cultural competence can change over time through formalized education on cultural competence (Jeffreys, 2006).

Evidence-based practice (EBP) is a problem-solving approach to the delivery of care that incorporates the best evidence from well-designed studies in combination with a clinician's expertise and patient preferences (Strauss et al., 2005). It is an established method for improving clinical practice (Richardson, Miller, & Potter, 2002) and has been shown to improve cost-effectiveness of patient care (Kitson, 2000; Madigan, 1998; Rosenfeld, Duthie, Bier, Bower-Ferres, Fulmer, Iervolino, McClure, McGivern, & Roncoli, 2000; Selig, 2000; Winch, Creedy, & Chaboyer, 2002). The effect of EBP on patient outcomes and cost has been discussed in the literature for years. Nursing practice based on evidence has been found to improve patient outcomes by 28% (Heater, Becker & Olson, 1988). Additionally, nursing care based on the best currently available evidence has been shown to decrease cost (Goode et al., 2000).

The purpose of this study is to answer the following questions:

Does the enhancement of cultural competence and evidence-based practice knowledge for faculty and Doctor of Nursing Practice Students in the Pace University, Lienhard School of Nursing, Department of Graduate Studies, improve faculty and students'

(1) transcultural self-efficacy
(2) beliefs about and confidence in knowledge of evidence-based practice, and
(3) evidence-based practice implementation behaviors?

Course

Close scrutiny at the course level (undergraduate and graduate) should assess whether cultural competency development is emphasized substantially, equally, and symmetrically in all dimensions and course components. This can begin by examining all components of the course outline: course description, course objectives, course topics, student expected outcomes, learning activities, course assignments, and methods of evaluation. Using the general questions depicted in Figure 6.3 and Jeffreys Toolkit 2010, Item 15, nurse educators can conduct a systematic inquiry, make a decision, choose an action, and then develop innovations. For example, if a nurse educator decides that "care of culturally diverse clients" mentioned in the course description is "barely visible" in the other course outline components, the action chosen should be to make major revisions, develop innovations, and reevaluate within a specified time period. Collaboration with other faculty teaching in the nursing program and outside experts will be essential to the overall curricular goals and process. As a second example, a nurse educator may decide that the course topics present cultural competence as an "add-on" or "disconnected attachment." Thereafter, the chosen action will be to connect together, or better still, to integrate as a horizontal thread.

Inquiry at the course level also includes all instructional media (e.g., textbooks, films, videos, movies, computer-assisted instruction, journal articles, Web page, and PowerPoint), course components (e.g., classroom, nursing skills laboratory, clinical, service learning, and/or immersion experience), teaching–learning activities, and methods of evaluation (e.g., written assignments, presentations, and examination questions). Each of the following sections will highlight several select course-level components, providing examples of course-specific innovations. It is beyond the scope of this chapter to detail all elements. Readers are encouraged to critique the innovations presented, modify, adapt, and create new innovations for the teaching and learning of cultural competence. TSET Research Exhibit 6.3 illustrates how the TSET can be used to evaluate the effectiveness of educational interventions implemented within a course.

TSET Research Exhibit 6.3   Evaluating the Effectiveness of a Transcultural Nursing Course on Students' Transcultural Self-Efficacy

Appraisal of BSN Students' Transcultural Self-Efficacy using Jeffreys' Transcultural Self-Efficacy Tool

Theresa M. Adams, RN, MSN, CSN
Assistant Professor of Nursing, Alvernia University
Doctoral student, PhD in Leadership, Alvernia University
Reading, PA
Kathleen M. Nevel, MEIE
Doctoral student, PhD in Leadership, Alvernia University

Abstract

The purpose of this study was to measure baccalaureate nursing students' transcultural self-efficacy (TSE) before and after an educational intervention during an academic semester. The 83-item Transcultural Self-Efficacy Tool (TSET) was administered to a purposive sample of 58 BSN students. A significant increase from pretest to posttest was found in all three subscales (cognitive, practical, and affective). The results of this study supported the assessment that transcultural self-efficacy is dynamic and changes following effective transcultural nursing educational strategies. A longitudinal study using the same design may provide additional supportive data to advocate using these teaching strategies in nursing education.

Research Report

Purpose: The purpose of this study was to examine the influence of a transcultural nursing course on baccalaureate nursing students' transcultural self-efficacy during an academic semester.

Research Question: Is there a significant change in the perceived self-efficacy of nursing students after the completion of the transcultural nursing course, as measured by the TSET tool?

Study Design: Quasi-experimental

Sample:
   Size: 58 nursing students
   Type of learner: BSN students
   Demographics: The demographics profile consisted of 97% female and 83% white; 9% Asian and 5% black. The age ranges were 67% between 20 and 29; 17% between 30 and 39; and 14% between 40 and 59. Sixty-two percent of the students had some previous health care experience. The generic nursing students took this course as a required course; however, the RN-BSN students took it as an elective.

TSET Data Collection
> *Pretest*: Data were collected at the beginning of the semester
> *Posttest*: Data were collected at the end of the semester

Educational interventions/teaching–learning strategies: Throughout the semester the following methods of instruction were implemented: Lecture, discussions, brainstorming, videos, and DVD (*The Multicultural Health Series, Part I and Part II* and *Cultural Issues in the Clinical Setting* (Kaiser Permanente, 2002, 2003, 2004) and *Hold Your Breath* (Grainger-Monsen & Haslett, 2005)), PowerPoint presentations by faculty and students, book review of *The Spirit Catches You and You Fall down* (Fadiman, 1997), cultural meal and guest speakers. Eshelman and Davihizar (2006) suggest integrating a cultural meal and guest speakers into the curriculum to promote cultural competency. Therefore, students were required to complete a variety of assignments including: self-heritage assessment, group cultural assessment, cultural film review, cultural educational pamphlet, and an interview of a client from another culture. In addition, the nursing students, course faculty, and the university's multicultural coordinator planned a cultural meal for junior and senior level nursing students, nursing faculty, and university administrators.

Using media, 20 multicultural case studies were shown to the students throughout the semester to simulate real-life scenarios the students may experience during their nursing careers. Moreover, *The Spirit Catches You and You Fall Down* was assigned to the students to assist them to recognize some barriers patients from diverse populations may face while implementing our health care system. This book was selected because Anderson (2004) reported students demonstrated an increase in cultural competence as evidenced in their short writing assignments after reading and discussing this book. Using the Wilcoxon signed rank test to assess differences in students' scores before and after reading the book, Anderson noted statistically significant increases in the students' responses to direct eye contact with patients ($z = -2.18, p - 0.29$).

TSET Reliability (Crohnbach's alpha)
> <u>Total TSET</u>: 0.969
> <u>Cognitive Subscale</u>: 0.966
> <u>Practical Subscale</u>: 0.976
> <u>Affective Subscale</u>: 0.870

Data Analysis
Results: Nursing students' transcultural self-efficacy (TSE) SEST scores changed significantly from pretest (beginning of course) to posttest (end of course) for nursing students.

TSE SEST scores (n = 58)

Subscale	Mean	Standard Deviation	t-test	Significance
Cognitive				
Pretest	5.62	1.79	−40.77	P < 0.000
Posttest	8.55	0.96		
Practical				
Pretest	5.62	1.98	−11.47	P < 0.000
Posttest	8.67	1.16		
Affective				
Pretest	7.91	1.29	−9.54	P < 0.000
Posttest	9.44	0.71		

SEL Scores grouping into High, Medium, and Low

Subscale	High	Medium	Low
Cognitive			
Pretest	12	46	0
Posttest	54	4	0
Practical			
Pretest	13	45	0
Posttest	53	5	0
Affective			
Pretest	44	14	0
Posttest	58	0	0

Discussion: There were no low scores reported in any subscale for either the pretest or posttest. The greatest percentage of pretest high scores occurred in the Affective subscale (76%) followed by the Practical subscale at 22% and Cognitive at 21%. The greatest percentage of posttest high scores occurred in the Affective subscale at 100% followed by Cognitive at 97% and Practical at 91%. No decline in SEL scores was noted. The greatest increase in SEL scores occurred on the Cognitive and Practical subscales while the least change in scores was noted in the Affective subscale. There was no decrease in scores in any subscale between the pretest and posttest. The SEL scores for the Cognitive subscale exhibited the greatest percentage point improvement as a result of the self-efficacy teaching interventions. Students' knowledge and awareness of cultural issues in nursing care were favorably influenced by the various teaching strategies, speakers, videos, book reviews, and cultural assessments.

Qualitative Data
Qualitative results were depicted in students' comments on their course evaluations at the end of the semester: "Videos were good examples of different scenarios a nurse may encounter"; "Movies related to the topic being taught"; "Multicultural videos portrayed cultural groups without over-exaggeration and showed important beliefs recognized to the cultures"; "I have become increasingly more confident in cultural compliance and awareness, the different teaching styles and material (videos, speakers, etc.) facilitated a higher degree of learning because it was a change in the curriculum and grasped students' attention"; "It allowed students who have not had experience with diversity to learn about other cultures and preventing them from stereotyping"; "I now have an appreciation of other cultures and it has moved me to want to go to the Dominican Republic trip to help there"; "I learned about other cultures which will help me to provide better care and avoid stereotyping and miscommunication with patients as future nurses or in everyday life."

Curricular Implications

1. Consider requiring transcultural nursing course at the beginning of the nursing course sequence for all baccalaureate nursing students
2. Continue collecting data using TSET

Dissemination of Results: Manuscript under review

Textbooks and Reading Assignments

Appraising textbooks carefully using preset criteria provides a systematic evaluation of textbook options (Schoolcraft & Novotny, 2000). Although evaluation of content areas, supplementary features, cost, date of publication, and usability are important considerations, nurse educators must consider other aspects, especially if the needs of academically diverse and culturally diverse students are to be met. Textbook selection must be guided by learner characteristics, type of course, intended purpose of reading assignments, textbook features, coordination with other course components, and connection with other courses (prerequisite, corequisite, and subsequent).

It is important to remember that it is not only the textbook that can make a difference in the learning process and the achievement of learning outcomes, but rather how the textbook is used (or not used). Accurate knowledge and comprehension about learner characteristics is a necessary precursor to textbook selection and the preparation of reading assignments. Exhibit 6.2 presents an overview of learner characteristics helpful in developing a profile of learner characteristics. For example, if many nursing students are financially challenged, it is unrealistic to expect that a supplementary textbook will be purchased to complete two required class

---

Exhibit 6.2   Innovations in Cultural Competence Development: Assessment of Learner Characteristics

Type of Course
_____Required _____Elective _____AAS _____BS generic _____RN-BS _____Masters _____Doctorate
Prerequisites _____Corequisites_____
_____Transcultural _____Clinical _____Theory _____Research _____Issues _____Leadership _____Community
_____Other_____

Learner Characteristics
Age   _____Adult Learners _____Traditional Age Students   Age Range_____Average_____
Gender   _____Female _____Male
Language   _____English as first language (EPL)   _____English as second (other) language (ESL)
ESL predominant languages _____
Prior educational experience _____U.S. High school diploma _____Foreign HS diploma _____GED
                                 _____general _____academic _____honors _____advanced placement _____vocational
Remedial education   _____reading _____writing _____math _____biology _____chemistry _____other
Prior college experience _____Transfer credits, no degree _____U.S. _____Foreign
                          _____Community College _____Senior College _____Graduate School
                          _____Associate degree _____Bachelor's degree _____Masters' degree _____Doctorate
                          _____Nursing degree _____Non-nursing degree
Enrollment history   _____Continuous _____Course withdrawals _____Stopouts
Enrollment status   _____full-time _____part-time _____matriculated _____non-matriculated
Prior health care experience _____Unlicensed health care personnel _____Licensed health care personnel
                          _____LPN _____RN _____Other
Prior work experience   _____None _____Displaced Homemaker _____Second career
Employment status   _____full-time _____part-time _____on-campus _____off-campus
Financial status   _____Disadvantaged _____Financial Aid _____Subsidized loans _____Work-study
Family Role Responsibilities _____single parent _____parent _____spouse _____caregiver _____other
Group Disparity   _____African American or Black _____Hispanic _____Native American
                        _____under-represented Asian _____other Asian _____White, disadvantaged
                        _____White
Ethnic Diversity   Predominant student groups_____
                        New immigrant student groups_____
                        New refugee student groups_____
                        Foreign student groups_____
                        Other student groups_____
Religious Diversity   Predominant student religions_____
                        Other student religions_____

Institutional Characteristics
_____Open enrollment _____Public_____Private, non-religious _____Religious (type)_____
_____Historically Black College or University (HBCU) _____Hispanic-serving _____Tribal College
_____Community College _____Senior College _____Graduate Degree College
_____Urban_____Suburban _____Rural _____Commuter _____Residential

Nursing Program Characteristics
_____Weekend program _____Evening program _____Day and evening program _____Cohort program
_____Cooperative-learning-work program _____Distance learning _____Web-based _____Web-enhanced

readings. In fact, such expectations may cause undue stress to financially challenged students. A better approach may be to supplement one main textbook with select journal articles available online with full-text access or on reserve in the library. Several brief journal articles, featuring select cultural topics can be used to enhance cultural competence development by creatively integrating the articles with other course activities. Optional readings concerning culture (or any topic) send a mixed message to students. For example, students may perceive that cultural considerations in nursing care is optional rather than an expected, integral component in providing quality nursing care and/or never complete the reading.

As another example, an academically diverse student group will need much guidance with how to become active readers, use tables and graphs effectively, analyze and synthesize material, formulate questions, and highlight important information (Mertig, 2003). A new student orientation or course orientation that customizes pre-reading strategies, time management, active reading strategies, note-taking, and study skills to the nursing course will be most beneficial in enhancing success. Without reinforced guidance, students may not see the importance of textbook case studies, research briefs, clinical snapshots, or other textbook chapter features concerning culturally diverse clients. As a result, students may neglect to read these sections. Consistent with trends in higher education, the numbers of academically diverse undergraduate nursing students, such as ESL students or students who completed remedial courses, have also increased. Nurse educators can further assist diverse students by:

- Selecting an easy-to-read appropriate textbook that is enhanced with visual aids
- Identifying reasonable number of reading assignments that students can complete
- Encouraging use of a dictionary to look up unfamiliar words
- Preparing advance organizers, discussion questions, or outline to focus reading
- Developing study guide that correlates with course and reading assignment
- Organizing weekly study groups to discuss readings and answer questions

Examining the textbook for the age, gender, and cultural diversity of registered nurses and other health professionals depicted in illustrations, photos, or case exemplars is another important consideration to promote inclusion and foster cultural competence development. Identifying gaps between learner characteristics and textbook case studies provides the opportunity for nurse educators to supplement readings with other

examples featuring cultures both similar and different from those of learners. Such supplements are valuable whether the course is an undergraduate medical-surgical nursing course, a required core course in the master's
degree curriculum, or any other course on any degree level.

Films, Movies, or Videos

Films, movies, or videos provide unique opportunities to enhance student cognitive, psychomotor, and affective learning. For the purposes of
this chapter, "films, movies, and videos" will be referred to simply as
"videos." Through videos, students are exposed to a combined audio
and visual medium that can enhance learning, especially among visual
learners. If used appropriately, videos can expose students to a wide variety of new situations and cultural groups in a short amount of time that,
ordinarily, they may not have the opportunity to encounter at all or for
some time. Unfortunately, videos also have the potential for perpetrating
stereotypes unless students are properly guided.

The best learning can take place if students are appropriately guided
toward what to focus on in the video. A set of guided objectives, expected
outcomes, and/or preset discussion questions can direct students' attention toward achieving the desired learning outcomes. Pausing the video
at strategic points is beneficial to maximize active learning (Ulrich &
Glendon, 1999). For example, the nurse educator can elaborate upon key
components, ask probing questions to stimulate further inquiry, direct
learners to reflect upon the last segment viewed, and provide opportunity for guided class questions and/or discussion before proceeding on
with film. Pauses permit self-reflection, class-dialogue, synthesis, clarification, and organized compartmentalization of learning "chunks" before
proceeding to new learning. New questions or areas of guided focus can
assist learners (especially novices) about what to look for, thereby serving
as a jump/start for critical thinking about cultural competence.

Cautioning viewers about the dangers of stereotyping based on the
scenarios depicted in the video recognizes limitations but permits a partial insight into a different, emic (insider's) view. An outsider from a
different culture may gain a new viewpoint. Through organized class discussion, a student who is an "insider" into the depicted culture may also
gain a new perspective on how outsiders (classmates) view certain CVB
while also being able to add his/her perspective on CVB presented in the
video. Every video should be evaluated as to how it potentially perpetu-
ates misperceptions, inaccuracies, and biases within nursing, health care,
and particular cultural groups. The instructor is empowered to make
a significant difference by developing cultural competence in students
concerning every topic. Stopping the video to describe application to

various cultural groups emphasizes the importance of culture and effectively links culture with other course components. When comparing and contrasting cultures, focused questions can assist students recognize subtle differences in various cultures (Ulrich & Glendon, 1999).

Whether or not videos viewed outside of class are required or supplemental can have a tremendous impact upon learning outcomes. For example, if a video on "Chinese healing" is supplemental rather than required, then the perception is that it is (a) unnecessary, (b) less important than "required" assignments, and/or (c) optional. Similarly, if a video is "required" but it is not connected to the other course components, assignments, or discussions, it is really a disconnected attachment that needs to be connected or integrated effectively throughout the course (or ideally the curriculum). (See Chapter 7 for an innovative strategy that integrates video within a multidimensional strategy design.)

Educational course videos may focus on varied topics such as (a) general transcultural nursing principles, (b) a particular cultural group, (c) comparison between several cultural groups, (d) multidisciplinary health care, (e) clinical topics with cultural competence addressed, (f) clinical topics without cultural competence addressed, (g) client-centered teaching, or (h) conferences and meetings. Creatively selecting fiction and/or nonfiction TV movies/clips and/or cinema films/clips can effectively complement and enhance course topics. Clinical topic videos should be critically appraised for relevance within and between cultural groups. For example, videos that include skin assessment should take into account differences based on physical appearance (e.g., variations in skin pigmentation, healing, and scar formation), cultural practices (e.g., tattoos, body-piercing, male and female circumcision), and cultural values (taboos, modesty in exposing skin to examiners of different genders, ages, cultures, and religions). Although the film may not address this, or may address these issues minimally, the nurse educator has the potential to make a difference by asking students to reflect on different client situations, asking questions, storytelling about actual clinical incidents, and presenting case studies (see Exhibit 6.3).

Computer-Assisted Instruction

Preparing computer-literate graduates of nursing programs who exercise critical thinking, clinical decision making, and reflection is an absolute necessity presently and in the future (Mueller, Pullen, & McGee, 2002). In particular, the future demands that nurses exercise critical thinking and clinical decision making that consider clients' cultural values, beliefs, and practices. Empirical evidence supports that computer-assisted instruction (CAI) can enhance self-efficacy in clinical decision making and create a link between theoretical and clinical learning without the fear of

Exhibit 6.3   Innovations in Cultural Competence Development:
In-Class Video Teaching–Learning Activities

1. Select videos that accurately depict culturally diverse clients, nurses, and other health care providers.
2. For all videos, but especially for clinically focused videos with little cultural diversity, note limitations and develop learning activities (questions, reflection, discussion, role-playing, and storytelling) to expand upon clinical focus by addressing cultural issues.
3. Create a guided set of objectives/learning outcomes that corresponds/ links with (or expands upon) other aspects of course content/ objectives, videos, patient care assignments, reading assignments, specific for the video teaching–learning experience.
4. Include objectives and learning outcomes for video teaching–learning activity in course outline and/or class handout. (Discussion questions and prerequisite reading can provide necessary background information to facilitate achievement of the desired learning outcomes).
5. Review objectives and learning outcomes with students, emphasizing learner centered feature aimed at developing cultural competence. Give students a guided "movie preview."
6. Prepare a set of guided questions, comments, alternate case scenario with different cultural dimensions within the same cultural group; alternate case scenario with different cultural dimensions among different cultural groups, and pause points for strategic points in the video. (Note that select questions and scenarios can also be divided among several small groups for a small group discussion that is followed by a large group discussion or debriefing session.)
7. Interject comments, questions, and invite student questions and comments.
8. Note areas of interested discussion, student questions and responses, weakness, strengths, and gaps.
9. Obtain students' verbal and/or written feedback concerning video teaching–learning activity.
10. Incorporate results from steps 8 and 9 into future course offerings and curricular revision.

jeopardizing client safety (Edwards et al., 2007; Madorin & Iwasiw, 1999; Mertig, 2003; Weis & Guyton-Simmons, 1998). Within the context of cultural competence development this means that students can potentially interact with a wide sampling of clients who are culturally different from the student without fear of making cultural mistakes. Students may have guided practice without the instructor present (Boyce & Winne, 2000), thereby decreasing the anxiety of being observed, judged, or graded. Especially for adult learners who are self-directed and desire immediate feedback for performance, CAI offers a forum for independent learning, immediate feedback, clinical decision making, and critical thinking in a nonthreatening environment; TSE perceptions will be positively influenced. In addition, computer-based learning tools can emphasize life-long learning (Zinatelli, Dube, Jovanovic, 2002), a quality necessary to keep pace with the ever-changing client populations and cultures.

Previous computer experience and faculty promotion of software programs has a direct impact on student use (Thede, Taft, Coeling, 1994). Previous computer experience may include a degree of comfort and familiarity with computer use, satisfaction with software programs, correlation of CAI material with course content and immediate goals, self-efficacy about computer skills, easy access to CAI, satisfaction, and support services associated with CAI use. For example, the quality of the software program can influence student learning, interest, and motivation. A high-quality program is one that is interactive, stimulating, uses multimedia format, permits user control, and enables immediate and descriptive feedback in questioning (Khoiny, 1995). If software programs are to be perceived as user-friendly, programs must be promoted consistently by faculty throughout the curriculum, beginning students must be introduced to CAI early in the curriculum, and software programs must complement and enhance learning via other educational media (e.g., film, video, reading, and lecture). Using a standardized, reliable, and valid evaluation tool for appraising instructional software can enhance the probability that programs will meet overall curricular objectives (Boyce & Winne, 2000). Adding several items that evaluate the capacity to enhance learning related to cultural competence development and accurate exposure to multicultural clients, families, communities, nurses, and health care professionals will provide comparative information. Such data will help with purchasing decisions, design of strategies to integrate programs systematically throughout the course (and curriculum), and development of supplementary materials as needed to further address cultural similarities and differences. Examples of strategy design innovations are presented in Exhibit 6.4.

Exhibit 6.4   Innovations in Cultural Competence Development: Computer-Assisted Instruction

Sample Programmed Instruction Guide
1. Click on the icon "Medical-Surgical Nursing."
2. Click on the case study "Care of the Client with_____.
3. Click on the CAI program option "Video with tutorial" and view segment 1.
4. What assumptions did you make about the client's cultural background in video segment 1? Why?

5. What assumptions did you make about the nurse's cultural background in video segment 1? Why?
6. What are the dangers of making assumptions based on physical characteristics, age, and/or gender?
7. Proceed to the video segment and tutorial CAI in segment 2–7.
8. What verbal and nonverbal communication techniques do the clients use?
9. What verbal and nonverbal communication techniques do the nurses use?
10. Are the communication patterns used effective? Why or why not?
11. What information concerning the client's cultural values, beliefs, and practices were presented?
12. How did the nurse incorporate the client's cultural values, beliefs, and practices into the plan of care?
13. To achieve culturally congruent care, what (else) should the nurse have done? Why?
14. Reflect upon the traditional elderly Chinese client presented in last week's class video. How would the nurse–client interaction and plan of care be the same (or different) to achieve culturally congruent care? Explain.
15. Reflect upon the case study about the Mexican American migrant worker presented in this week's assigned reading (Chapter 12). How would the nurse–client interaction and plan of care be the same to achieve culturally congruent care? Explain.
16. Proceed to video segment and tutorial CAI number 8–15.
17. To achieve culturally congruent care, how would the nurse's discharge teaching and home care plan be the same (or different), if the client held the dominant (traditional) values, beliefs, and practices consistent with the _____ culture. (Examples: Egyptian, Filipino, Nigerian, Lakota, Jamaican, etc.). Explain.
18. To achieve culturally congruent care, how would the nurse's discharge teaching and home care plan be the same (or different) if the clients in the above-listed ethnic groups were also _____ (Examples: female, Muslim, Jehovah Witness, Catholic, Jewish, Mormon, indigent, wealthy, illiterate, deaf, unemployed, unmarried, etc.). Explain.
19. Proceed to complete the review questions and check your answers and rationale.
20. Reflect on your experience completing this CAI and programmed instruction guide questions. What did you like best? Discuss.

Unfortunately, the growing numbers of minority students and new immigrants in higher education have limited resources. Furthermore, limited access to computer technology will be characteristic of many minority and lower income students (Burr, Burr, & Novak, 1999). The "nontraditional" student is older with multiple role responsibilities competing with academic demands; their organized study time and ability to use educational resources is often limited. Frequently, students are ineffica-cious in their ability to use computers and other educational resources. Consequently, integrating computer technology throughout the nursing curriculum must be accompanied by strategies to enhance nursing stu-dents' computer technology access, skills, use, and values (Jeffreys, 2004; Pressler & Kenner, 2009).

Unless CAI is valued, expected (required) throughout the curriculum, many students opt out of the "optional" CAI programs. Unfortunately, this will create a greater gap between those students who are computer literate or computer comfortable and the potential values of CAI will never be realized. Faculty-run workshops at the beginning of each nurs-ing course, designed to introduce small groups of students to CAI use, functions, and benefits, should be supplemented by opportunities for short workshops throughout the semester and by advanced student peers and mentors. Adult learners respond best and are most motivated by per-ceived direct applicability to learning needs and long-term career goals. Highlighting the benefits within this context and introducing students to CAI programs most relevant to the course currently enrolled in will reap the greatest results. Results can be maximized by providing a warm, relaxed environment or place for students to use CAI, such as a nursing student resource center (nursing neighborhood) in which peer mentors (advanced students) serve as role models, resources, and guides to less advanced students (Jeffreys, 2004).

Web Page or Web Site

The course Web page or Web site has a unique opportunity to expand stu-dents' horizons in cultural competence development beyond geographic limitations. Because there are no geographic boundaries in cyberspace, students have the potential opportunity to venture out into worlds previ-ously foreign, unknown, and undiscovered. Although the advantages are many, there are also disadvantages. One of the biggest disadvantages is that inaccurate information can be transmitted widely. Discriminating be-tween reputable and reliable sites and questionable sites is often confusing to the novice (Andrews, Burr, & Janetos, 2004; Wink, 2009). Assisting students to access scholarly and reliable sites related to culture, health care, and nursing is an essential responsibility of educators. One way to do this is to create a course or program Web page with direct links to reputable Internet sites and peer-reviewed professional literature (Wink, 2009; Xiao, 2005) (see Chapter 7, Exhibit 7.2). Full-text journal articles increase access to reputable information. Web page features, particularly important to the development of cultural competence, are presented in Exhibit 6.5.

Exhibit 6.5 Innovations in Cultural Competence Development:
Course Web Page

- Course Announcements: Cultural events, holidays, meetings, conferences, food festival, newly published articles, discussion board invitation, brown-bag roundtable discussion lunch meeting, check other part of webpage

- Graphics, Photos, Slides Culturally diverse clients, students, nurses, and other health care providers in various settings. Graphics describing picture, event, date, individuals

- Virtual Tour Campus, nursing student resource center, nursing skills lab, depicting culturally diverse students, faculty, and staff

- Video Clip Above examples

- Calendar Cultural holidays and events

- How to Use Web page General information about Blackboard features, support services for students who need assistance on-line, Workshops, in-person support at Nursing Student Resource Center or College Library/Computer Lab Center, Finding Web page Resources related to cultural competence.

- Web site Links: Local cultural agencies and resources, Ethnic Nursing Organizations, Transcultural Nursing Society (TCNS), local TCNS Chapter, Healthy People 2010, Office of Minority Health, US Census, Patient Education

- Full-Text Articles Organized by cultural group (CINAHL, ERIC, Psychlit)

- Discussion Board Weekly discussion (asynchronous or synchronous) about a cultural clinical case study, assigned reading, video, computer-assisted instructional program, or other course component or outside assigned activity

- Reading Assignments Questions posted to prompt reflection and guide reading concerning to address cultural competency development

- Course Documents Highlight cultural components in yellow for the following documents: Course outline, program outcomes, characteristics of the graduate, Code of Ethics from ANA, ICN, NSNA. Transcultural Nursing Code of Ethics, Cultural Linguistics

- E-mail Individual, select, and all user communication to send personalized messages in addition to course announcements

Students, especially nontraditional students, will need ongoing guidance about computer technology, literature and Web searches, and the computer-assistance services available via the nursing department and the college (Dorrian & Wache, 2008; Mertig, 2003; Pressler & Kenner, 2009). By enhancing the ease with which students can access known reputable information, students can become more confident (efficacious) about developing their transcultural nursing skills. For example, a student who retrieves known reputable information about a particular cultural group and clinical topic will be better prepared to conduct a culturally congruent health history in the clinical setting and most likely will be realistically efficacious. Optimally, a workshop designed and conducted by the course instructor, librarian, or nursing support personnel will maximize student use by increasing knowledge, computer skills, and appreciation of computer technology (Xiao, 2005). (See Chapter 7 for library orientation and computer workshop interactive, integrative component.) Often, students are inefficacious about computer skills, library searches, or resources available. Strategies that expand on instructor workshops, especially ones that incorporate peer mentors and role modeling will enhance student use, persistence, satisfaction, and self-efficacy concerning computer use and research skills (Jeffreys, 2004).

Ciesielka (2008) described an innovative strategy for using wiki to meet graduate nursing education competencies in collaboration and community health. Different from discussion board, authorized users may post and edit content directly on the closed Web site. Wikis can build collaborative networks of learners and professionals and have the potential to include the ongoing development of cultural competence amongst the group members. Other strategies for enhancing cultural competence development may include problem-based learning hybrid courses that involve case studies and small group participation with instructor guidance (O'Neill et al., 2009; Rash, 2008), online reflective journaling (Kessler & Lund, 2004), and the virtual hospital (Edwards et al., 2007) (see Exhibit 6.1).

Nursing Skills Laboratory

Traditionally, the main purpose of the nursing skills laboratory (NSL) was to permit the teaching and practicing of clinical skills via a nonthreatening, controlled environment and simulation. *Simulation* has been defined as a situation or event made to resemble clinical practice (Rauen, 2001). Simulation permits the student to practice clinical skills prior to implementation on a real patient. Whether the NSL contains the new high-technology human patient simulators, simulated patient actors, or rubber mannequins, it is simulation as a teaching method that has much potential in enhancing learning. Simulation can increase knowledge, critical thinking, and confidence; it has been used successfully in nursing education for clinical skills (Hodge et al., 2008; Medley & Horne, 2005; Morton & Rauen, 2004; Nehring & Lashley, 2004; Ulrich & Glendon, 1999).

Nurse educators have a wonderful opportunity to further develop students' cultural competence by creating simulated patient case scenarios that incorporate cultural dimensions. Simulated patient case scenarios build self-efficacy, critical thinking, and clinical decision making (Dearman, 2003; Hodge et al., 2008; Ravert, 2008). First, the NSL environment can be modeled (or remodeled) to outwardly embrace and emphasize cultural diversity. Although the purchase of culturally diverse mannequins may be one option, the market options for mannequins are limited to a few differences in physical characteristics, neglecting the more important variations in CVB. There are more detailed and inexpensive strategies to make the NSL more "culturally friendly" and inclusive. For example, each mannequin can be given a name and background information representing different ethnic, racial, gender, socioeconomic, age, and religious groups (see Figure 6.4). Corresponding patient charts, bed tags,

151

Patient Name: Maria Lopez Age: 45 Sex: Female Marital Status: Widowed Religion: Roman Catholic Ed. Level: GED Occupation: Cashier in supermarket Health Insurance: BC/BS Significant Other: Daughter Elena Lopez-Ruiz Significant Cultural Factors: 1) Prefers traditional Mexican foods; 2) Daily Communion 3) Participation in Mass on Sundays in hospital chapel; 4) Daughter be informed of medical diagnoses and must be consulted for medical decision-making; 5) Female physician or female nurse practitioner for gynecological exams 6) Patient education literature in English and Spanish 7) Prefers extended visitation to include members of extended family & church network	Patient Name: Andrew O'Leary Age: 34 Sex: Male Marital Status: Single, lives with partner Religion: Methodist Ed. Level: Junior college (AS degree) Occupation: x-ray technician Health Insurance: Blue Cross/Blue Shield Significant Other: Mario LaRosa Significant Cultural Factors: 1) Significant other is domestic partner and has power of attorney in case of emergency 2) Requests visitation privileges to include members of Gay Men Health Crisis support group
Patient Name: Ming Chen Age: 53 Sex: Male Marital Status: Married Religion: Buddhist Ed. Level: Foreign HS Occupation: grocer, self-employed Health Insurance: Medicaid Significant Other: Lily Chen (wife) Significant Cultural Factors: 1) Prefers traditional Chinese foods 2) Daily tai-chi exercises and meditation 3) Patient education literature in Chinese and English 4) Prefers hot beverages with meals and when taking medications 5) Uses tiger balm to rub on sore muscles 6) Uses traditional Chinese herbal teas to regulate bowels	Patient Name: Dev Patel Age: 53 Sex: Male Marital Status: Married Religion: Hindu Ed. Level: Bachelor's degree Occupation: accountant Health Insurance: Medicaid Significant Other: Sandi Patel (wife) Significant Cultural Factors: 1) Prefers traditional Asian Indian foods that are vegetarian 2) Daily yoga and meditation 3) Patient education literature in English 4) Prefers hot beverages with meals and when taking medications 5) Uses traditional herbal teas to regulate bowels and promote sleep
Patient Name: Konstantine Stamos Age: 33 Sex: Male Marital Status: Single Religion: Greek Orthodox Ed. Level: Foreign HS Occupation: waiter Health Insurance: Medicaid Significant Other: (sister) Significant Cultural Factors: 1) Prefers traditional Greek foods 2) Patient education literature in Greek and English 3) Only family visitor is sister, Kristina. Most of family lives in Greece.	

Figure 6.4 Demographic Data

Patient Name: __LaToya Jones__ Age: __72__ Sex: __Female__	Patient Name: __Joshua Redfeather__ Age: __47__ Sex: __Male__
Marital Status: __Married__ Religion: __Jehovah Witness__	Marital Status: __Divorced__ Religion: __Lutheran__
Ed. Level: __Master's degree__ Occupation: __retired high school English teacher__	Ed. Level: __High school__ Occupation: __construction worker__
Health Insurance: __Medicare; GHI__ Significant Other: __Bernard Jones (husband)__	Health Insurance: __HIP__ Significant Other: __Linda Crow (girlfriend)__
<u>Significant Cultural Factors:</u>	<u>Significant Cultural Factors:</u>
1) No blood transfusions or blood products 2) Daily prayers 3) Participation in Jehovah Witness meetings 3 times weekly 4) Prefers extended visitation to include members of extended family & church network	1) Prefers traditional Navajo and Southwestern US foods 2) Seeks guidance from tribal leaders 3) Uses traditional tribal remedies (teas, ointments, sweat lodges, prayers, dance) for health promotion 4) Extended family and extended visiting hours 5) Communication patterns include periods of silence and avoidance of direct eye contact as preferred
Patient Name: __Omar Ali__ Age: __63__ Sex: __Male__	Patient Name: __Harry Greenfield__ Age: __62__ Sex: __Male__
Marital Status: __Married__ Religion: __Muslim__	Marital Status: __Married__ Religion: __Jewish__
Ed. Level: __Master's degree__ Occupation: __High school physics teacher__	Ed. Level: __Bachelor's degree__ Occupation: __clothing salesman__
Health Insurance: __HIP__ Significant Other: __Amina Hassan (wife)__	Health Insurance: __HIP__ Significant Other: __Sara Greenfield (wife)__
<u>Significant Cultural Factors:</u>	<u>Significant Cultural Factors:</u>
1) Prefers traditional Egyptian foods 2) Prayers five times daily facing Mecca 3) Patient education literature in English 4) Use right hand to place medications, food, or beverages in patient's mouth 5) Avoid use of food and products made with pork or alcohol 6) Prefers halal meats	1) Kosher food 2) Prayers five times daily 3) Requests weekly visit from rabbi 4) Visitation to include immediate and extended family as well as members of synagogue 5) No tests and procedures on Sabbath and holy days
Patient Name: __Lucienne Rabideau__ Age: __82__ Sex: __Female__	
Marital Status: __Widowed__ Religion: __Roman Catholic__	
Ed. Level: __grade 10, Montreal__ Occupation: __homemaker__	
Health Insurance: __Aetna__ Significant Other: __Jean-Pierre Rabideau (son)__	
<u>Significant Cultural Factors:</u>	
1) Prefers traditional French foods 2) Daily Communion 3) Participation in Mass on Sundays in hospital chapel; 4) Son must be informed of medical diagnoses and must be consulted for medical decision-making; 5) Patient education literature in French and English 6) Prefers regular visitations to include only members of immediate family	

Figure 6.4 Demographic Data (*continued*)

152

patient identification tags, ethnic clothing, religious articles, non-English reading materials, ethnic menus, and other items can be placed on or near the mannequins. Clinical case scenarios, incorporating various cultural data along with the clinical topics relevant to previous class sessions and the current week's class can be developed into a large group discussion, small group activity, role play, case exemplar, care plan, and/or other learner-centered activity (see Exhibit 6.6 – Educator-In-Action Vignette).

Exhibit 6.6   Educator-In-Action Vignette

Coordinating course components and optimizing learning outcomes among culturally and academically diverse students who must care for many groups of diverse patient populations is challenging. Attempting coordinated synthesis and consistency between nursing skills lab sections taught by different full-time and part-time faculty with different types of clinical expertise and preparation as an educator contributes to the challenge. Professor Quest receives faculty support for designing and group piloting of an Integrated Skills (IS) laboratory session during the last nursing skills lab class. After reviewing course materials, available resources, and nursing and educational literature, Professor Quest designs the educational strategy. A written instruction packet is reviewed with course instructors and laboratory technicians at a course meeting (see below). Feedback from faculty and students concerning the strategy will guide future IS lab sessions.

Integrated Skills (IS) Lab: Instructions for Lab Instructors

The IS strategy aims to integrate and synthesize key concepts, skills, and professional values addressed throughout the semester in lecture/theory, college lab, and clinical. Cultural competence is an integral component. Accordingly, the IS strategy incorporates several strategy components essential for maximizing learning outcomes, including:

Prerequisite Assignment: During the previous week, students should be told to bring drug book, AIDS and pneumonia drug handouts to IS class, and to review course components, especially skills and medications.
   (Please note that times listed are approximate.)

1. Pre-conference and background information (teachers highlight and assign) [5 minutes]
   (a) Introduction to objectives, plan, and expectations for the day
   (b) Assignment of students into teacher-selected pairs
2. Data-gathering (initial) [15 minutes]
   (a) Taped nurse's report
   (b) Immediate initial assessment of patient
   (c) Review of chart (health history, lab data, progress notes, doctor's order sheet), medication sheet, and flow sheets

3. Culturally congruent nursing actions within appropriate time frame [2 hours]
    (a) Diagnostic interventions (assessment)
    (b) Therapeutic interventions
    (c) Teaching interventions
    (d) Referral/collaboration
    (e) Delegation
    (f) Report
    (g) Nursing diagnoses
    (h) Documentation
4. Debriefing session (large group discussion)
    (a) Sample verbal reports by at least two student groups with group discussion [15 minutes]
    (b) Guided discussion, questions, and answers [5 minutes]
5. Reflection about IS learning experience
    (a) Individual written (1 page); then collect [5 minutes]
    (b) Large group discussion about learning experience [5 minutes]
6. Summary (Teachers synthesize and highlight major components [5 minutes])

Instructors: To assist with class preparation, please review the following materials *prior to* the IS class (**BUT DO NOT DISTRIBUTE OR SHARE WITH STUDENTS**):

1. IS instructor template (see Figure 6.5)
2. IS patient demographic (cultural) information (see Figure 6.4)
3. Patient charts and patient report (see Exhibit 6.7)
4. AIDS and pneumonia drug handouts (previously distributed to students in class)
5. Any other necessary materials to enhance student learning outcomes

Please note that the IS strategy example below should incorporate learning in each area:

1. Cognitive domain (knowledge, comprehension, application, analysis about such areas as the patient's disease, health problems, nursing diagnoses, nursing process, cultural competence, skills, medications, delegation, collaboration, documentation, etc.)
2. Psychomotor domain (vital signs, apical pulse, BP, breath sounds, bowel sounds, dressing changes, injections, IV meds, oral meds, eye drops, pulse oximeter, oxygen therapy, pulmonary toilet, turning and positioning, communication, report, etc.)
3. Affective domain (professional attitudes, values and beliefs related to patient care, culture, ethics, professional standards, etc.)
4. Teaching (meds, diet, pulmonary toilet, infection control, health promotion, etc.)
5. Collaboration (physician and other health professionals as needed, other nurses)
6. Documentation (flow sheet, med sheet, progress notes, controlled substance record, etc.)

Integrated Skills Template

(Specific orders and prescriptions would be added and match with patient chart)

		Medical Diagnosis #1 Scenario	Medical Diagnosis #2 Scenario
1	**General Medical Information**		
	Admitting Diagnosis		
	History of		
	Wound # 1		
	Wound #2		
	Allergy: PCN (anaphylactic shock)		
2	**Daily Medications**		
	Anti-infective IVPB #1		
	Anti-infective IVPB #2		
	Stool softener		
	MVI PO		
	Narcotic IV lock 30 minutes before dressing change (QID)		
	Inhaler med		
	Other meds		
	IV		
3	**PRN Medications**		
	NSAID		
	Narcotic analgesic		
	Sedative hypnotic		
	Laxative		
	Antidiarrheal		
	Antipyretic		
	Antiemetic		
	Antipruritic		
	Natural tears		
4	**Diet**		
	Nutritional supplement: Protein shake 3X daily		
5	**Oxygen & Respiratory Care**		
	Oxygen delivery		
	Pulse oximeter Q shift and prn		
6	**Expected Assessments**		
	Apical radial pulse		
	BP		
	Breath sounds		
	Lung sounds		
	Wounds		
	General head to toe		
	IV bags, tubing, IV lock, site		
	Lab data		
	Oxygen equipment		
	Dressings		

Figure 6.5   Integrated Skills Template

	Doctor's orders		
	Medication sheet		
	Patient ID band		
	Patient chart		
	Kardex		
7	**Nursing Orders (Practice Delegation)**		
	Bed bath		
	Oral care Q 2hrs		
	TCDB q 2hrs while awake		
	CBR		
	Obtain U/A		
	Daily weight		
	Monitor and record BM		
	Encourage fluids		
	Meals with assistance		
	Wound care #1		
	Wound care #2		
	Diet teaching		
	Teach pursed lip breathing		
	Fingersticks Q 6 hours		
	I and O Q 8 hours		
8	**Documentation**		
	Flow sheet with pain scale		
	Medication sheet		
	Progress note		
	NANDA, NIC, NOC		
9	**Collaboration/Referral**		
	Physician		
	Dietician		
	CNS		
10	**Ethical, Legal, and Cultural Issues**		
	DNR status		
	Patient cultural requests		
	Other		

Figure 6.5   Integrated Skills Template (*continued*)

Exhibit 6.7   Integrated Skills: Report Script

_____ is a-year-old woman/man with AIDS, PCP, CMV retinitis, a right heel wound, SOB, DOE, and S/P abdominal surgery for small bowel obstruction. She/he has an h/o asthma that was well-managed with prn medications only up until 2 days before admission. _____ had increasing SOB with a nonproductive cough and was admitted. A bronchoscopy 3 days ago confirmed PCP. She/he still c/o pleuritic pain when coughing and has some hemoptysis. Although she/he received a sleeping pill last night, she/he woke up coughing. She/he received guafenesin last at 2AM with relief of coughing episode. 7 AM oral T = 98.9, P = 87, R = 24 with wheezes noted in lower right and left lobes upon auscultation. Pulse oximeter reading was 98% at 7 AM while on Oxygen 35% via Venti mask. She/he is due for her/his morning peak expiratory flow meter reading at 9 AM. Please compare with lab data results in her/his chart.

While at home, she/he noticed decreased peripheral vision and blurriness; opthalmoscopic examination confirmed CMV retinitis. While walking barefoot, _____ stepped on a tack and now has a dime-sized superficial right heel wound with healing tissue noted. She/he gets a DSD to her/his heel three times a day and is due for wound care at 10:30 AM. She/he had abdominal surgery about two weeks ago for a small bowel obstruction and her/his wound opened. The abdominal wound is approximately 5 inch long, 1/2 inch deep mid-abdominal wound with small amounts of thick, yellow drainage and granulation tissue present. She/he gets a DSD dressing to the abdomen three times a day and is due for wound care at 10:30 AM.

_____ c/o severe pain during the dressing change, therefore she/he has morphine 1 mg via IV lock 30 minutes before the dressing change. Because her/his abdominal pain is more severe than her/his heel pain, it is best to change the heel dressing first and allow for the peak action of morphine to occur.

_____ c/o decreased appetite and receives a can of ensure with each meal. She/he needs much encouragement to eat. Yesterday, the nurse began teaching _____ about foods with high protein and vitamin C to promote healing as well as the increased caloric needs to fight off infection with a weakened immune system; however, _____ needs follow-up teaching.

Insert appropriate cultural considerations information:

Mrs. Lopez prefers traditional Mexican foods so her daughter usually brings in home-cooked foods at lunchtime. As per Mrs. Lopez' request, her daughter Elena Lopez-Ruiz must be informed of any new medical diagnoses and must be consulted for medical decision making. Please note the culture-specific care documented on her chart. The Catholic priest stops by every day around 11:30 AM so Mrs. Lopez becomes very anxious if her morning care and dressings are not completed on time. Also, it is important for her to receive Communion so she must fast for at least 1 hour; therefore, her oral medications need to be administered by 10:30 AM.

Mr. O'Leary prefers home-cooked meals, so his partner usually brings in home-cooked foods at lunchtime. As per Mr. O'Leary's request, his partner Mario LaRosa has power of attorney. Please note the culture-specific care documented on his chart. Some of his support group members from the Gay Men Health Crisis Center stop by every day around 11:30 AM, so Mr. O'Leary becomes very anxious if his morning care and dressings are not completed on time. Also, it is important for him to be able to verbalize his feelings with them so we make every effort to complete his oral medications and inhaler meds prior to this time.

Mr. Chen prefers traditional Chinese foods, so his wife Lily Chen usually brings in home-cooked foods around 11:30 AM. Although Mr. Chen rarely complains about anything, Mr. Chen becomes very happy and verbalizes his appreciation if his morning care and dressings are completed on time, so we make every effort to complete his oral medications and inhaler meds prior to this time. Please note the culture-specific care documented on his chart.

Mr. Patel—Please note the culture-specific care documented on his chart. He prefers traditional Asian-Indian vegetarian foods, so his wife Sandi Patel usually brings in home-cooked foods around 11:30 AM. Although Mr. Patel rarely complains about anything, he becomes very happy and verbalizes his appreciation if his morning care and dressings are completed on time, so we make every effort to complete his oral medications and inhaler meds prior to this time.

Mr. Stamos—Please note the culture-specific care documented on his chart. He prefers traditional Greek foods and his sister Kristina Stamos usually brings in home-cooked foods around 11:30 AM, so Mr. Stamos becomes very anxious if his morning care and dressings are not completed on time. Also, it is important for him to be able to verbalize his feelings with her, so we make every effort to complete his oral medications and inhaler meds prior to this time.

As with any teaching strategy, it will be beneficial to explain the purpose, objectives, activities, and time frame before the onset. Supplementing verbal information with a brief outline or handout can be used as a reference for students periodically throughout the activity to keep students on target. A debriefing session will help summarize and clarify key points, giving the nurse educator another opportunity to emphasize cultural competence development as an expected component to any clinical skill. To further enhance affective learning and self-discovery (as well as provide feedback to the nurse educator), students can be asked to reflect on the case scenario, group discussion, or other activity. Written student comments and feedback will provide new insight into the teaching strategy's perceived benefits, limitations, and learning associated with furthering cultural competence development; student feedback will be valuable in modifying or continuing with strategy components.

Other strategies for making the NSL "culturally friendly" and inclusive extend toward making culturally diverse students feel welcome. NSL posters, bulletin boards, and journal article postings that celebrate cultural diversity and emphasize the nursing professional's role in culture-specific nursing care is one strategy. Creating situational questions that address cultural issues as new clinical skills are introduced or previously learned skills are refreshed to supplement and enhance learning.

Awareness that covert or subtle racism can consciously or unconsciously create feelings of isolation, stress, and cultural pain must also acknowledge that these unwanted feelings can adversely influence learning. One example of subtle racism in nursing and health care is the prevalence of physical examination "norms" that are based on the assessment of a "white" individual (Barbee & Gibson, 2001; Bosher & Pharris, 2009). Discussing and demonstrating physical assessment skills to accurately assess patients with dark skin pigmentation for stage I decubitus ulcers, cyanosis, jaundice, petechiae, Kaposi's sarcoma, melanoma, and other assessments should be integrated as an expected component within the appropriate clinical topics; these assessment skills should not be presented as afterthought.

Prior to the implementation of skills with patients in clinical settings, students may be observed or tested to assure a minimum level of proficiency. Although the purpose of the NSL is to enhance learning and develop confidence via a nonthreatening environment, the testing and retesting of nursing skills can greatly increase stress, thereby decreasing learning and satisfaction (Delgado & Mack, 2002). This is particularly true if students' CVB perceive learning performance to be a direct reflection on the teacher, demanding proficiency and excellence after initial instructor demonstration. Nurse educators must learn to adapt teaching styles to accommodate students' diverse CVB concerning learning and the teacher–student role if culturally congruent teaching is to be achieved. Culturally congruent teaching–learning strategies must be integrated within all components of nursing education. Table 6.3 presents several examples contrasting culturally congruent and culturally incongruent teacher–student interactions. Creating a caring, nurturing community through "care groups" for enhancing cognitive, psychomotor, and affective learning in the NSL is one successfully implemented strategy (Pullen, Murray, & McGee, 2001, 2003).

Clinical Settings

Although great differences in types of clinical settings, learning experiences, and instructor involvement exist, there are certain criteria that should be considered. One consideration is the clinical setting's cultural diversity of clients, nurses, and other agency personnel in relation to the surrounding community and to the nursing student population. A second consideration involves students' perceptions concerning diversity. Routine collection and analysis of data from a "student evaluation of clinical experience" questionnaire can provide valuable insight, especially if items solicit information concerning client characteristics and the students' perception about the clinical setting's cultural diversity (Jeffreys, Massoni, O'Donnell, & Smodlaka, 1997) (see also Jeffreys 2010 Toolkit Item 7).

Interaction with culturally diverse patients, families, communities, and health care providers in the clinical setting offers a wealth of learning opportunities for students. Providing opportunities for students to

Table 6.3 Faculty Helpfulness in the Nursing Skills Laboratory, Clinical Setting, and Classroom: Examples of Culturally Incongruent and Culturally Congruent Approaches

SITUATION	CULTURALLY INCONGRUENT	CULTURALLY CONGRUENT
Nursing Skills Laboratory After a detailed skills laboratory class on injections, it is now Lee's turn to administer an intramuscular injection into the skill's laboratory mannequin for the first time. Lee's CVB view the teacher as an authority figure. Less than perfect performance would poorly reflect on the teacher and cause embarrassment for the teacher in front of the other students. Lee is fearful that she will not demonstrate the skill perfectly and feels that she must "save face," yet Lee does not want to refuse the professor's request to "inject." Anxiously, she asks if she can first practice with her peers.	Professor wants to help all students equally and aims to "treat all students alike." Professor insists that Lee administer the injection. Result: Lee feels increasingly anxious and pressured that she must perform the injection perfectly. Additionally, she feels cultural pain because she believes that she initiated conflict with an authority figure. Lee attempts the injection but when she forgets to aspirate, she becomes even more anxious and experiences cultural pain because she has now "embarrassed her teacher." Lee feels much dissatisfaction and stress; she questions her ability to complete the nursing program.	Professor recognizes that Lee's anxiety may not be related to lack of academic readiness, but due to underlying CVB. Professor reassures Lee that she does not expect perfection on the first attempt, however, still notes nonverbal cues of anxiety (facial tension, shaking hands, flushed appearance). Professor pairs Lee with a strong student who has already performed the injection and allows privacy for several practice injections. Result: Lee does not feel pressured to "save face" and can relax enough with her peer to perfect her skill prior to observation by the instructor. After demonstrating the injection to the professor accurately, Lee experiences satisfaction.
Clinical During clinical post-conference, one student (Jane) assertively questions the clinical instructor's statement about a medication. Jane's CVB openly encourage assertiveness and equally view teachers and learners as co-participants in the teaching–learning process. Several students with different CVB are obviously uncomfortable by the perceived confrontation.	Professor's CVB consider the preservation of group harmony and "saving face" as a priority. She sees the discomfort of two other students in the group and aims to help the group avoid conflict. Professor's response is to evade answering Jane's question and dismiss the post-conference early. Result: Jane is still confused and feels stressed about the medication. She is dissatisfied with the professor's actions.	Professor recognizes differences between an individual versus group orientation. Although her own CVB are group orientation, Professor realizes that Jane's behavior is appropriate. Professor answers Jane's question and uses this opportunity to discuss various differences in communication patterns, values, and beliefs among different cultures. Result: Jane and the other students receive clarification about the statement and receive new information about culture and values clarification, enhancing academic outcomes and promoting positive psychological outcomes.

Table 6.3   Faculty Helpfulness in the Nursing Skills Laboratory, Clinical
             Setting, and Classroom: Examples of Culturally Incongruent and
             Culturally Congruent Approaches (*continued*)

SITUATION	CULTURALLY INCONGRUENT	CULTURALLY CONGRUENT
Classroom Lou performed excellently on an examination, achieving the highest grade. Lou has group orientation rather than individual orientation, therefore is uncomfortable with individual praise.	Professor intends to be helpful, acknowledge strong performance, and motivate other students. Professor verbally praises Lou's performance in the classroom, announcing her name and exceptional performance. Result: Lou is embarrassed and feels ashamed over being singled out in the class.	Professor intends to be helpful and acknowledges strong performance and motivates other students, yet is aware of CVB that impact upon a culturally congruent approach. Professor verbally acknowledges the outstanding performance demonstrated by several students without mentioning their names. Result: Lou feels satisfied and comfortable with the knowledge that her performance and that of others in the group has been appreciated.

Adapted from Jeffreys, M.R. (2004). *Nursing Student Retention: Understanding the Process and Making a Difference*, New York: Springer.

interact with culturally diverse clients and personnel must be appropriately partnered with cultural competence development as an integral course and curricular component. Students must have the general transcultural nursing skills, knowledge, and values to successfully achieve positive learning outcomes for cultural competence development. As mentioned previously, TSE (confidence) perceptions will directly influence student's commitment, motivation, and persistence with transcultural skills. Because interactions may result in "cultural mistakes," inefficacious students may avoid cultural considerations when planning and implementing care. Overly confident students may never exercise the task of "preparing" to engage in culturally congruent patient interactions, assessments, planning, or interventions. Without appropriate guidance and feedback, students' TSE perceptions may adversely affect student learning, performance, and outcomes as well as cause negative effects on patient care and patient outcomes (Figure 3.2).

Initial and ongoing student assessment must include transcultural knowledge, skills, values, and confidence. Nurse educators can develop individual and group diagnostic-prescriptive educational interventions based on assessment findings. Anecdotal notes should include regular entries describing student strengths, weaknesses, and client description (Oermann & Gaberson, 2009; Schoolcraft & Novotny, 2000). Often clinical instructors keep anecdotal notes detailing clinical skills or tasks performed by students and patient's medical diagnosis. This information is then used to rotate students through various clinical skills, tasks, and medical diagnoses. A proactive action for enhancing cultural competence development expands anecdotal notes to include details about patient's cultural dimensions and the transcultural skills learned and/or performed by the student.

Clinical instructors have unlimited opportunities to effectively weave cultural competence development throughout the clinical learning experience. Although some learning experiences may be preplanned, clinical instructors must be prepared to be flexible and to adapt learning objectives to the ever-changing situation. Because the clinical setting is not a "controlled" environment, clinical instructors must always be ready to expect the unexpected. Unexpected situations will present new learning opportunities for students' professional growth; some of these unexpected situations may be rich opportunities for expanding cultural competence. Despite the cultural diversity within a clinical setting, the instructor is pivotal to guide students to new levels of cultural competence development. The clinical instructor can supplement actual clinical experiences with case studies representing different cultural groups, values, beliefs, behaviors, and/or practices. A guided post-clinical conference whereby students work together or in small groups to critically appraise information and propose a culturally congruent plan of care is another option.

Preplanned learning objectives that incorporate cultural competence development may or may not be shared with students at the onset of the clinical experience. For example, if self-discovery or group learning through discovery is an intended outcome, telling students about the desired outcomes would be inappropriate. Guided discussion and shared information during a clinical post-conference can help students discover the diverse patient groups represented that day and how similar or different CVB affected the implementation of culturally congruent nursing care, clinical skills, and actual/potential patient outcomes (see Educator-In-Action Vignette, Exhibit 2.1). Post-conference summary of student's cognitive, practical, and affective learning outcomes will be beneficial to future learning activities designed to incorporate this prerequisite learning. Besides comparison of the same clinical skill, other possibilities are cultural similarities and differences between patients with the same signs, symptoms, medical diagnoses, nursing diagnoses, diagnostic procedures, treatments, or prognoses. Positive, realistic instructor feedback and vicarious learning (by observing others) will help improve TSE perceptions.

In clinical settings where the clinical instructor is not present (such as home visits or internship), preset learning objectives, including cultural competence, must be clearly delineated. Instructor comments on weekly journal entries, peer comments on course Web page discussion boards, and/or post-clinical conferences and seminars will further assist students connect together experiences in their cultural competence development. E-mentoring has the potential to connect nurses, students, and instructors "to a learning, sharing environment while crossing the barriers of distance, agency isolation, and busy schedules" (Miller et al., 2008).

Positive learning experiences have been reported from immersion experiences, international public health exchange projects, service-learning, and community-placements (Campbell-Heider et al., 2006; Colling & Wilson, 1998; Critchley et al., 2009; Cummings, 1998; Gomez & White, 2002; Haloburdo & Thompson, 1998; Hughes & Hood, 2007; Kollar & Ailinger, 2002; Leininger & McFarland, 2002; Moch, Long, Jones, Shadlick, & Solheim, 1999; Pickerell, 2001; Ryan, Twibell, Brigham, & Bennett, 2000; Sandin, Grahn, & Kronvall, 2004; Stevens, 1998; St. Clair & McKenry, 1999; Tabi & Mukherjee, 2003). Despite the reported benefits, it is crucial that immersion experiences in cultural communities or international clinical experiences are sufficiently linked with prerequisite and on-site comprehensive learning about the host culture. In addition, experiences should contain sufficient patient–nurse interaction and should be followed with a reflective component to enhance long-term positive learning impact on students (Kollar & Ailinger, 2002; Leininger & McFarland, 2002; Sandin et al., 2004; St. Clair & McKenry, 1999). Adequate preparation and support during the immersion experience must incorporate effective coping strategies (Ryan et al., 2000).

Students can also benefit by the awareness that faculty are also learning and developing cultural competency skills within ethnic communities (Leininger & McFarland, 2002; Moch et al., 1999). By reaching out to surrounding communities, community-based curricula have the potential to provide students with a wealth of valuable experiences if accompanied by other substantial curricular components that embrace a wide diversity of cultures. "Tacking on" culture courses or course components or the "adopt-a-community" approach alone is insufficient for preparing nurses and nursing students to provide culturally congruent care (Baldwin, 1999). TSET Research Exhibits 6.4 and 6.5 illustrate how the TSET has been used to evaluate the effectiveness of immersion experiences and service learning.

TSET Research Exhibit 6.4   Evaluating the Effectiveness of an Immersion Experience on Cultural Competence

Developing and Measuring Cultural Competence in Nursing Students
Rachelle Parsons, PhD, RN, Associate Professor;
LuAnn Reif, PhD, RN, Associate Professor
College of St. Benedict/St. John's University
St. Joseph, MN

Abstract

The purpose of this study was to determine the impact of immersion experiences on nursing student's transcultural competence. Fourteen baccalaureate nursing students who were participating in a study abroad experience completed the Transcultural Self-Efficacy Tool (TSET) online 1 week before and immediately following their immersion experiences. Nursing students not participating in a study abroad experience (n = 25) acted as a control group and completed the instrument at the same times. Findings from the study indicate students who participated in an immersion experience had significantly higher posttest transcultural self-efficacy scores (p < .001); and when compared with the control group the immersion students had significantly higher posttest scores (p < .001). Data collected from seven student journals revealed four themes, insight into the culture, insight into the migrant journey, how will I explain this experience, and rollercoaster of emotions. Recommendations for faculty include encouraging student participation in immersion experiences to enhance transcultural competence.

Purpose: To determine the impact of immersion experiences on nursing student's transcultural competence.

Research Questions

1. Nursing students who participate in a May term cultural immersion experience will have increased transcultural self-efficacy scores
2. Nursing students who participate in a May term cultural immersion experience will have higher change scores when compared with those who do not participate in this experience
3. What is the relationship of number of cultures interacted with and number of cultural classes taken to pretest and posttest subscales scores

Study Design: Quasi-experimental nonequivalent control group, cross-sectional

Sample:
   Size: 39 junior nursing students: 14 students were in the intervention (immersion group) and 25 were in the control group (those who did not participate in an immersion)
   Type of learner: BSN students
   Demographics: Caucasian n = 39, female n = 33, participated in an immersion experience n = 15. Age data were not collected; all students were traditional nursing students between the ages of 20 and 21.

TSET Data Collection
    Pretest: Data were collected online prior to the May term immersion experience
    Posttest: Data were collected online immediately following the immersion experience

Educational interventions/teaching–learning strategies: The 14 students participating in an immersion completed a one credit cultural selective class to prepare for the immersion experience. These students then either spent 2 weeks in El Paso, Texas/Juarez, Mexico, or 2 and $^1/_2$ weeks in South Africa. Both groups of students experienced the culture by living in the communities and providing health care to the population. The control group did not participate in either the classroom preparation or the immersion experience.

TSET Reliability (Crohnbach's alpha)
    Total TSET: 0.994
    Cognitive Subscale: 0.982
    Practical Subscale: 0.989
    Affective Subscale: 0.990

Data Analysis
Results Question 1: Transcultural self-efficacy (TSE) scores increased significantly from pretest to posttest for nursing students who completed a May term cultural immersion experience.

TSE scores (n = 14)

Subscale	Mean	Standard Deviation	t-test	Significance
Cognitive				
Pretest	169.5	34.9	5.48	P < 0.001
Posttest	206.4	31.0		
Practical				
Pretest	196.0	36.0	4.38	P < 0.001
Posttest	230.5	37.3		
Affective				
Pretest	257.7	21.2	2.50	P < 0.027
Posttest	271.4	25.3		

Results Question 2: Nursing students who participated in a May term cultural immersion experience had significantly greater positive change scores on each subscale when compared with those students not participating in a May term experience.

	Control (n = 25)	Treatment (n = 14)		
Subscale	Mean	Standard Deviation	t-test	Significance
Cognitive				
Control	0.96	34.15	−3.44	p < 0.001
Treatment	36.86	35.18		
Practical				
Control	6.44	29.71	−2.84	P < 0.007
Treatment	34.50	29.46		
Affective				
Control	0.84	17.31	−2.09	P < 0.044
Treatment	13.71	20.52		

Change Scores

Results Question 3:

- Total number of cultures the students reported interacting with was not correlated with pretest TSE scores on the Cognitive or Practical Subscale, but was correlated with the Affective Subscale ($r = 0.40$, $p = 0.011$). (The more cultures a student reported working with the greater their pretest confidence in their cultural values, beliefs, and attitudes.)
- Total number of cultures the students reported interacting with was not correlated with posttest TSE scores on the Cognitive Subscale, but was correlated with the Practical Subscale ($r = 0.33$, $p = 0.042$) and Affective Subscale ($r = 0.45$, $p = 0.004$). (The more cultures a student reported working with the greater their post test confidence in their ability to interview clients of different cultural backgrounds and in their cultural values, beliefs, and attitudes.)
- There is no correlation between the number of cultural classes a student completes and TSET pretest or posttest scores.

Qualitative data analysis of journals completed by 7 of the students revealed 4 themes:

- Insight into the culture
- Insight into the migrant journey
- How will I explain this to someone else
- Rollercoaster of emotions

Curricular Implications

1. Change the method of offering cultural education classes to include immersion experiences for all students.
2. Continue collecting data using TSET.

Dissemination of Results:

Parsons, R. & Reif, L. (2008, September). *Developing nursing student cultural care knowledge through an immersion experience.* 34th Annual Conference of the Transcultural Nursing Society, Minneapolis, Minnesota.

Parsons, R. & Reif, L. (2008, October). *Developing and Measuring Cultural Competence in Nursing Students.* Symposium conducted at Creating Jazz; Transforming Exchanges in Education & Practice 35th National Conference on Professional Nursing Education and Development, Kansas City, Missouri.

TSET Research Exhibit 6.5   Evaluating the Effectiveness of a Community Health Course and Service-Learning on Students' Transcultural Self-Efficacy

Assessment of Transcultural Self-Efficacy of Senior Level Nursing Students Enrolled in a Baccalaureate Nursing Program
Roxanne Amerson, PhD, RN, BC, CTN-A
Clemson University
Clemson, SC

Abstract

Service-learning introduces students to clients of different cultural backgrounds, facilitates the awareness of issues these clients face related to culture and health care, and provides opportunities to teach culturally appropriate care. The Transcultural Self-Efficacy Tool (TSET) was used to evaluate self-perceived cultural competence in a convenience sample of 60 baccalaureate nursing students enrolled in a community health nursing course following the completion of service-learning projects with local and international communities. Pre- and post-surveys were analyzed based on total scores and subscale (cognitive, practical, and affective) scores. Paired-samples t tests demonstrated a significant increase between the mean of pre-test and post-test total scores. In addition, paired-samples t tests demonstrated a significant increase in each subscale. A one-way MANOVA was calculated examining the effect of clinical section on each subscale pre- and post-score. A significant effect was found for the cognitive scores, although no significant effect was found with practical, affective scores, or total scores.

Research Report

Purpose: To evaluate self-perceived cultural competence in a convenience sample of 60 baccalaureate nursing students enrolled in a community health nursing course following the completion of service-learning projects with local and international communities.

Research Question: What is the effect of a community health nursing course with a service-learning component on senior student' perceived confidence for performing general transcultural nursing skills among diverse populations?

Study Design: Pretest and Posttest design

Sample:
  Size: 60 nursing students
  Type of learner: BSN students enrolled in a community health nursing course
  Demographics: The demographics profile consisted of 56 females, 4 males; 62% = 21 yrs age; 32% = 22 yrs; 6% > 23 yrs; 92% White; 5% African American; 2% Asian; 1% Other

TSET Data Collection
  Pretest: Data were collected at the beginning of the semester on first day of class
  Posttest: Data were collected at the end of the semester following completion of service-learning projects with local and international communities.

Educational interventions/teaching–learning strategies: The study involved a community health nursing course with a service-learning component (local and international communities). Each clinical section worked with a selected subpopulation to conduct a community assessment including windshield surveys, statistical data, and interviews with community leaders. Based on the findings from the assessment, a health education need was identified. Students worked with community leaders to provide health education programs based on the unique needs of the target population. The students worked with local communities over a 7-week period, while the international clinical section worked a very intensive 1 week in remote villages of Guatemala.

Six clinical sections completed service-learning projects with local communities. One additional clinical section completed an international service-learning project. All students enrolled in the course were required to meet the same service-learning objectives, although the specific health education program varied based on the community's need.

Clinical Group A conducted a community assessment in a local, urban area at the request of a community taskforce to address the health needs of a predominantly African American neighborhood. Students interviewed community leaders and attended the monthly taskforce meeting to meet with participants. Articles from nursing literature related to health and diet practices of African Americans were required reading. Statistical data were obtained related to the community to include population trends, education levels, socioeconomic status, religious influences, occupation rates, birth and death rates, morbidity and mortality rates, infectious diseases, health agencies, governmental influences, and recreational facilities. Based on the information gained from statistical data and community informants, a health fair was planned and implemented at a local school for a Saturday morning. The health fair provided screenings for glucose, height/weight and body mass index, and blood pressure. In addition, health education tips to control blood pressure and heart disease along with nutrition information were made available. Students from the university's nutritional science and public health departments assisted with door prizes and preparing healthy food choices. The health fair was perceived as a success by community leaders, although the number of participants was relatively low. The community leaders requested that nursing students repeat the health fair next year.

Clinical Group B participated in a short-term medical mission trip to Guatemala. Students conducted similar community assessments using statistical data available via the internet and library resources. Key informant interviews were conducted with members of previous medical missions. The cost of phone calls was prohibitive for interviews with community leaders in Guatemala. The availability of technology remains very limited and sometimes non-existent in remote regions of Guatemala, so interviews via the Internet were not feasible as well. Students were required to read several articles from nursing and medical literature that explored current health problems in Guatemala. Based on the information obtained, students prepared educational materials to focus on basic hygiene, handwashing, food and water safety, and dental care.

Students collected toothbrushes, soap, and other hygiene products to be distributed during the trip. As part of the preparation for the trip, students participated in introductory sessions of medical Spanish. All of the students had previous experience with high school or college level Spanish. No student was considered fluent in Spanish. The trip took place over the spring break vacation and consisted of a total of 8 days. Three days were spent in travel via airline and personal vehicles. Four days were spent conducting medical clinics in remote regions, many of which were only accessible by 4-wheel drive. Once in-country, students conducted cultural assessments and interviews with community leaders to learn their perceptions of current health problems within their villages. Each clinical day involved setting up a make-shift clinic, providing triage, administering de-worming medications and vitamins, preparing prescriptions in pharmacy, assisting physicians with procedures, making house calls to people unable to walk to the clinic site, and teaching basic hygiene and dental care. Each clinic day began at 6:00 AM and came to a close at approximately 10:00 PM. An additional day was spent sight-seeing in Antigua. The sight-seeing opportunities included visiting local cathedrals; shopping in a local, native market; touring historical sites; and dinner in a former convent, which has been converted to a restaurant and hotel.

TSET Reliability (Crohnbach's alpha)
  Total TSET:
    Pretest = 0.974
    Posttest = 0.986

Data Analysis
Results: Transcultural self-efficacy (TSE) SEST scores changed significantly from pretest (beginning of course) to posttest (end of course) for nursing students.

TSE SEST scores (n = 60)

Subscale	Mean	Standard Deviation	t-test	Significance
Total TSET score				
Pretest	606.68	76.44	−9.995	$p < 0.001$
Posttest	719.20	65.44		
Cognitive				
Pretest	6.60	1.29	−10.96	$p < 0.001$
Posttest	8.43	0.96		
Practical				
Pretest	6.70	1.28	−8.03	$p < 0.001$
Posttest	8.34	1.08		
Affective				
Pretest	8.46	0.95	−5.40	$p < 0.001$
Posttest	9.16	0.65		

Multivariate analysis was used to evaluate the effect of clinical section on pre- and post-scores. A one-way MANOVA was calculated examining the effect of clinical section on each subscale pre- and post-score. A significant effect was found for the cognitive scores (Lambda(12104) = 0.661, p = 0.032), although the follow-up ANOVAs for pre- and post-cognitive score demonstrated no significant effect ($F(6,53) = 1.787$, p > 0.05). No significant effects were found for practical, affective, or total scores.

Curricular Implications

1. Continue with service-learning components within the senior level community health course.
2. Continue collecting data using TSET
3. Replicate study while adding a qualitative component to evaluate outcomes that may not be evident through quantitative methods

Dissemination of Results:

The Impact of Service-Learning on Cultural Competence, *Nursing Education Perspectives* (2010, Jan/Feb).

Teaching Culturally Competent Care through Service-Learning Projects—Paper Presentation Education Summit 2007, Sponsored by National League of Nursing, Phoenix, AZ, September 28, 2007.

Incorporating an International Perspective of Community Health Nursing into a Baccalaureate Nursing Program—Oral Presentation, 39th Biennial Convention, Sponsored by Sigma Theta Tau International, Baltimore, MD, November 4, 2007.

Promoting Cultural Competence in Nursing Students through International Service-Learning—Oral Presentation—Best Practice, ACC-IAC Conference, Sponsored by NC State University, Raleigh, NC, February 2, 2008.

The Impact of Service-Learning on Cultural Competence—Oral presentation, SouthEastern Association of Education Studies, Sponsored by The Graduate School of USC and The College of Education at USC, Columbia, SC, February 23, 2008.

Written Assignments

Written assignments may be differentiated between low-stakes and high-stakes assignments. Each type has a potentially valuable role in cultural competence development, if used effectively. Low-stakes writing minimizes the pressure of "grading" associated with high-stakes writing (Elbow, 1997) and optimizes affective learning outcomes. Unfortunately, because low-stakes writing assignments have the potential to be unvalued or undervalued by both students and faculty, low-stakes writing assignments are often underutilized. Affective learning is an important component in cultural competence development; therefore, the design of carefully planned low-stakes writing assignments targeting cultural issues should be an integral component in various dimensions of the course (clinical, classroom, NSL, and immersion components). Known teaching–learning strategies that strongly enhance affective learning must be incorporated within written assignments. Reflection is one strategy that enhances affective learning (Schön, 1987). Engaging the student via in-class or out-of-class written assignments can easily include an individual reflective component. For example, students can be asked to write a "low-stakes" written reflection about:

- In-class group discussion about culturally competent ethical decision making for the assigned case study
- Feelings experienced after viewing a film on racism
- Changes in views on transcultural nursing since the beginning of the semester
- Feelings experienced before, during, and after interviewing a culturally different person about their cultural values, beliefs, and practices.
- Changes in perceived confidence for providing culturally congruent care for culturally different patients
- New feelings of appreciation for cultural diversity within the nursing profession
- Most valuable learning from the process of completing a review of literature paper on a specific cultural group
- Feelings experienced after reading a journal article on health disparities and health care disparities among diverse populations

The benefits of transferring reflective thoughts into written format have the potential to further develop students' affective learning. The exercise of writing encourages students to reflect, organize, and synthesize thoughts before writing, thus assisting students in gaining new insights and self-discovery. Students can reread and then reflect upon written ideas, thus leading to higher levels of thoughtful synthesized inquiry, reflection, insight, and learning. The nurse educator who skillfully reviews written low-stakes writing assignments has the unique benefit of gaining insight into another dimension of students' thought process, learning, beliefs, values, strengths, weaknesses, and confidence. Nurse educators' positive written feedback and nonthreatening written questions serve to further guide or mentor students' affective learning and cultural competence development. For example, mentored clinical journals have been identified to enhance the process of reflection and critical thinking (Bilinski, 2002; Kessler & Lund, 2004; Lasater & Nielsen, 2009); such an approach can be adapted to focus students on culture-specific care and issues. Preparing a series of questions and objectives for written journal reflections can assist students in their self-discovery experienced during an immersion experience (Gomez & White, 2002; St. Clair & McKenry, 1999).

High-stakes written assignments or papers have the potential to achieve positive learning outcomes if strategically linked with other course components. Unfortunately, many students (and some educators) view written papers, such as term papers, as a final end product. The real value of a written assignment is the process of completing the assignment rather than the mere product (paper). Such a philosophy corresponds with the Writing-to-Learn strategy in which various in-class and out-of-class writing activities aim to further develop thinking and learning (Luthy et al., 2009; Schmidt, 2004a, 2004b). For example, written "term" papers that can be and are completed in 1–2 days rather than over an extended period do not achieve desirable outcomes. Exhaustion, dislike, and short-term memory predominate, hindering the long-term goal of building a repertoire of skills, values, and knowledge needed for developing cultural competence and confidence.

If a written assignment is to have any real effect on the ongoing development of cultural competence, then the emphasis of the assignment should be on the process of completing the assignment. Elements that favor the achievement of long-term learning outcomes include:

- Stagger over a period of time with periodic in-class discussion over the process of the paper
- Link with other course components and course topics
- Demonstrate evidence of long-term benefits to students' future professional role
- Distribute a written guide to the "process" of completing the assignment
- Collect drafts or portions of the paper throughout the semester and provide constructive feedback
- Integrate several different learning activities
- Include a reflective component that targets affective learning
- Define evaluative criteria with appropriately weighted grading distribution components
- Publicize easily accessible resources for completing the assignment

Within the context of papers aimed at cultural issues and developing cultural competence, long-term effects plus the potential for expanding knowledge, skills, and values through synthesis is desirable. This involves commitment, time, and coordinated planning among faculty in an effort to link various approaches. One example, an innovative philosophy for creative learning activities called *"Cultural Discovery,"* included a written paper assignment in conjunction with several other components (see Chapter 7). Background reading assignments, classroom activity components (lecture and discussion), clinical post-conference discussions, a collaborative library introductory program, a videotape program, an interview of a culturally different elderly person, a cultural assessment, Leininger's Acculturation Health Care Assessment Enabler for Cultural Patterns in Traditional and Nontraditional Lifeways (Leininger, 1991c), a literature review, and a reflection were used. *Cultural Discovery* assisted first semester associate degree students to systematically conduct a basic cultural assessment, identify similarities and differences among individuals within cultural groups, distinguish between varying dimensions of acculturation, discover the importance of culturally congruent nursing care, and recognize cultural competence development as an ongoing process (Jeffreys & O'Donnell, 1997). The "process" of the written assignment was multidimensional with various learner-centered activities connecting clinical and classroom topics and incorporating cognitive, psychomotor/practical (communication), and affective skills. The "product" of the written assignment (paper) provided concrete evidence of the connection between the components.

Weekly written care plans that incorporate cultural assessment data into the plan of care is another strategy to develop cultural competence. A written weekly journal and then a summary journal entry focusing on cultural issues and culturally congruent care can provide a measure of the type of cognitive, practical, and affective learning within the context of cultural competence development. Written reports following observational experiences in various settings with clients of different ethnic, racial, cultural, and socioeconomic groups is another approach. Every written assignment has the potential to have a cultural component integrated substantially within it. One important question is, Does it? A second question is, How is the cultural component piece perceived by students? Inclusion of a reflective component, an anonymous survey with open-ended questions and/or a comment section, and/or focus groups will provide nurse educators with valuable information about student perceptions and learning that can guide strategy modifications.

Because adult learners are most motivated to engage in activities that they perceive are most relevant, it is important to truly capture the students' interest in the written paper. For example, many students enrolled in a master's program with an adult health clinical nurse specialist focus do not enter the master's program with the primary goal of developing cultural competency. Typically, clinical nurse specialist (CNS) students are interested in developing clinical competencies in a clinical specialty and obtaining certification in a clinical specialty; therefore, nurse educators are challenged to invigorate zeal and instill interest among these adult learners. The same phenomena would apply to DNP students who typically enter a DNP program. A foundational required course in transcultural nursing offers the best approach, because students will similarly be introduced to the knowledge, skills, and values for developing cultural competence (Jeffreys, 2002; Leininger, 1995b). To capture student's interest and to develop cultural competencies at the CNS level, students enrolled in a required transcultural core course in the CNS curriculum were asked to write two papers that would help develop the selected area of the adult health clinical nurse specialist role (Jeffreys, 2002). The following strategies assisted students with the process of writing and with conducting a review of literature on cultural and clinical topics:

- The "Guide to Writing" handbook included strategies for selecting topics, narrowing topics, writing an introduction, method of literature search, synthesizing ideas, and so forth.
- Course Web page contained bibliography and links to relevant cultural and clinical resources
- Weekly (brief) end-of-class group discussion concerning process of assignment and ongoing reflection
- Individual or small group meetings with instructor as needed
- Submission of designated paper components over the semester
- Incorporation of instructor comments into revision

Sharing information during the process of writing assisted students with developing knowledge, skills, and values necessary for culturally competent advanced practice nursing, writing, and research. During the graduate seminars, students discussed the "lived experience" about the process involved with the paper. Peers as role models presented both the achievements and struggles; vicarious learning and role modeling can effectively increase self-efficacy, motivation, learning, and persistence (Bandura, 1986). For hybrid courses or totally online courses, students can discuss their lived experience about the process and offer suggestions via course discussion board or chat rooms. Another valuable teaching–learning strategy for writing development includes structured peer review. Assigning and rotating students weekly or biweekly to critique a peer's written work provides feedback to the student author while also assisting the critiquing student with writing skills and exposure to other students' cultural paper topics. Disseminating information to others after "product" or paper is completed helps synthesize information and broadens the learning beyond one's own research and paper to gain insight into other perspectives, recognizing similarities and differences within and between cultural groups. Dissemination may be done via newsletter, journal, Web site, video, oral presentation, poster presentation, and/or PowerPoint presentation.

Presentations

The presentations discussed in this chapter include oral, poster, and PowerPoint presentation. Individually or in combination with each other, these types of presentation have great power in disseminating information, views, skills, feelings, attitudes, and resources about cultural competence that can positively influence cultural competence and confidence. Nurse educators need to be astute in guiding students so that stereotypes and misperceptions are not perpetuated intentionally or inadvertently. For example, if an undergraduate "introduction to research" small group class assignment includes reading a research article, preparing a poster, and presenting orally to the class, students should be reminded to mention study limitations, especially sampling and generalizability. Although the main focus of the research class is understanding the steps of the research process, critically appraising research for utilization in clinical practice, and identifying areas for further research, nurse educators have many creative opportunities for introducing cultural issues related to research. One approach may be that several presentations include any one or more of the combinations below:

- Different methodology with the same cultural group
- The same methodology with different cultural groups
- The same research topic with different cultural groups
- The same methodology with the same cultural group but different socioeconomic status, gender, age, or level of acculturation
- Different conceptual frameworks and the same cultural group
- The same conceptual framework and different cultural groups

Allocating brief question/answer and comment session after each presentation permits students to clarify information and feelings, as well as to discover similarities and differences within and between groups. A summary dialogue and discussion can further compare and contrast information about cultures.

To enhance cultural learning while also promoting positive feelings about the overall "presentation" experience, several additional strategies may be employed. The sharing of cultural foods, beverages, and music of presented cultural groups promotes sensory stimulation and learning through sight, taste, touch, smell, and sound. Compilation of presenters' abstracts into a professional looking "Book of Abstracts" organized alphabetically by cultural group, topic, or presenter provides a mechanism for ongoing networks, shared information, long-term learning, and validation. Opportunities for students to display posters or present information at a nursing student club meeting, professional meeting, recruitment event, local ethnic nursing meeting, Transcultural Nursing Society local chapter meeting, or Sigma Theta Tau chapter meeting is beneficial for the audience as well as for the presenters. Professional events that encourage students' active participation offer students validation for their achievements so far in their professional development and their educational process. Validation is important and helps increase self-efficacy. Validation is especially important for nontraditional students (older, commuter, and/or minority) and has been positively linked with persistence behaviors (Rendon, 1994; Rendon, Jalomo, & Nora, 2000). Students who are recognized and thanked by members of the professional community for their presentation as well as their time receive positive feedback for their professional nursing actions to enhance cultural competence development in self and in others.

Examinations

Unfortunately, many students associate the importance of learning and information based on what will be on an upcoming examination. Multiple-choice test questions, short answer examination questions, and/or essay questions concerning culturally congruent care have the potential to further demonstrate the importance of cultural competence and to provide valuable feedback about learning (and teaching). A quantitative award (test item points or test grade) that directly impacts upon the course grade validates cultural competence as significant enough to award a quantitative measure that will affect the immediate course grade and progression in the nursing curriculum. In contrast, testing in which cultural diversity and cultural competence is invisible may inadvertently reinforce students' misperception that cultural competence is nonessential, cosmetic, optional, irrelevant, or a time waster. Furthermore, absence of testing results in the lack of empirical data necessary to identify learner strengths and weaknesses, guide teaching–learning interventions, and direct course and curricular revision.

Views on testing, type of testing, and comfort and familiarity with different test formats and procedures varies among culturally diverse and academically diverse students. Assessing students' familiarity with test formats, concerns, anxiety, confidence, strengths, weaknesses, and past test experiences is a necessary first step when designing culturally congruent test items and examinations. A general overview of learner characteristics within the student cohort group provides valuable information (Exhibit 6.2 and Table 1.2). Although the topic of testing is quite complicated, several key considerations will be mentioned in this chapter. First, students with primary and/or secondary education in foreign countries may be unfamiliar with multiple-choice questions, especially those that require decision making and critical thinking. Some foreign-educated individuals are more familiar with essay questions or questions requiring rote memorization. Second, students educated within at-risk school districts within the United States are at risk for poor test-taking skills and low confidence for taking examinations. Third, older students or students with substantial gaps in their educational experience may benefit from "refresher" techniques for taking tests. Fourth, multiple-choice examinations may require a different approach to thinking and communicating than typically used within the students' cultural group. Fifth, computerized examinations require familiarity and comfort with computers as well as adapting test-taking strategies preventing the return to previous questions and changing answers. Finally, examinations should be free of overt and covert cultural biases. For example, among traditional Native American students, Crow (1993) recommends incorporating both individual and family into the keyed multiple-choice response rather than demanding that a choice be made between family and individual.

It is challenging to create examinations that are fair, valid, and culturally congruent with respect to cultural knowledge, skills, and values tested as well as to the culturally diverse learner. Offering test preparation workshops periodically throughout the semester and incorporating learner characteristics and ongoing assessments into the workshops can make a positive difference by enhancing learning, test success, and confidence. Recognizing that students' responses to types of instructor feedback may vary based on CVB, nurse educators are challenged to develop culturally congruent approaches for advice, feedback, helpfulness, and recognition.

Workshops can identify additional strengths, weaknesses, and gaps, thereby providing valuable information to guide subsequent workshops and teaching strategies within the present student cohort and future student groups. As part of the formative evaluation, administration of a workshop evaluation survey after each workshop will provide feedback concerning students' perceptions. A summative evaluation may include administration of a survey to evaluate students' perceptions about test preparation workshops and test-taking skills at the end of the semester, year, and/or program.

Supplementary Resources

Within the academic setting, supplementary resources have the potential to support or restrict cultural competence development. Examples of supplementary resources include the library, enrichment programs (EPs), nursing student resource center (NSRC), nursing student club (NSC), bulletin boards, local Sigma Theta Tau International (STTI) Honor Society in Nursing Chapter, local chapters of specialty and ethnic nursing organizations, and invited guest speakers. Resources that embrace cultural diversity by being culturally friendly and inclusive of culturally diverse and academically diverse nursing students create caring environments that foster student feelings of social integration, satisfaction, and cultural congruence with the nursing profession and educational institution. For example, the aforementioned supplementary resources outwardly display a celebration of diversity if respective brochures, posters, mentors, employees, workshops, invited guest speakers, events, meetings, and student participants appropriately represent a variety of cultural groups.

Appraising existing supplementary resources beyond their superficial appearance may uncover untapped areas necessitating further action, expansion, inclusiveness, and innovation. Similarly, discovery that supplementary resources do not exist suggests the need for immediate action and innovation. Several ideas follow:

- Develop collaborative partnerships with librarians
- Obtain new library resources for cultural competence development
- Foster cross-cultural student interaction via EP study groups led by peer mentor-tutors
- Revise NSRC brochures to feature students of different age, gender, and cultural groups
- Advertise upcoming cultural events, holidays, and workshops on bulletin boards
- Host an international food festival organized by the NSC
- Cosponsor a cultural workshop with STTI chapter and involve students as volunteers
- Sponsor student(s) for participation in cultural nursing conference
- Establish networks with local ethnic nursing organizations

- Form a local chapter of the transcultural nursing society
- Raffle a student membership in the Transcultural Nursing Society and local chapter
- Invite guest speakers from different cultural backgrounds to speak about cultural topics

Nurse educators are challenged to expand the web of student inclusion beyond the traditionally required educational curriculum and setting through professional events and memberships. The web of inclusion refers to an interwoven professional network that embraces culturally diverse students and strives to promote professional integration and cultural competence development through participation in professional events and memberships (Jeffreys, 2004). Participation in professional events and memberships is viewed as an essential activity for professional growth and career mobility by providing unique opportunities for professional socialization, networking, skill enhancement, knowledge expansion, and professional attitude development (Betts & Cherry, 2002; Bosher & Pharris, 2009; Joel & Kelly, 2002). Strategies that enhance student opportunities to actively use supplementary resources and participate in cultural competence development outside of nursing courses will ultimately benefit students and the nursing profession.

KEY POINT SUMMARY

- The academic setting has the potential to make enormous strides in cultural competence development, especially through entry-level education.
- Cultural competence development can only occur with well-qualified, committed nursing faculty and through the use of culturally congruent teaching–learning strategies that address students' diverse cultural values and beliefs.
- Each individual faculty member is empowered to make a positive difference; however, the greatest impact will be achieved through a coordinated, holistic group effort that thoughtfully weaves together nursing course components, nursing curriculum, and supplementary resources.
- Promoting optimal cultural competence in academia requires considerable, sincere effort that begins with faculty self-assessment.
- Resilient TSE (confidence) is the integral component necessary in the process of cultural competence development (of self and in others).

- Resilient TSE perceptions embrace lifelong learning in the quest to become "more" culturally competent and in the quest to assist others (learners) to become more culturally competent.
- At the undergraduate and graduate setting, it becomes increasingly urgent to closely examine how visible (or invisible) cultural competence development is actively present.
- Examination at the curricular, program, school, and course level requires courage, commitment, time, energy, and a systematic plan.
- Inquiry, action, and innovation at the curriculum level involve the philosophy, conceptual framework, program objectives, program outcomes, courses, course components, horizontal threads, and vertical threads.
- Inquiry, action, and innovation at the course level involve the course outline, instructional media, learning activities, course components, and clinical settings.
- Inquiry, action, and innovation at the supplementary resource level involve the library, enrichment programs, nursing student club, nursing student resource center, bulletin boards, honor society chapter, local organizations, and guest speakers.
- Cultural competence development must be introduced early, integrated purposely, and intricately woven within the academic setting to create a durable fabric that provides long-lasting learning and desirable educational, professional, and patient outcomes.

CHAPTER 7

Case Exemplar: Linking Strategies—Spotlight on the *Cultural Discovery* Integrated Approach

Marianne R. Jeffreys, EdD, RN

Mary O'Donnell, PhD, RN

Judy Xiao, MA, MS

This chapter describes an innovative philosophical approach and learning activities for integrating general transcultural nursing concepts and skills within a first semester introductory nursing course. The approach and activity design will assist novice nursing students to achieve the following objectives: (a) systematically conduct a basic general cultural assessment; (b) identify some similarities and differences among individuals within cultural groups; (c) distinguish between varying dimensions of acculturation (nontraditional and traditional values, beliefs, and practices); and (d) discover the importance of culture in nursing care.

This chapter was excerpted and adapted from Jeffreys, M.R. & O'Donnell, M. (1997). Cultural Discovery: An innovative philosophy for creative learning activities. *Journal of Transcultural Nursing, 8* (2), 17–22. By permission, Sage.

"Cultural competence in nursing education is receiving renewed emphasis. Cultural competence is linked increasingly to reducing health care disparities among racial, ethnic, uninsured, and underserved U.S. populations" (Lipson & DeSantis, 2007, p. 10S). This activity design was developed to assist the beginning student on the journey toward cultural competence. (Figure 7.1).

The nurse educators also wanted to enhance a course that would provide meaningful experiences and stimulate critical thinking among nontraditional, culturally diverse students who need to care for many clients of culturally diverse backgrounds. Gilchrist & Rector (2007) recognize "the great need for a culturally representative workforce as our population continues to become diverse. In order to serve our diverse population, our RN's should mirror that diverse U.S. population" of (p. 277). The philosophy and activity designed in this course are imperative steps in helping the nontraditional student to develop those skills necessary to effectively take place in this workplace. The need to create a learner-centered philosophy and activities to develop critical thinking skills has long been supported in the literature (Alien, 1990; Bevis & Murray, 1990; Beyer, 1987; Brookfield, 1987; Chinn, 1990; deTornyay, 1990; Diekelmann, 1990; Leininger, 1995b; Moccia, 1989; Tanner, 1990; Waters, 1990).

In their effort to complement course topics, the nurse educators developed an approach called *Cultural Discovery,* which focuses on the concepts of culture, aging, and health. These learner-centered activities emphasized learning outcomes in both the cognitive, affective, and experiential (practical or psychomotor) domains. The cognitive domain focuses on knowledge outcomes, intellectual abilities, and skills (Bloom, 1956) while the affective domain involves attitudes, interests, appreciation, and modes of adjustment (Krathwohl, 1964). Of these, the affective domain needs the most attention because affective outcomes include students' professional values, motives, and attitudes (King, 1993; Waltz, 1988). The experiential approach of learning directly about cultures was also important here. Without challenges such as encountering people with different worldviews and social norms, "Lindgren notes . . . students often see culture as something out there, irrelevant, and not affecting their practice. They tend to judge their client's belief and practices from their own perception of reality" (Lipson & DeSantis, 2007, p. 19S).

The learning activities included several components in conjunction with the Leininger Acculturation Health Care Assessment Enabler[1] for Cultural Patterns in Traditional and Nontraditional Lifeways (Leininger, 1991a). The activities were: (a) background reading assignments; (b) classroom activity component; (c) collaborative library introductory program; (d) videotape program; (e) interview; (f) literature review;

CULTURAL DISCOVERY:
An Innovative Approach for Creative Learning Activities

Marianne R. Jeffreys, EdD RN & Mary O'Donnell, PhD, RN
The City University of New York College of Staten Island

PURPOSE

To describe an innovative philosophical approach and learning activities for integrating general transcultural nursing concepts and skills within a first semester associate degree nursing course.

OBJECTIVES

To assist students to:

1) systematically conduct a basic cultural assessment
2) identify similarities and differences among individuals within cultural groups
3) distinguish between varying dimensions of acculturation
4) discover the importance of culture in nursing care

STRATEGY COMPONENTS

1) **Background Reading Assignment**
   Biological changes of aging
   Basic human needs (Maslow)
   Universal human experience
   Culture & spirituality
2) **Classroom Activity Component**
   Transcultural nursing
   Discussion
   Reflective shared experience
3) **Librarian Collaboration Program**
   Hands-on experience
   Cultural literature search

4) **Videotape Program**
   Leininger interview of the American-Polish client
5) **Interview** culturally different elder
   Leininger acculturation health care assessment enabler for cultural patterns in traditional and nontraditional lifeways
6) **Literature Review**
7) **Reflection**
8) **Written Paper Assignment**

LEARNING OUTCOMES

Cognitive

Knowledge, Intellectual Abilities, & Skills

Communication Process
Culture
Aging
Health
Aims of Nursing
Holistic Care

Experiential (Psychomotor)

Cultural Assessment Interview
Literature Search

Affective

Awareness
Self-awareness
Awareness of others
Acceptance
Point of view from a person of a different culture
What is important to others
Appreciation
Culturally diverse beliefs, values, and practices
Recognition
Similarities & differences within & between cultures
Ethnocentric tendencies
Cultural imposition

IMPLICATIONS FOR PRACTICE, EDUCATION, AND RESEARCH

1. Expand the use of Leininger theory and enabler as an organizing framework
2. Increase opportunities to learn about other cultures and own culture
3. Support ongoing advocacy for cultural congruent care
4. Explore the significance of guided "cultural discovery" experiences in cultural competency development
5. Integrate cultural care competencies within all aspects of the nursing profession
6. Promote higher levels of cultural competency development
7. Develop a seminar series on cultural competence that builds on previous learning
8. Foster opportunities for interaction between culturally diverse groups
9. Create active learning strategies that target cognitive and affective outcomes
10. Encourage networking and mentoring experiences between transcultural nursing experts, nursing students, and other nurses

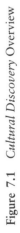

Figure 7.1 *Cultural Discovery Overview*

(g) reflection; and (h) written paper assignment. Basic principles of transcultural nursing (Leininger, 1995) and andrology (Knowles, 1984) were integrated throughout the students' learning. Several goals were sought and carried through the course. They incorporated the relevancy of cultural assessment to immediate career goals, discovery, immediate feedback by interaction with a culturally different client, and collaborative relationships between nursing student and client and nursing student and instructor as well as ongoing collaboration with the librarian.

The *Cultural Discovery* learning activities have been implemented over an 8-week period with associate degree nursing students enrolled in the first nursing course at a large, northeastern urban public college. Typically, 140–200 first semester students are enrolled annually yielding diverse demographic profiles such as: 68% women; 32% men; mean age 32; 61% white; 20% black; 11% Latino; 4% Asian; 4% other; and 12%–30% non-native English speakers. Within each demographic category, numerous cultural groups are represented. *Cultural Discovery* has direct relevance and easy application for entry-level baccalaureate students. Components of *Cultural Discovery* are easily adaptable to other target audiences such as graduate nursing students, students in health science professions, nurses in practice settings, and other health care professionals. The chapter will present background information, learning activity components, and implications for future use in a variety of settings. Two "Application to Health Care Institutions" exhibits will conclude the chapter.

BACKGROUND

Leininger's transcultural care model (2006) offers nurse educators a conceptual framework from which to guide transcultural nursing practice, research, and education. Consideration of student background characteristics is also important (Tuck & Harris, 1988). Background variables describe student characteristics upon entry into college. Such characteristics provide information on the composition of the student group that is integral to determining the special needs of the students and individualizing learning (Hansen, 1988). Background characteristics may include the cultural identity and background of the students as well as their beliefs, values, and practices.

It is well-documented that the applicant pool for nursing is changing with more nontraditional students entering nursing (Leininger, 1995b). Furthermore, nontraditional students are seeking increased, as typical, entry into associate degree nursing programs (Garcia, 1987; Grosset, 1991; Nora, 1987; Quintilian, 1985; Spanard, 1990, Vorhees, 1987; Woloshin,

1981). As associate degree programs prepare the greatest number of nurses for entry into practice, it is imperative to address the needs of this group (Rubini, 1988). Hansen (1988) described the associate degree student population as traditionally older students, men, and minority students. Moccia (1989) defined the nontraditional student population as adults with family responsibilities, of different cultures where English is a second language, having more varied educational preparation, and more likely to attend school part-time. Grosset (1991) identified age as a student characteristic that often distinguished the associate degree student from the baccalaureate student. Today, associate degree programs continue to reflect great diversity in academic preparedness, age, immigration, economic, and cultural diversity with predictions that anticipate similar demographics in the near future.

Clearly, this student composition reflects a change from the traditional nursing student. This is consistent with Montag and Gotkin's expectations that associate degree nursing programs would attract individuals who could not otherwise enter nursing (Montag & Gotkin, 1959). Merrill et al. (2006) noted in their baccalaureate student population that, "Nontraditional students are multitask individuals who are forced to become self-directed learners with limits on time available for course and personal family responsibilities" (p. 109) and so it is with associate degree students. Associate degree nursing programs, therefore, are challenged to accommodate the needs of such a diverse student population (Jeffreys, 2004; Tagliareni, 2008; Waters, 1990). Moreover, the time constraints imposed by the two-year programs inspire the design of innovative philosophical approaches and learning activities that: (a) aim to provide nurses with a beginning foundation of transcultural nursing knowledge, skills, and values; (b) stimulate a desire to pursue advanced learning in transcultural nursing; and (c) motivate learners to actively advocate culture-specific nursing care in practice settings.

To disregard the various cultures and needs of these nontraditional students may result in inadequately preparing nurses to function holistically in a multicultural society. Leininger (1995b) stated that the time has come for the nursing profession to commit to major changes in all aspects of nursing as it shifts from a unicultural to multicultural focus. For nurse educators, the focus must turn to meeting the different needs of diverse student groups and to transform nursing through the preparation of culturally competent nurses. Not only must nurse educators recognize the diversity in students, they must develop interventions targeted at enhancing transcultural nursing skills. Furthermore, accreditation guidelines specifically stipulate the inclusion of educational activities and experiences designed to prepare associate degree nursing students in meeting the needs of culturally diverse patients, families, and communities and in working productively and harmoniously within a multicultural workforce (NLNAC, 2008d). Such stipulations are also evidenced in baccalaureate program guidelines by the AACN and NLN with clear expectations to build upon foundational cultural competence knowledge and skills in nursing graduate education (AACN, 2008, 2009; NLNAC 2008a, 2008b, 2008c; NLN, 2009).

SIGNIFICANCE OF LEININGER'S ACCULTURATION ENABLER

With the use of Leininger's Acculturation Health Care Assessment Enabler[1] for Cultural Patterns in Traditional and Nontraditional Lifeways, (Leininger, 1991a, 2006), nurse educators can stimulate cultural awareness and implementation of a focused and complete cultural assessment technique. The beginning associate degree nursing student is often overwhelmed by performing a cultural assessment on any client, especially with an individual of a different cultural background. Even more difficult may be their addressing multiple aspects of cultural influences. For example, there is the need to distinguish between universal similarities and differences in individuals and cultures as well as the degree to which clients may be quite traditional in some aspects, yet nontraditional in other instances. Beginning students often have difficulty knowing how to effectively approach a culturally different client and conduct a systematic assessment.

Cultural assessment skills, if not introduced in the first nursing course, may limit an effective integration throughout the curriculum and ultimately throughout later nursing practice. Because a strong commitment to transcultural nursing is integral to providing quality health care to culturally diverse individuals and to student learning, the inability to perform a basic cultural assessment may lead to an avoidance of cultural considerations in planning and implementing nursing care. Beginning associate degree nursing students often have great difficulty focusing on all dimensions of the assessment when using Leininger's Sunrise Model (Leininger, 1988) or a broad holistic nursing theory and then sorting through seemingly overwhelming amounts of patient information to identify client needs. Without help at this initial stage, students find it extremely difficult to learn transcultural nursing principles and concepts and the opportunity to provide holistic care for their clients is impeded.

As students enter nursing, their journey of discovery begins. Faculty and professional nursing staff guide the students' experiences through innovative strategies to assist them to reach the threshold of their own personal discoveries. The major aim of the *Cultural Discovery* philo-sophical approach and related learning activities was to facilitate student self-discovery regarding the interplay of culture, aging, and health. To facilitate this discovery, the student's interview and cultural assessment of a healthy, noninstitutionalized elderly person utilizing Leininger's en-abler was used (Leininger, 1991a). Additionally, students were instructed to interview individuals of different cultural backgrounds and identities other than their own.

BEGINNING THE COURSE: READING AND CLASSROOM COMPONENT

Beginning with an introduction to necessary theoretical principles and skills, the first part of the course focused on the cognitive domain through the background reading assignment. The desired cognitive learning out-comes included basic knowledge and skills concerning communication, culture, aging, and health. First, an understanding of the normal bio-logical changes of aging as well as basic human needs as described by Maslow and others contributed other dimensions of learning to this dis-covery experience. According to Andrews (1995), "To achieve an appro-priate balance, nurse educators ought to begin by emphasizing the uni-versal human experience and common needs of all people of the world" (p. 7). Secondly, an understanding of the nursing goals of health promo-tion, maintenance of health, and prevention of illness added impetus and significance to this experience. Thirdly, holistic care is another concept introduced at the beginning of the nursing experience. Inherent in this concept is the deliverance of culturally congruent care. Familiarity with broad transcultural principles, concepts, theories, and research findings for clients of diverse cultures is essential.

Completion of select reading assignments on culture, aging, and health and wellness promotion provided these nontraditional adult learn-ers with common background knowledge. Through lecture and classroom discussion, students were encouraged to explore the interaction of cul-ture, aging, and health and wellness promotion. The faculty facilitated expansion of this knowledge base by further emphasizing the relevance of cultural assessment to the students' career goal of professional nurs-ing. The role of transcultural nursing in meeting the health care needs of culturally diverse client populations was discussed. Dialogue included a sharing of cultural beliefs and traditional health and caring practices that the students and their families practiced. Additionally, students de-scribed some of their experiences with culturally diverse clients in the clinical setting. Because the student group reflected much diversity in cultural background and previous health care experience, much reflection, collaboration, and sharing ensued.

Through this reflective sharing process, students became more aware of their own cultural similarities and differences. Guided by Leininger's Theory of Culture Care Diversity and Universality (Leininger, 1991a), similarities and differences between their own beliefs, values, and practices and that of their family members or members of their own cultural group were also recognized. This awareness and recognition suggested that affective learning outcomes were achieved through the classroom activity component and use of the general theory to examine cultural differences and similarities (Leininger, 1991a). Once affect was aroused, students were eager to learn how to accurately assess cultural beliefs, values, practices, and needs of clients.

Next, Leininger's enabler,[1] the Culture Care Theory, and the Sunrise Model were used to assess health care influencers in such categories as worldview, language, cultural values, kinship, religion, politics, technology, education, and environmental context (Leininger, 1991a). A description of each category, followed by sample questions, provided the framework for beginning discovery. The importance of asking questions using culturally acceptable verbal and nonverbal communication skills was emphasized in discussion sessions. Students participated by sharing their own similarities and differences in acceptable communication behavior.

USE OF VIDEOTAPE, LIBRARY, AND COLLABORATION TO INCREASE UNDERSTANDING

Next, students were encouraged to view the videotape Transcultural Nursing: Cultural Care Assessment of an American Polish Client (Leininger, 1991c). The film provides a guide to cultural assessment and serves to illustrate the use of Leininger's enabler while also providing a succinct yet comprehensive overview of the underlying theoretical principles that guide its practical application. Student feedback concerning the film was positive, suggesting that this instructional medium constituted a transitional bridge between theory and practical application. Initially, the film was shown at set times in the Nursing Skills Laboratory outside of class time; however, in recent years, advanced technology provided an innovative solution to accommodate students' multiple role responsibilities outside class time. Collaboration with media specialists in the library yielded a well-received solution. After receiving permission from the film's copyright holder, the media specialists digitalized the video onto a DVD format, created a password protected link via the course's Web page (Blackboard) so that students could access the video via the Internet within a specified 4-week period. Written reflective statements from students following the pilot of this new initiative indicated that overall students were pleased with the flexibility of viewing times and option to individually pause the film, take notes, and/or review essential points again.

In order to further prepare the student for this discovery experience, collaboration of faculty is necessary. As Leininger (1995b) recommends, students and faculty should be co-participants in the learning and teaching process. All nursing faculty involved should be conversant with Leininger's enabler that provides a basis for student discovery of a culture other than their own. Prior to meeting, all course instructors reviewed Leininger's Culture Care Theory (Leininger, 1988, 1991c; Reynolds & Leininger, 1993), Leininger's Acculturation Health Care Assessment Enabler for Cultural Patterns in Traditional and Nontraditional Life-ways (Leininger, 1991a), course objectives, and student prerequisite assignments. During the meeting, the role of the faculty in facilitating the *Cultural Discovery* was discussed and agreed upon. Full-time classroom faculty and adjunct clinical faculty work together and with the students. Together, faculty guide students in learning the knowledge, skills, and values necessary for the discoveries that lead to culturally sensitive care.

An added dimension to this collaborative approach involved support and assistance from the librarian. Students attended a library orientation program designed by nursing faculty and the librarian. The program has two major components: (a) one-hour library instruction to help students gain knowledge and skills necessary for cultural and transcultural nursing research; and (b) the use of Blackboard to extend library instruction in support of *Cultural Discovery* (Exhibit 7.1). Several library instruction sessions were available to allow for small group work and hands-on experience with the computer and database search. The small class size of 20 students enabled the librarian to answer students' questions and respond to those who needed extra help. The use of the Blackboard Learning System helped support students' cultural discovery beyond the limited one-hour library instruction. Web pages containing course-related resources, including transcultural nursing resources, tutorial for searching Cumulative Index to Nursing and Allied Health Literature (CINAHL), and writing resources were developed and integrated into the Nursing Blackboard course Web site. These resources, accessible anytime, helped reinforce what was taught in the library instruction session, and allowed students, especially those who needed extra help, to learn at their own pace. Library instruction continued with students posting their research questions on the discussion board, and seeking help for information sources for specific cultures. The online discussion forum became a learning community where the students, professors, and the librarian came together to help each other, and to share their experiences in *Cultural Discovery*.

Exhibit 7.1   Components of the Library Orientation Program

(a) One-hour library instruction to help students gain knowledge and skills necessary for cultural and transcultural nursing research. Topics and activities include:
- Introduction of cultural and transcultural nursing resources posted on the Nursing Blackboard course Web site.
- Library databases available to search for cultural and transcultural nursing information, with major emphasis on CINAHL.
- Demo by the librarian of how to search CINAHL on a select cultural topic, and methods of obtaining articles selected from CINAHL search.
- Hands-on practice by students in conducting a CINAHL search on the culture and health of an ethnic group of his or her choice.
- Methods of locating books related to culture and transcultural nursing: library catalogs, books on reserve, and interlibrary loan.
- Use of reliable Web sites for cultural and transcultural nursing research.
- How to access library's electronic resources off-campus.

(b) Use of Blackboard to extend library instruction in support of *Cultural Discovery*
- Develop course-related library resources and integrate them into the Nursing Blackboard course Web site. These include library databases related to nursing, tutorials, bibliography of books and articles on specific cultures, Web sites of interest in transcultural nursing, APA style guides, and plagiarism prevention resources.
- Create discussion forums to provide opportunities for students to discuss their work, and ask questions related to library research and finding resources for their cultural discovery research paper.
- Provide research assistance to students at their point of need via discussion board, email, phone, and in-person consultation.

Several institutional review board (IRB) approved research studies evaluating the program's effectiveness indicated that the library orientation program was helpful, and that students became more skilled in utilizing the resources of the library for cultural research, and in writing a literature-supported research paper. Faculty–librarian collaboration helped create positive and effective learning experiences for students. The "field trip" students took to the library not only helped improve their skills for transcultural nursing research, but also gave them the opportunity to interact with librarians and the library environment so that they were comfortable coming to the library or seeking librarians' help online and in person (Xiao, 2005). The first library orientation program survey drew 80 respondents (a 92% response rate), with three closed-ended questions, and two open-ended questions with room for qualitative comments. Responses to the library program were largely positive, and majority of the respondents agreed that the library program made them more aware of the resources available for nursing, especially transcultural nursing research (Xiao, 2005, pp. 61–62). Evaluation of the program's effectiveness continued using a variety of methods, including library instruction pretest and posttest survey at the end of the library instruction session, and survey at the end of students' 8-week cultural discovery. Survey questions were distributed in print format, but also made available online and via the Nursing 110 Blackboard course Web site. Nursing faculty encouraged their students to participate, and helped with the in-classroom data collection, which greatly improved student response rates. Data continue to provide empirical support for ongoing and revised strategies and to guide curricular and library program development.

Merrill et al. (2006) state that "the use of technology in nursing education in the 21st century is a permanent change that will continue to impact learning outcomes of the non-traditional students as well as the traditional student" (p. 109). The use of the technology in this activity is an important aspect of this activity and introduces the student to valuable resources for the course.

INTERVIEW AND LITERATURE REVIEW

Kurz (1993) notes that experiential approaches have an important role in changing attitudes and increasing sensitivity to problems stemming from cross-cultural misunderstanding. During the interview, culture care, values, expressions, patterns, and health beliefs become apparent to the student. Students were instructed to write a paper based on two main components. These components were: (a) an interview with a healthy, noninstitutionalized elderly person of a different cultural background and identity than their own; and (b) a review of current nursing (including transcultural nursing) and allied health literature related to the culture of the person being interviewed. Typically, students have interviewed neighbors, senior citizen club members, friends, relatives, and elderly college students. Because the interview often took place in the client's home where symbols of the culture might be evident, this added yet another dimension of discovery to the experience. Use of Leininger's enabler assisted the student to assess all dimensions of culture systematically. To address the issue of aging, students examined the individual's perceptions, feelings, and attitudes of aging as well as noting any physical signs of aging. Recognizing that the primary aims of nursing include the promotion of health, prevention of disease, maintenance of health and consolation of the dying—students explored the elder person's experience with health. Waters (2007) states that "using community and culturally based strategies that fit into the context of peoples' everyday lives may increase the quality and duration of a healthy life and eliminate health disparities . . . it gives voice to the people" (pp. 66, 67S). Cognitive, affective, and practical (psychomotor) learning outcomes were achieved through the interview experience (see Figure 7.1).

Following each interview, the student reviewed the literature concerning the cultural heritage of each person. For persons of multiple cultures, students were referred to resources concerning multicultural individuals. Due to the limited available information concerning multicultural individuals, students also had the option of researching one of the interviewee's cultural groups. Students were encouraged to review resources from nursing and other disciplines. Collaboration between faculty, students, and librarian often occurred during the literature search and review, because many students were inexperienced in writing a literature-supported paper. Ongoing communication occurred in person, telephone, e-mail, and/or discussion board. Student peer mentor-tutors were also available to assist students individually and/or in small group sessions in the Nursing Student Resource Center (NSRC) and the Nursing Student Test Prep Center (NSTPC) (Jeffreys, 2004). Additionally, an online tutorial, specifically designed by the librarian, helped students not only find relevant literature for their research, but also integrate these sources effectively and ethically into their paper (Exhibit 7.2).

Exhibit 7.2 *Cultural Discovery* Research Paper Tutorial

Follow this tutorial to find professional literature for your research paper, cite your sources in APA style, and avoid plagiarism.

1. **Start by reading an essay on the specific culture group you want to research**
   Gale Encyclopedia of Multicultural America, part of the Gale Virtual Reference Library database is a good place to start your research. This three-volume online encyclopedia contains 8,000 to 12,000 word

essays on specific culture groups in the United States, emphasizing religions, customs, and languages in addition to providing information on historical background and settlement patterns. Search the database by culture group, such as Norwegian Americans, Jamaican Americans, Jewish Americans, or Italian Americans.

2. Search library databases for articles on the health beliefs, values, and practices predominant for this ethnic group. Related databases include:

   a) *CINAHL PLUS with Full Text*
   b) *Health Source: Nursing/Academic Edition*
   c) *SAGE Health Sciences Collection:*
   d) *Health & Wellness Resource Center:*
   e) *MEDLINE*
   f) *Academic Search Premier*
   g) *ScienceDirect*

   Search Strategy: Keyword searching is possible; however, searching by subject terms will make your searching more precise, and enable you to retrieve more relevant articles. Try Arabs and culture, blacks and transcultural nursing, Hispanics and culture values, Chinese and transcultural care. More subject terms are provided below.

Ethnic Groups	Subject Terms
Amish	Transcultural Nursing
Arabs	Transcultural Care
Asians	Culture
Cambodians	Cultural Diversity
Chinese	Cultural Sensitivity
Filipinos	Cultural Values
Japanese	Ethnic Groups
Koreans	Ethnology
Laotians	Medicine, Arabic
Vietnamese	Medicine, Herbal
Blacks	Medicine, Traditional
Gypsies	Faith Healing
Hispanics	Complementary Therapies
Jews	Medicine, Chinese Traditional
Whites	Drugs, Chinese Herbal
American Indians	Medicine, Native American

3. Search the library catalog for books related to transcultural nursing and ethnic groups.

   The books listed below contain information about specific culture and ethnic groups.

   Andrews, M.M., & Boyle, J.S. (2008). *Transcultural Concepts in Nursing Care.* Philadelphia: Wolters Kluwer Health/Lippincott Williams & Wilkins.

Crouch, N. (2004). *Mexicans & Americans: Cracking the Cultural Code.* London: Nicholas Brealey Pub.

D'Avanzo, C.E. (2008). *Pocket Guide to Cultural Health Assessment* (4th ed.). St. Louis: Mosby.

Galanti, G. (2004). *Caring for Patients from Different Cultures* (3rd ed.). Philadelphia: University of Pennsylvania Press.

Ghosh, P. (2005). *Transcultural Geriatrics: Caring for the Elderly of Indo-Asian Origin.* Oxford: Radcliffe.

Giger, J.N., & Davidhizar, R.E. (2008). *Transcultural Nursing: Assessment and Intervention* (5th edition). St. Louis: Mosby.

Hill, P.S., Lipson, J.G., & Meleis, A.I. (2003). *Caring for Women Cross-Culturally* (3rd ed.). Philadelphia, PA: Davis.

LaGumina, S.J. (Ed.). (2000). *The Italian American Experience: An Encyclopedia.* New York: Garland Publications.

Leininger, M., & McFarland, M. (2002). *Transcultural Nursing: Concepts, Theories, Research, & Practice.* New York: McGraw-Hill.

Purnell, L.D., & Paulanka, B.J. (2008). *Transcultural Health Care: A Culturally Competent Approach.* Philadelphia: Davis.

Satcher, D. (2006). *Multicultural Medicine and Health Disparities.* New York: McGraw-Hill.

Schaefer, R.T. (2006). *Racial and Ethnic Groups.* New Jersey: Pearson Prentice Hall.

Spector, R. (2004). *Cultural Diversity in Health & Illness* (6th ed.). Norwalk, CT: Appleton & Lange.

Srivastava, R. (2007). *The Healthcare Professional's Guide to Clinical Cultural Competence.* Toronto: Mosby Elsevier.

4. **Web sites that provide useful and reliable information on different cultures**
   - *Background Notes (http://www.state.gov/r/pa/ei/bgn/)*
     Contain information on all the countries of the world with which the United States has relations.
   - *CIA World Factbook (https://www.cia.gov/library/publications/the-world-factbook/countrylisting.html)*
     The U.S. government's complete geographical handbook for all nations.
   - *Center for Disease Control and Prevention (http://www.cdc.gov)*
     Provides extensive statistical information on health problems affecting minority groups in the United States. *Fastats A to Z* is a government database on Asian and Pacific Islander, Hispanic, Black, and American Indian health.
   - *EthnoMed (http://www.ethnomed.org)*
     Provides information on cultural beliefs, and medical issues of recent immigrants.
   - *MEDLINEplus Health Information (http://www.nlm.nih.gov/medlineplus/populationgroups.html)*

Includes links to Web sites dealing with health issues for various ethnic groups and special populations including Hispanic Americans, Asian Americans, African Americans, Native Americans, and seniors.

- *Office of Alternative Medicine (http://altmed.od.nih.gov)*
  This federal office focuses on complementary and alternative medicine, which covers a broad range of healing philosophies, approaches, and therapies.
- *Office of Minority Health and Health Disparities (http://www.cdc. gov/omhd/Populations/populations.htm)*
  The racial and ethnic populations section of the Web site provides information for many ethnic groups regarding demographics, health statistics, leading causes of death, and high prevalence health issues.
- *Office of Minority Health (http://www.omhrc.gov)*
  Provides data/statistics for ethnic groups, including African American profile, Asian American profile, Hispanic/Latino profile, Native Hawaiian/other Pacific Islander profile.

5. **Cite your sources and avoid plagiarism**
   - Research and Documentation Online: *http://www.dianahacker. com/resdoc/*
     Diana Hacker, author of *A Pocket Style Manual*, provides guidelines for documenting print and online sources, as well as sample student papers using APA style.
   - Consult style guides such as the *Publication Manual of the American Psychological Association*, and *A Pocket Style Manual* by Diana Hacker. They are available in the library.
   - Read College Policy on Academic Integrity *(http://www1.cuny. edu/portal_ur/content/2004/policies/policies.html)*.
     Provides definitions and examples of academic dishonesty, including plagiarism and internet plagiarism.
   - Plagiarism Prevention and Citation Resources from Plagiarism.org *(http://www.plagiarism.org)*
     Defines plagiarism in easy-to-understand terms, offers tips on how to avoid both internet-based and conventional plagiarism, and provides guidelines for proper citation.

As the student analyzed and integrated the research and experience, discovery of how an individual's culture influences health care beliefs, needs, and practices emerged. Students were encouraged to draw upon their theoretical knowledge concerning the cultural group to further enhance their ability to examine similarities and differences. In this way, awareness and sensitivity to individuals from a particular cultural group can be enhanced.

REFLECTION AND WRITTEN PAPER

Reflection has been cited as an essential component to critical thinking (Beyer, 1987; Schön, 1987). For the final segment of the paper "Culture, Aging and Health," students were asked to reflect upon the experience. In order to evaluate learning outcomes, the creators of the *Cultural Discovery* learning activities reviewed student papers. Students consistently wrote that they developed a satisfying relationship with the elder of a different culture, and were frequently privy to cultural practices not "... casually shared with strangers" (Bartz, Bowles, & Underwood, 1993). Many students described their experience as helping them develop an open mind toward the beliefs and practices of others. The theme of an open mind was frequently referred to in the reflection part of the paper and illustrated the affective learning outcomes resulting from the overall *Cultural Discovery* teaching approach. These affective learning outcomes were categorized by the *Cultural Discovery* creators as awareness, acceptance, appreciation, and recognition (Figure 7.1).

Themes of awareness could be further subdivided between self-awareness and the awareness of others. Self-awareness referred to the student becoming more aware of one's own cultural beliefs, values, and practices and the impact these had within the student's own life. Several students reported that although they might not think of or speak of preconceptions about other cultural groups and/or the elderly population, their mind was actually filled with underlying assumptions. In this way, students discovered that they possessed personal biases that would have prevented open-mindedness and severely limited holistic nursing care.

Awareness of others was broadly reflected by one student who commented, "I learned that not everyone is like me." Students noted that they learned that they could not determine what a person was like by looking at them or just reading about his/her culture in a book. Use of Leininger's enabler assisted in the discovery that one needed to effectively communicate with an individual to learn just what cultural beliefs, practices, and values a person possessed. Comments indicated that students discovered the varying degrees of nontraditional and traditional cultural practices, beliefs, and values possible within one individual. One student described this blend and acculturation as giving richness to both cultures.

Further reflection on the learning accrued by completing Leininger's enabler revealed that students not only began to discover cultural patterns but became enthusiastic about the meaning of such patterns. Students tended to examine their own cultural beliefs, noting similarities and differences. After these experiences, students believed that they would be less inclined to impose their own beliefs upon the client. A deeper appreciation for culturally diverse beliefs, values, and practices was reported.

The acceptance of the point of view from a person of a different culture was further demonstrated by statements that indicated that students had developed respect for what is important to others.

IMPLICATIONS

The literature reveals an alarming gap in conceptually and empirically supported teaching strategies, especially those targeting cultural competence development in diverse nursing students who must care for many different groups of culturally diverse patients. Time constraints of two-year nursing programs, student diversity in academic preparedness, cultural background, experiential background, and age have contributed to the challenge of teaching transcultural nursing to associate degree students. Time constraints, prioritization of content, and lack of nurse educators prepared in transcultural nursing also pose challenges in baccalaureate programs, graduate programs, and health care institutions.

This chapter described a philosophical approach for integrating general transcultural nursing concepts and skills within a first semester associate degree nursing course. With a focus on culture, aging, and health, the *Cultural Discovery* approach assisted beginning nursing students to systematically conduct a basic cultural assessment, identify similarities and differences among individuals within cultural groups, distinguish between varying levels of acculturation, and discover the importance of culturally congruent nursing care. Initially, curiosity concerning other cultures was experienced by students. Following the *Cultural Discovery* learning activities, this curiosity often evolved to advocacy for culturally congruent care. Notably, students were stimulated to critically identify ways that their client's cultural health care practices, values, and beliefs could be preserved, accommodated, or restructured for optimal health results. For example, students identified potential health problems that could arise from their client's reluctant use of the professional health care system and prescribed treatment regimens and then suggested nursing strategies for providing culturally congruent care.

Leininger's theory and the acculturation enabler not only provide a framework that is readily usable but also provides a framework for collaboration between peers and instructors. The framework also enhances understanding of the student's beliefs and practices, and many verbalized that they recognize they must understand and value their own cultural beliefs and practices as well as their client's in order to carry out effective nursing care. The opportunity to learn about cultures, approach people from cultures other than their own, and analyze the experiences provided learning in the cognitive as well as the affective domain. This guided experience of *Cultural Discovery* provided a basis for further cultural assessment and enhanced holistic care.

Seminars in which learning outcomes, cultural discoveries, insights, and worldviews can be additionally shared and explored will further expand the ways in which *Cultural Discovery* and its various components can be adapted and applied. Future research recommendations include a qualitative study investigating the phenomenon of *Cultural Discovery* with a variety of learners in various settings. Other recommended implications for practice, education, and research are:

1. Expand the use of Leininger's theory and enabler as an organizing framework
2. Increase opportunities to learn about other cultures and own culture
3. Support ongoing advocacy for cultural congruent care
4. Explore the significance of guided *Cultural Discovery* in cultural competence development
5. Integrate culture care competencies within all aspects of the nursing profession
6. Promote higher levels of cultural competency development beyond the introductory level
7. Develop a seminar series on cultural competence that builds on previous learning
8. Foster opportunities for interaction between culturally diverse groups
9. Create active learning strategies that target cognitive and affective outcomes
10. Encourage networking and mentoring experiences between transcultural nursing experts, nursing students, other nurses, and other health professionals

APPLICATION TO HEALTH CARE INSTITUTIONS

Cultural Discovery is easily adaptable to health care institutions (HCI). Using the COMPETENCE acronym and framework described in Chapter 2, a multidimensional integrated 15-step approach is illustrated in Exhibit 7.3 and Exhibit 7.4. Time constraints of working nurses amidst different shifts coupled with varying levels of motivation challenge HCIs to use multiple, flexible, yet interactive and scaffolded teaching–learning strategies. Because continuing education units may be required for salary increases, RN license renewal, continued employment, and/or promotion, the awarding of continuing education units serves as a powerful incentive. Other key features include direct relevance to unit-based patient care, guided cultural assessment, independent study and flexible time via the online learning environment, and opportunities to develop networking communities. One important network for nurses is establishing collaborative relationships with librarians (Billings & Kowalski, 2009). An underlying assumption of the adapted *Cultural Discovery* approach is that it is adapted, implemented, and evaluated by a qualified nurse educator/researcher. The nurse educator serves as a facilitator and guide throughout the various steps, offering ongoing feedback throughout the ongoing online discussion board. Additionally, proper workshop planning and implementation is essential for optimizing desired outcomes (Horsfall & Cleary, 2008). (See Chapters 10, 11, and 12 for more information on cultural competence education in the HCI.)

Exhibit 7.3   *Cultural Discovery* for Health Care Institutions: A COMPETENCE approach

	Learning Strategy Description	Step	Min.
Caring	Background reading assignment: Leininger's theory & model "Caring and culture care is the essence of nursing"—Leininger Discussion board	4	60
Ongoing	Bimonthly paper and online newsletter: Cultural competence: Meeting the needs of (insert name of cultural group) patients Discussion board, CE quiz	10–14	60 × 4
Multidimensional	Background reading assignment: Use of Leininger's acculturation enabler Videotape program via closed hospital web site: Leininger interview of the American-Polish client	5 6	60 60
Proactive	Cultural assessment incorporated within admission assessment— interview patients Discussion board	8	60

	Learning Strategy Description	Step	Min.
Ethics	Background reading	2	30
	Patient Bill of Rights		
	ANA Code of Ethics		
	Transcultural care principles, human rights, ethics (Leininger, 1991b)		
Trust	Developing trust among multicultural staff and patients: Diversity awareness (Jeffreys, 2008a & 2006a article or Jeffreys 2010, chapter 2)	2	30
	Staff meeting or workshop discussion – sharing cultural values and beliefs	3	30
	Developing trust with culturally diverse patients (workshop 1 & 2)		
Education	Introductory workshop 1: Cultural Competence theory & action	7	90
	Discussion board over 1 week following each strategy		
	Unit-based workshop 2: Meeting the needs of culturally diverse patients on the (insert name) unit (Also videotaped and posted on Blackboard)	9	60
Networks	Language interpreter services	7	60
	Transcultural nursing society: List of experts and scholars		
	Local professional and community resources		
	Librarian		
	Guest presenter(s)		
Confidence	Staff meeting to discuss *Cultural Discovery*	1	10
	TSET pretest, demographic questionnaire	1	20
	TSET post-test, reflection	15	30
*Evaluation**	Data Collection		
	Formative: Learning Strategy Evaluation	2–14	
	Tool	1, 15	
	Summative: TSET pretest and post-test and		
	demographics, reflection	16–20	
	Data analysis and research results report*		

*Data analysis and research results report conducted by health care institution's evaluation team

Exhibit 7.4   *Cultural Discovery* for Health Care Institutions: A 15-Step Plan

	Content Description	Strategy	Min*
1	Staff meeting to discuss *Cultural Discovery*	Lecture	10
	TSET pretest, demographic questionnaire	Discussion	20
		Group	
		Questionnaires	
2	Background reading	Reading	60
	Patient Bill of Rights	Online	
	ANA Code of Ethics	Discussion	
	Transcultural care principles, human rights, ethics (Leininger, 1991a)		
	Developing trust among multicultural staff and patients: Diversity awareness (Jeffreys, 2008a & 2006a article or Jeffreys 2010, chapter 2)		
3	Sharing cultural values and beliefs: Enhancing Diversity Awareness (Staff meeting or workshop discussion)	Lecture	30
		Discussion	
		Group	
4	Leininger's theory & model	Reading	60
		Online	
		Discussion	
		Video	
		PowerPoint	
5	Use of Leininger's acculturation enabler	Reading	60
		Online	
		Discussion	
6	Application of theory, model, and assessment enabler: Videotape program via closed hospital web site (Leininger interview of the American-Polish client)	Videotape	
		Online	
		Discussion	
7	Introductory workshop 1: Cultural Competence theory & action	Lecture	150
	Language interpreter services	Discussion	
	Transcultural nursing society: List of experts and scholars	PowerPoint	
	Local professional and community resources	Group	
	Librarian	Gaming	
	Guest presenter(s)	Reflection	

	Content Description	Strategy	Min*
8	Cultural assessment incorporated within admission assessment—interview patients Discussion board	Online Discussion	60
9	Unit-based workshop 2: Meeting the needs of culturally diverse patients on the (insert name) unit (Also videotaped and posted on Blackboard)	Lecture Discussion PowerPoint Group Gaming Reflection	60
10 to 14	Bi monthly paper and online newsletter: Cultural competence: Meeting the needs of (insert name of cultural group) patients Discussion board, CE quiz	Reading Online Discussion CE quiz Reflection	300
15	TSET post-test Reflection	Questionnaire Reflection	20 10

Total CE Time = 14 hours

KEY POINT SUMMARY

- *Cultural Discovery* is an innovative philosophical approach and learning activities for integrating general transcultural nursing concepts and skills within a first semester nursing course.
- *Cultural Discovery* includes several components in conjunction with the Leininger Acculturation Health Care Assessment Enabler for Cultural patterns in Traditional and Nontraditional Lifeways, specifically: background reading assignments, classroom activity component, collaborative library introductory program, video-tape program, interview, literature review, reflection, and written paper assignment.
- Implemented over an 8-week period, *Cultural Discovery* assisted beginning nursing students to systematically conduct a basic general cultural assessment, identify some similarities and differences among individuals within cultural groups, distinguish between varying dimensions of acculturation, and discover the importance of culturally congruent nursing care.

- Using the COMPETENCE acronym and framework, a multidimensional integrated 15-step approach for use in health care institutions includes: background reading assignments, workshop and unit-based activity components, collaborative networking, videotape program, interview, reflection, online interactive learning, and continuing education (CE) quizzes.

ENDNOTE

1. The authors would like to note that in recent publications Leininger uses the term "enabler" rather than the concept of "tool". Tool is considered too impersonal and mechanistic while enabler more readily fits ethnonursing research philosophy.

CHAPTER 8

Case Exemplar: Linking Strategies—Spotlight on the Innovative Field Trip Experience

Marianne R. Jeffreys, EdD, RN

Lenore Bertone, MS, RN

Jo-Ann Douglas, MS, RN

Vivien Li, BS, RN

Sara Newman, MS, RN

This chapter describes a multidimensional strategy for teaching and learning cultural competence in graduate nursing education with a specific focus on the innovative field trip experience (IFTE). First, a brief overview of the literature in nursing and higher education provides the essential background information underlying strategy development, implementation, and evaluation, including a discussion of how the Cultural Competence

This chapter was excerpted and adapted from Jeffreys, M. R.; Bertone, L.; Douglas, J-A.; Li, V.; and Newman, S. (2007). A multidimensional strategy for teaching cultural competence: Spotlight on an innovative field trip experience. (In: Oermann, M. & Heinrich, K. ed). *Annual Review of Nursing Education, Volume V*, New York: Springer, 101–134. By permission, Springer.

and Confidence (CCC) model guided development. Next, an overview of the transcultural nursing core course within the Clinical Nurse Specialist (CNS) curriculum is highlighted. Four case exemplars, supplemented by detailed tables and figures, demonstrate easy application. A discussion of cognitive, practical, and affective learning outcomes and implications for nurse educators conclude the chapter.

BACKGROUND

Transcultural nursing is "a formal area of humanistic and scientific knowledge and practices focused on holistic culture care (caring) phenomena and competence to assist individuals or groups to maintain or regain their health (or well-being) and to deal with disabilities, dying, or other human conditions in culturally congruent and beneficial ways" (Leininger, 2002d, p. 84). Leininger's theory of culture care diversity and universality and her illustrative sunrise model (Leininger, 1991a, 1994a, 2002a) provides a valuable resource and guide for preparing advanced practice nurses to care for culturally diverse populations. The desired outcome of the model is care customized to fit with the patient's cultural values, beliefs, and practices. Attaining this outcome requires a systematic assessment of the dynamic patterns and cultural dimensions of a particular culture (subculture or society), including religious, kinship (social), political (and legal), economic, educational, technologic, and cultural values, and how these factors may be interrelated and function to influence behavior in various environmental contexts. Culturally congruent care, however, can only occur when culture care values, expressions, or patterns are known and used competently (Leininger, 2002a).

Two other frequently used conceptual frameworks include models by Campinha-Bacote (2003) and Purnell (2008). Campinha-Bacote's "Culturally Competent Model of Care" presents cultural awareness, knowledge, skill, desire, and encounters as necessary components of cultural competence. Cultural desire is the key, pivotal element in the ongoing process of cultural competence development (Campinha-Bacote, 2003). Purnell's model of cultural competence identifies areas of assessment (of clients) that will provide nurses and health care professionals with the information needed to provide culturally specific and congruent care (Purnell, 2003). The model depicts a nonlinear continuum of cultural competency ranging from the categories of unconsciously incompetent, consciously incompetent, consciously competent, and unconsciously competent. Conscious competence occurs when one seeks and obtains general knowledge about another culture, verifies generalizations about the client, and then provides culturally specific care.

These models acknowledge that cultural competency is an ongoing, complex learning process that involves continual skill acquisition and refinement. Although scholars support that all individuals, regardless of cultural background, need formalized preparation in transcultural nursing, this goal is not equally valued by all nurses (Andrews, 1995; Leininger, 1995b; Leininger & McFarland, 2002). Because adult learners are most motivated to engage in activities that they perceive are most relevant, it is important to truly capture students' interest in cultural competence development. For example, students enrolled in an adult health CNS master's program generally do not enter the master's program with the primary goal of developing cultural competency. "The essence of CNS practice is clinical nursing expertise in diagnosing and treatments to prevent, remediate, or alleviate illness and promote health with a defined specialty population. . . " (NACNS, 2005, p. 5). CNS practice aims to achieve quality, cost-effective patient-focused outcomes across three spheres of influence: (a) patient/client, (b) nurses and nursing practice, and (c) organization/system (NACNS, 2005). Typically, CNS students are interested in developing clinical competencies in a clinical specialty and obtaining certification in a clinical specialty; therefore, nurse educators are challenged to invigorate zeal and instill interest among these adult learners.

Proponents of adult learning theory attest to the marked influence of educational enterprises, motivation, and commitment in relation to immediate career goals (Brookfield, 1986; Knowles, 1984). Adult learners will be most motivated and interested in learning if immediate benefits to career goals and daily professional responsibilities are clearly evident and learning goals are realistic (Brookfield, 1986; Knowles, 1984). With increased globalization and the changing demographics and characteristics within and between cultural groups, it is unrealistic to expect that nurses will become specialists in caring for (or working with) all of the many different cultural groups that they may encounter. To become a specialist in one or more select cultural groups requires a series of specialized transcultural courses and concentrated fieldwork at the graduate level (Leininger, 1989; Leininger & McFarland, 2002). It is realistic to expect that all nurses acquire the basic or generalist transcultural nursing skills needed to provide care for culturally diverse and different patients. A transcultural generalist approach emphasizes broad transcultural principles, concepts, theories, and research findings to care for patients of many different cultures (Leininger, 1989). It is also reasonable to expect nurses who have been prepared as generalists demonstrate commitment and participate in ongoing cultural competence education. Especially pertinent are educational programs designed to expand learning with direct application to specific, targeted priority cultural groups dwelling in surrounding communities.

Despite the numerous educational opportunities available, some nurses are more actively engaged in cultural competence development and direct clinical application while others are not. Some nurses are more motivated to pursue cultural competence development and are more committed to the goal of culturally congruent care than others. Therefore, the consideration of factors that may influence motivation, persistence, and commitment is necessary. Confidence (self-efficacy) is one such factor. According to Bandura (1986), the construct of self-efficacy is the individuals' perceived confidence for learning or performing specific tasks or skills necessary to achieve a particular goal. In learning tasks, inefficacious learners are at risk for decreased motivation, lack of commitment, and/or avoidance of tasks. Learners with a resilient (strong) sense of self-efficacy in a specific domain demonstrate high levels of commitment, persistence at skill development, view difficult skills as challenges to be overcome, and expend extra energy to overcome obstacles. In contrast, supremely efficacious (overly confident) learners view tasks as insignificant and/or requiring little preparation, increasing the risk for poor outcomes. In clinical practice, avoidance of culture considerations, lack of adequate preparation, and/or rendering culturally incongruent care jeopardizes patient safety and health.

CONCEPTUAL FRAMEWORK

The Cultural Competence and Confidence (CCC) model (Figure 3.1) aims to interrelate concepts that explain, describe, influence, and/or predict the phenomenon of learning (developing) cultural competence and incorporates the construct of transcultural self-efficacy. Transcultural self-efficacy (TSE) is the perceived confidence for performing or learning general transcultural nursing skills among culturally different patients. Transcultural nursing skills are those skills necessary for assessing, planning, implementing, and evaluating culturally congruent nursing care. The performance of transcultural nursing skill competencies is directly influenced by the adequate learning of such skills and by transcultural self-efficacy perceptions (Jeffreys, 2000, 2006).

Within the CCC model, cultural competence is defined as a multidimensional learning process that integrates transcultural skills in all three dimensions (cognitive, practical, and affective), involves transcultural self-efficacy (confidence) as a major influencing factor, and aims to achieve culturally congruent care. The term "learning process" emphasizes that the cognitive, practical, and affective dimensions of transcultural self-efficacy and transcultural skill development can change over time as a result of formalized education and other learning experiences. Within the context of transcultural learning, cognitive learning skills include knowledge and comprehension about ways in which cultural factors may influence professional nursing care among clients of different cultural backgrounds and throughout various phases of the life cycle. The practical learning dimension is similar to the psychomotor learning domain and focuses on motor skills or practical application of skills. Within the context of transcultural learning, practical learning skills refer to communication skills (verbal and nonverbal) needed to interview clients of different cultural backgrounds about their values and beliefs. The affective learning dimension is a learning dimension concerned with attitudes, values, and beliefs and is considered to be the most important in developing professional values and attitudes. Affective learning includes self-awareness, awareness of cultural gap (differences), acceptance, appreciation, recognition, and advocacy (Jeffreys, 2000, 2006b).

Formalized educational experiences and other learning experiences that: (a) carefully weave cognitive, practical, and affective transcultural nursing skills; (b) encompass assessment, planning, implementation, and evaluation; and (c) integrate self-efficacy appraisals and diagnostic-specific interventions are considered essential in cultural competence education (Jeffreys, 2006b). Because transcultural self-efficacy perceptions influence a learner's actions, performance, and persistence for learning tasks associated with cultural competence development, it is important that educators fully understand the vital role of self-efficacy appraisal. Self-efficacy appraisal is an individualized process influenced by four information sources: actual performances, vicarious experiences (observing role models), forms of persuasion (receiving encouragement and judicious praise), and emotional arousal (physiological indices). Actual performances are the strongest source of efficacy information (Bandura, 1986). Successful performances can raise efficacy while unsuccessful performances lower it. Lowered self-efficacy can be psychologically stressful and dissatisfying to nurses, thereby adversely affecting motivation, persistence, and cultural competency development. Individuals with low self-efficacy initially can feel devastated by failure or poor performance and further lowered self-efficacy can cause avoidance behaviors (Bandura, 1986, 1997). Formalized teaching strategies that provide essential background information and facilitate varied opportunities for self-directed, learner-centered interactive activities and experiential learning will be most beneficial. Combining several strategies to create empowering learning environments will promote a stronger sense of meaningfulness in task accomplishment, resilient confidence, and greater control over choices in the learning process in a truly learning-centered curricula (Candela, Dally, & Benzel-Lindley, 2006; Siu, Laschinger, & Vingilis, 2005).

COURSE OVERVIEW

"Transcultural Concepts and Issues in Health Care," a 3-credit 15-week graduate core course within the adult health CNS curriculum, was taught at a large urban, public college that serves various student and client cultural groups. The course aimed to provide students with a strong foundation in transcultural nursing that permits purposeful integration of transcultural nursing concepts and skills at higher levels of complexity throughout the curriculum and advanced practice role development. (After completion of the CNS, students may choose to pursue the NP option). Based on current recommendations in the literature, the course focuses on the general philosophy, ethics, concepts, skills, theory, research, and practices underlying transcultural care. Current issues in pluralism, diversity, and health care are explored in relationship to culturally competent care of advanced practitioners in multiple health care settings. Leininger's theory of Culture Care (1991a) and other selected theories and research studies are critically appraised for utilization in various practice and management settings. Future directions of transcultural care are discussed with special emphasis on advanced practice roles and how to effectively create the needed transformational changes in health care, education, practice, research, and policy. Course objectives are specifically linked to the course description, course topics, and curriculum objectives, and program outcomes. (See Jeffreys, 2002b, for specific details on transcultural course.)

Following an introduction to Leininger's theory, ethnonursing research methodology, and other conceptual models, students are introduced to various topics concerning health disparities, cultural assessment, ethnicity, race, class, gender, sexual orientation, religion, ethnopharmacology, discrimination and bias, multiple heritage individuals, female circumcision, complementary and alternative medicine, physical assessment, spirituality, and mental health. Students are expected to be active, well-prepared graduate seminar participants who critically discuss assigned chapters, journal articles, class films, lectures, and PowerPoint presentations. Other teaching-learning strategies involve conducting a review of literature (ROL) on a select transcultural topic and a clinical topic (usually chosen to develop the CNS targeted area of specialty); writing a ROL paper, connecting ROL paper to future CNS role, and writing a CNS paper. Students have a choice of several CNS paper options: (a) cultural assessment enabler; (b) sphere of influence, (c) professional development: conference; (d) leadership: letter to the editor or author; or (e) innovative field trip experience. Methods of evaluation comprise seminar participation (30%), ROL paper (40%), and CNS paper (30%). The selection of multidimensional teaching and evaluation strategies is twofold: first, to address varied learning styles among diverse learners, and second, to stimulate learning in the cognitive, psychomotor (practical), and affective domains.

THE INNOVATIVE FIELD TRIP EXPERIENCE

The IFTE is a learner-centered, creative strategy that was implemented during the second half of a required transcultural core course in the CNS/NP curriculum. IFTE included prerequisite components (background reading assignments, classroom seminar and films, literature review, and written paper), general required components (student-initiated field trip selection, purpose and objectives, instructor approval, plan, implementation, and written paper), and information-sharing/dissemination components (storytelling and cultural food buffet). Figure 8.1 presents the IFTE components as formal and informal educational experiences within the context of the CCC model.

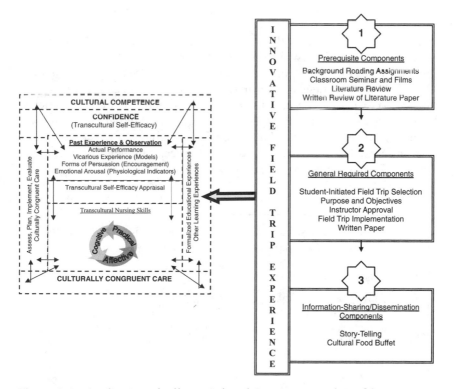

Figure 8.1 Application of Jeffreys' Cultural Competence and Confidence (CCC) model: Innovative Field Trip Experience

The prerequisite components were designed to provide students with beginning foundational knowledge in transcultural nursing and in the expected role competencies of the CNS. The background reading assignments provided a common framework for seminar discussion. Films expanded upon reading and prior learning, presenting students with the opportunity to gain a different perspective into the emic (insider) perspective of different cultural groups. By the third week, students selected their own review of literature topics. The process of searching the literature and available resources on both selected clinical and transcultural topics provided students with some essential "holding" knowledge. Leininger (2002b) described the powerful value of "holding" knowledge prior to interacting with members of a cultural community or engaging in other "immersion" experiences to enhance understanding of the culture.

The student's self-selection of the field trip option, formulation of purpose and objectives, and planning of the intended experience (Exhibit 8.1) is consistent with principles of adult learning theory. This process involves reflection. When used appropriately, reflection is an effective teaching method that enhances nursing practice (Ruth-Sahd, 2003). "When students are challenged to choose topics about which they are passionate and reflect on their application of research-based evidence to clinical practice, their work reflects scholarly effort" (Sevean, Poole, & Shane Strickland, 2005, p. 475). Students must reflect upon their prior learning, present stage as a learner, and future advanced practice role in order to create one's own, individualized, and highly relevant practicum. "A reflective practicum is an experience of high interpersonal intensity. The learning predicament, the students' vulnerability, and the behavioral worlds created by coaches and students critically influence learning outcomes" (Schön, 1987, p. 171).

Exhibit 8.1   Topics, Field Trip Selection, and Purposes/Objectives: Comparison of 4 Case Exemplars

Review of Literature Paper Title

| Promoting Prenatal Care for Asian Indian Women through Culture-Specific Care | Exploring Amish Cultural Beliefs and Immunization Practices | Helping Orthodox Jewish Families Cope with the End-of-Life Process in the Intensive Care Unit | Exploring Complementary and Alternative Medicine (CAM) for the Management of Arthritic Pain in African American (AA) Women. |

Transcultural Topic Focus

Asian Indian American women	Amish culture	Orthodox Jewish community	African American women

Clinical Topic Focus

Prenatal care	Immunization beliefs and practices	End-of-life care decisions	Arthritic pain management

Reason for Interest in Topic

Asian Indian women have a high incidence of low birth weight infants	With some general knowledge of the Amish, was intrigued to learn more	Limited knowledge in caring for the Orthodox Jew during end-of-life	Future CNS role in pain management Limited knowledge about AA culture

Reason for Selecting Field Trip Experience Instead of Other Options

A chance to explore Asian Indian culture	To fully appreciate and explore the world of the Amish in greater detail and obtain firsthand knowledge of the Amish way of life	To obtain firsthand experience and knowledge directly from members of the Orthodox Jewish community	Increase understanding of major historical and political events that shaped African American life and culture

Name of Field Trip Selected

Deepavali festival Asian Indian neighborhood	Amish community in Pennsylvania	Workshop on Bikur Cholim: A Prescription for Life (end-of-life care) held in an Orthodox Jewish high school in New York City	Exhibit on slavery in New York at a large local historical society

How the Field Trip Was Selected

Association of Indians in America Web site	Review of Internet sites	Recommendation of rabbi from the work setting	Internet research

Location of Field Trip

South Street Seaport (NYC) and 2 Asian Indian neighborhoods in Queens, NY	Amish community in Lancaster, PA	New York, NY	New York, NY

Purposes/Objective of Field Trip

1. Gain a personal experience of Asian Indian culture 2. Gain an insider's view into Asian Indian lifestyle 3. Gain knowledge on Asian Indian prenatal practices	1. Gain firsthand knowledge of the Amish culture 2. Explore the Amish culture's health care beliefs 3. Gain an understanding of Amish immunization practices	1. Gain knowledge on end-of-life care of the Orthodox Jew 2. Extrapolate what health care professionals can do individually and at the institutional level to provide culturally sensitive care 3. Tap into community resources	1. Gain a better understanding of AA culture from an emic perspective 2. To corroborate the importance of spirituality and religion on AA life 3. To acquire more background information in order to provide culturally congruent care as a CNS

Although instructor approval suggests a simple dichotomous approach—the proposed field trip and objectives are approved or they are not—it is not really this simple. Within the context of adult learning theory and reflection-in-action, the role of the instructor is to guide (coach) students to further explore, shape, modify, or revise their intended experience, purposes, and/or objectives and seek a deeper level of potential learning. According to Schön (1987), professional education should be focused on enhancing the professional's ability for "reflection-in-action" or the learning by doing and preparing professionals for lifelong learning and problem solving throughout professional practice. Certainly, cultural competence development involves lifelong learning and nurse educators are in a key position to guide students.

Students' implementation of the planned field trip experience permitted further opportunity to shape the experience and engage in ongoing reflect-in-action (Exhibit 8.2). For example, interviews, eating traditional foods, wearing traditional clothing, and other components were not preplanned but added a valuable dimension to the experience and further enhanced cognitive, practical, and affective learning. The process of writing the CNS paper encouraged students to further reflect on and evaluate the experience and explore the connections between the field trip experience, prior learning, future learning, and application to future CNS role (Exhibit 8.3). Preestablished paper grading criteria provided students with a common framework for focus and reflection, such as discussing the most significant field trip experience component to: (a) course topics,

(b) ROL paper, (c) CNS competencies, and (d) future advanced practice nurse role. Additionally, this aimed to validate learning via the field trip experience by demonstrating immediate and future application to the achievement of an important career goal.

Exhibit 8.2   Select Field Trip Components: Comparison of 4 Case Exemplars

Asian Indian Women and Prenatal Care	Amish Culture and Immunization Beliefs and Practices	Orthodox Jewish Community and End-of-Life Care	African-American Women and Arthritic Pain Management Using Complementary and Alternative Medicine (CAM)

Components of Field Trip

Asterisk (*) Placed in Front of Those Components That Were Not Pre-Planned

1. Deepavali festival 2. *Hindu Temples 3. Asian Indian Bridal shops 4. Asian Indian restaurant	1. Mennonite Information Center 2. Amish museum – *dressed in Amish attire 3. Amish farmhouse 4. *Amish cuisine 5. *Amish quilt shops	1. Workshop on "The Role of the Visitor—the How To's" 2. Workshop on "Being Present at Life's End" 3. *Kosher breakfast and lunch 4. *Interviews with project manager and rabbi	1. Historical perspective and exhibits 2. Spirituality, religion, church, and community exhibits 3. *Artifacts and clothing of the era 4. *Short movies and audiotaped documentaries

Interviewed Persons

*An Asian-Indian female physician at the Deepvali festival regarding traditional health practices and implications for health professionals	1. *Woman from Mennonite Information Center 2. *Amish elderly man at the Amish farmhouse	1. *Project manager 2. *Rabbi	N/A

Interaction with Others

*Conversations with bridal shop owners and workers in 2 Indian neighborhoods. *Worshippers in Hindu temple	*Many members of the Amish faith throughout field trip (farmhouse, quilt shops, Mennonite Center, church service)	Workshop participants mainly comprise Orthodox Jewish men and women in the 50–60-year age group. *Workshops were held in semi-circles and small groups to answer discussion questions of experiences with a loved one during the end-of-life and for one member to share with the group.	*It was interesting to observe the different groups from various backgrounds and ages who were visiting the exhibit

*Senses involved in the experience

Dance and music performances, food at the festival. Different smells and taste of spices used in food at the festival and restaurant.	Sounds of church service. Various smells at the Amish farmhouse and restaurant. Taste of different ethnic foods at restaurant. Sight and touch at museum, quilt shops, and tours.	During breakfast and lunch, the atmosphere was social and jovial with many people greeting long-time friends and socializing.	Audiotaped documentaries The artifacts and clothing of the era were a great part of the exhibit. Finally, the cafeteria had good food and refreshments

Methods Used to Record/Remember Experience Details

Pamphlets, camera	Notes, pamphlets, photos	Notes and pamphlets	Notes, pamphlets, and newspapers

---

Exhibit 8.3   Significance of Field Trip Experience: Comparison of 4 Case Exemplars

Asian Indian Women and Prenatal Care	Amish Culture and Immunization Beliefs and Practices	Orthodox Jewish Community and End-of-Life Care	African-American Women and Arthritic Pain Management Using Complementary and Alternative Medicine (CAM)

Most Significant Component of Field Trip to ROL Paper

Role of women in Asian Indian culture	Personal interview with an elderly Amish man who spoke about his culture's health care beliefs and immunization practices	Recurrent themes throughout the workshop of the importance of family and community being present during end-of-life. As stated in the *Book of Genesis*, Judaism centers on the family as a unit.	Spirituality and religion are major components of African American (AA) life, profoundly influencing health care practices and beliefs

Most Significant Component of Field Trip to Course Topics

Visiting Deepavali festival and exploring the Asian Indian culture	The opportunity to explore the Amish way of life experientially and speak to members of the Amish faith.	One-on-one communication with the Orthodox Jewish community as well as authorities on the culture	To gain a sense of the hardships African Americans encountered during slavery time and how this affects the present day

Most Significant Component of Field Trip to Future CNS Role

To understand the lifestyle and practices of a different culture in order to provide culturally appropriate care	Formulate a teaching plan to facilitate preventative healthcare using a culturally congruent approach	Formulate teaching plan to facilitate change at the institutional level	To provide culturally congruent care for African-Americans in general as well as specialized focus on AA women with arthritic pain

Desired Future CNS Role

Critical care/ Educator	Educator	Educator in cardiac care/ critical care	Pain management

Three Most Relevant CNS Competencies Further Developed Through Field Trip

Leadership Collaboration Clinical expertise in the specialty	Research Leadership Collaboration	Research Leadership Collaboration	Educator Researcher Partnership with faith-based centers

The final component of the IFTE (information-sharing/dissemination through storytelling and cultural food buffet) aimed to further develop several CNS competencies: collaboration, leadership, and education, specifically within the "nurses and nursing practice" sphere of influence. Reflective storytelling is a valuable strategy that facilitates reflective analysis, enhances self-esteem, and enriches cultural sensitivity and understanding (Davidhizar & Lonzer, 2003; Spence, 2005). The cultural food buffet setting provided a relaxed, informal atmosphere to share stories about the ROL topic and IFTE. After reviewing Leininger's chapter concerning the cultural meaning of food (Leininger, 2002c), students took great pride in sharing traditional cultural foods (from either their own culture or researched culture) and in sharing the cultural meanings and significance of the foods. The different tastes, smells, feels, sounds, and looks of the ethnic food evoked sensory stimulation and cultural learning while also promoting positive feelings about the overall "informal presentation" experience. The brief question and answer session encouraged participation and dialogue between students and thereby enhanced opportunities for clarification, collaboration, education, and critical thinking. Distribution of presenters' abstracts with name and contact information provided a mechanism for ongoing networks, shared information, long-term learning, and validation.

CASE EXEMPLARS: IFTE STRATEGY IN ACTION

The following actual case exemplars demonstrate application of the IFTE and present select highlights of the learning experience from the student perspective. In addition, Exhibits 8.1–8.3 enhance the text by providing easy comparison between the four case exemplars.

Asian Indian Women and Prenatal Care

Concern over the prevalence of low birth weight infants and the low rate of early prenatal care among Asian Indian women in the United States sparked interest in further understanding the traditional cultural values, beliefs, and health care practices. Initially, the field trip plan included participant observation at a Deepavali festival. The Deepavali festival is a festival of lights that fights off the darkness in human lives; it signifies both the beginning of the Asian Indian New Year and the victory of good over evil. The celebration is spread over one month. Music and dancing in traditional clothing in bright colors such as red and gold are essential in celebrations and spiritual devotions for special occasions, because its purpose is to bring in peace and prosperity, and to keep evil and disease away. At the festival, I (V. L.) had the opportunity to talk to a physician regarding the health practices of Asian Indians. During this informal interview and discussion, we spoke about health promotion and women's roles. In an Asian Indian family, men are the decision makers of the family and usually make decisions for their wives. Language barrier, access to health care, and other health practices may hinder their access to early prenatal care.

Next, the field trip expanded to include an exploration of an Asian Indian neighborhood in New York City. The neighborhood contained many bridal shops, because weddings are big occasions in the Asian Indian community. As I was visiting the various bridal shops, I thought of the idea that prenatal teaching should be made available here; it is most logical as it is the place where future brides would be sure to visit. Because the majority of Asian Indians are Hindu, I also visited two Hindu temples. I learned that before entering the temples, I needed to remove my shoes and placed them on the shoe racks located outside. Because Hindu temples are places of worship, shoe racks are placed outside for worshippers to take off their shoes before entering. Shoes are viewed as unclean and cleanliness must be preserved within the temple. The field trip enabled me to gain a personal experience of Asian Indian culture, gain an insider's view into Asian Indian lifestyle, and gain knowledge about Asian Indian prenatal practices. Through the various components of the field trip experience, I further developed competencies in collaboration, leadership, and clinical expertise. By further understanding the lifestyle and practices of a different culture, I will be better prepared to provide culturally appropriate care. Future potential networks include collaboration with physicians within the cultural community and proactively providing women's health teaching through cooperative alliances at bridal shops.

Amish Culture and Immunization Beliefs and Practices

Recent concerns over the outbreak of infectious disease occurring in Amish communities first prompted a review of the literature about the Amish and immunization practices. The desire to appreciate and explore the world of the Amish in greater detail and obtain firsthand knowledge about the Amish culture, particularly immunization practices and health care beliefs inspired an overnight trip to Lancaster, Pennsylvania. To accomplish these objectives, the following visits were planned: Mennonite Information Center, tour of a functional Amish farmhouse, driving tours, and the Lancaster County History Museum. The most powerful sensory experiences of the trip were the:

- the lull of streets without automobiles,
- a clear sky missing the chaos of telephone lines,
- the sweet smell of wheat and tobacco fields,

- the heavy taste of shoofly pie and
- the soft feel of handmade quilts skillfully crafted by the community over many hours juxtaposed to the stiff, constricting feel that I experienced while dressed in traditional Amish attire

Although not originally planned, my (L.B.) personal interviews with a woman from the Mennonite Center and an elderly Amish man at the farmhouse proved to be the most significant and compelling component of the trip. As we conversed, they enlightened me about the constant need to relate cultural beliefs, values, and customs to nursing practice. For example, the Amish man spoke about his culture's health care beliefs and immunization practices. Through a personal interview with the Amish man, I was provided with the fundamental framework on why and how Amish immunization practices are upheld. To my surprise, I learned that a major factor of underimmunization is financial issues—most Amish do not receive immunizations because it is costly to provide the whole family with this illness prevention measure. Furthermore, in relation to the Amish striving for autonomy, I discovered that when the state of Pennsylvania announced that immunizations would be provided free of charge, church bishops informed the Amish community that this would be accepting charity from the modern world—an unacceptable action. Although the church does not restrict immunizations, it is not a recommended practice; church leaders greatly influence health practice within the community. As a future CNS within the desired educator role, the field trip experience will assist me to formulate a teaching plan to facilitate preventive health care using a culturally congruent approach.

Orthodox Jewish Community and End-of-Life Care

Providing culturally competent end-of-life care for Orthodox Jewish patients and their families first required an in-depth comprehension of Orthodox Jewish values and beliefs. Based on my (J.D.) hospital rabbi's recommendation, participation at a Bikur Cholim (visiting the sick) workshop was ideal. The experience gave me an in depth understanding of the roles and responsibilities of the Orthodox Jewish community when a member of the community is sick or dying.

Although initial objectives targeted workshop attendance and information gathering, other learning and networking opportunities emerged. Through workshop attendance, contacts were made with professionals in the Orthodox Jewish community who had programs in place for meeting their community's end-of-life needs. These programs could be helpful blueprints that health care professionals can adapt and incorporate into their plan of care when working with the Orthodox Jewish community during end-of-life care. Future networking can provide links to assist nurses, other health professionals, and organizations in planning and providing culturally specific care to Orthodox Jews.

African American Women and Arthritic Pain Management Using Complementary and Alternative Medicine (CAM)

Pain perception and pain management involves highly personalized experiences that are greatly influenced by culture. My (S.N.) broad aim was to learn more about African American (AA) women and arthritic pain management using complementary and alternative medicine (CAM). Recognizing that the choice and use of CAM and Western medicine options are often influenced by ethnohistorical, social, and political factors, especially among minority groups historically suffering discrimination and oppression, the "Slavery in New York" exhibit at the local historical society provided a unique opportunity to gain further insight. The exhibit gave a great understanding of the major events that shaped AA life and culture.

Consistent with my ROL, the church proved once more to be the center of life for African Americans and a trusted social network. I learned that despite all adversities that AA women encountered, they shared "a community invisible to most whites, meeting secretly, burying their dead with dignity and preserving traces of Africa" (museum exhibit statement by Professor James Oliver Horton, chief historian, 2005). Today, many AA churches have become quite structured with leaders who can influence every aspect of life. Although churches are not traditional health care settings, faith communities have been long involved in providing health care. The field trip gave me a deeper understanding of AA culture, and helped me identify the elements that will make a difference on providing culturally congruent care for the AA client. As evidenced in the museum exhibits, pamphlets, and other literature, African Americans apply their religious and spiritual beliefs and practices to cope with some of life's most challenging circumstances. Church, spirituality, and prayer were found to be the factors that profoundly influence health care practices and beliefs of AA women. I realized that the CNS should attempt to work in partnership with faith-based centers in order to enhance health promotion and provide health education for AA women on how to cope with chronic diseases and symptoms, such as arthritic pain. Also, the CNS can improve quality of care by gaining culture-specific knowledge and by disseminating information and research findings to nurses, other health professionals, and health care organizations.

LEARNING OUTCOMES

Evaluation of a multidimensional teaching strategy involves a multidimensional evaluation plan that assesses cognitive, practical, and affective learning. To systematically appraise learning outcomes for presentation in this chapter, students completed surveys about their perceived learning outcomes as a result of the field trip experiences mentioned in this chapter. The instructor adapted a learning outcome survey from the Transcultural Self-Efficacy Tool (TSET) (Jeffreys, 1994, 2006b). To evaluate different levels of cognitive learning outcomes, students were first asked whether they "gained new knowledge, comprehended knowledge better, learned to apply knowledge, learned how to analyze information differently, or synthesize (repattern) information differently for a selection of 53 items. Next, to evaluate practical learning, students identified interview topics among the same 53 items. Formal interviews or conversations with people within the specific culture were included. Finally, affective learning outcomes were assessed by asking students whether they gained "new attitudes, values, or beliefs" or further developed "attitudes, values, and beliefs" concerning 30 items.

Although self-report findings must be viewed cautiously, evaluation of cultural competence behaviors in the clinical setting would be difficult. Self-report measures provide valuable insight into the student experience, perceptions of learning, and confidence (self-efficacy)—factors that influence cultural competence development and provision of culturally congruent care, therefore, a further discussion is justified. As anticipated, student cognitive and practical learning outcomes varied based on topics and setting. For example, only one student reported comprehension about "life support and resuscitation"; this student's field trip concerned end-of-life issues for Orthodox Jewish patients. In contrast, all students reported cognitive learning for "religious background and identity," "religious practices and beliefs," and "traditional health and illness beliefs."

Comparison of perceived cognitive, practical, and affective learning outcomes identified several interesting findings:

- All students reported cognitive and affective learning outcomes.
- The three participatory–observation experiences resulted in cognitive, practical, and affective learning outcomes; these experiences involved direct interaction and interview with informants within the selected culture.
- The museum experience resulted in the highest number of cognitive learning items.

- Cognitive learning occurred mainly on knowledge and comprehension levels.
- About members of different cultural groups, all students reported affective learning outcomes across several categories: awareness, acceptance, appreciation, recognition, and advocacy.

DEVELOPING PROFESSIONAL ROLES BEYOND THE COURSE: PUBLICATION, PRESENTATIONS, AND NETWORKING

To further develop professional roles beyond the course, the four students accepted the invitation of the course instructor to contribute as an author to a book chapter and submit an abstract to the international conference of the Transcultural Nursing Society (TCNS). Once the abstract was accepted for an oral presentation at the TCNS conference, students agreed to independently prepare a PowerPoint presentation, critique and revise each other's work, and practice the presentation together prior to the international conference. Students reported that the process of contributing to the book chapter facilitated professional growth and development, fostered independence, and provided the opportunity to share the experience with others reaching a broader audience. Through the preparation of the presentation, students learned the importance of following a particular format, meeting the needs of a particular target audience within the specified time frame, teamwork and rehearsal, and open communication with colleagues. The delivery of the actual presentation to an international audience offered an opportunity for active sharing, questions and answers, dialogue post-presentation, and validation that their learning experience was valued by varying levels of novice and experienced researchers and clinicians worldwide.

IMPLICATIONS FOR NURSE EDUCATORS

The literature reveals an alarming gap in conceptually and empirically supported teaching strategies, especially those targeting cultural competence development within clinically focused graduate nursing programs. Furthermore, teaching strategies designed to address the holistic learner—incorporating cognitive, practical (psychomotor), and affective skills—are grossly underrepresented in the literature. The Innovative Field Trip Experience (IFTE) is a learner-centered, creative strategy that involves a carefully orchestrated integration of cognitive, practical, and affective skills. Implemented during the second half of a required transcultural core course in the CNS/NP curriculum, the IFTE assisted beginning graduate students to enrich their cultural competence, gain insight into the emic (insider) perspective, and develop clinical expertise through formalized and informal, self-directed educational experiences. Positive student responses for the IFTE as well as positive learner outcomes support its continued use. The four case exemplars demonstrate easy application for use in various settings, list methods to evaluate learning, and identify learning outcomes achieved. Future empirical investigation of the IFTE, adapted to various student populations and settings, are recommended. To expand the repertoire of conceptually and empirically supported teaching strategies, nurse educators must exert an active role in the scholarship of teaching, participate in the ongoing dissemination of educational scholarship, challenge the status quo when appropriate, advocate for positive change, and replace teacher-centered pedagogy with learner-centered approaches.

KEY POINT SUMMARY

- The Innovative Field Trip Experience (IFTE) is a learner-centered, creative strategy that was implemented during the second half of a 15-week required transcultural core course in the CNS/NP curriculum.
- IFTE included prerequisite components (background reading assignments, classroom seminar and films, literature review, and written paper), general required components (student-initiated field trip selection, purpose and objectives, instructor approval, plan, implementation, and written paper), and information-sharing/dissemination components (storytelling and cultural food buffet).
- Four actual case exemplars demonstrate easy application of the IFTE in a variety of settings and present select highlights of the learning experience from the student perspective including: (a) Asian Indian women and prenatal care; (b) Amish culture and immunization beliefs and practices; (c) Orthodox Jewish community and end-of-life care; and (d) African American women and arthritic pain management using complementary and alternative medicines.
- Learning outcomes in the cognitive, practical, and affective dimensions were reported.

CHAPTER 9

Faculty Advisement and Helpfulness: A Culturally Congruent Approach

Marianne R. Jeffreys, EdD, RN

The active involvement of nursing faculty in the student's academic endeavors, career goals, and professional socialization is a well regarded professional value. It is manifested by faculty encouraging realistic educational and career goals, promoting positive feelings of self-worth, verbalizing belief in the student's ability to succeed, listening to problems and concerns, expressing interest in academic progress, showing optimism, offering assistance, and presence. Presence means caring about the student as a whole person, being available as a resource person, and making appropriate referrals when needed.

Considering the student as a whole person demands a culturally congruent approach to advisement and helpfulness. The inclusion of cultural values and beliefs (CVB) in the Nursing Undergraduate Retention and Success (NURS) model recognizes that a student's CVB unconsciously and consciously guide thinking, decisions, and actions that ultimately affect nursing student retention (Figure 9.1). The NURS model proposes

---

This chapter was excerpted and adapted from Jeffreys, M.R. (2004). Faculty Advisement and helpfulness: A culturally congruent approach. (In: Jeffreys, M.R.). *Nursing Student Retention: Understanding the Process and Making a Difference*. New York: Springer. By permission, Springer.

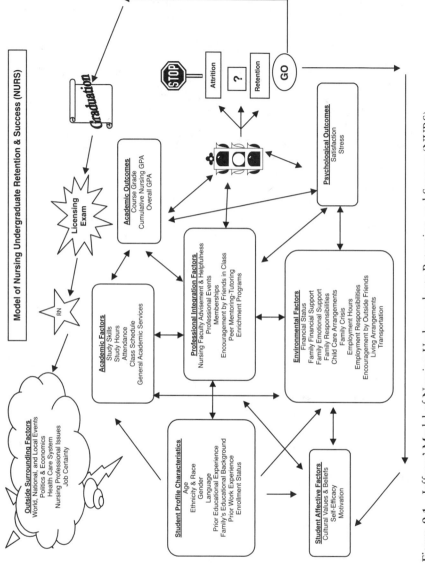

Figure 9.1   Jeffreys' Model of Nursing Undergraduate Retention and Success (NURS)

that high levels of cultural congruence will serve as a bridge to promoting positive academic and psychological outcomes, thus enhancing persistence behaviors and retention (see Chapter 1). Cultural congruence here is the degree of fit between the student's values and beliefs and those of their surrounding environment; that is, nursing education within the educational institution and the nursing profession. The term "cultural congruent (nursing) care," which was first coined by Leininger (1991a, p. 49) to describe her view of nursing care with clients, can be adapted to the educational setting. In this book, a culturally congruent approach to faculty advisement and helpfulness refers to those faculty actions that are tailored to fit with the student's CVB in order to promote, facilitate, or support academic endeavors, career goals, and professional socialization.

A culturally congruent approach to faculty advisement and helpfulness requires commitment and engagement in developing cultural congruence and becoming "culturally competent" as faculty advisors and helpful teachers. The process includes self-assessment, literature review, consultation and collaboration, student assessment, analysis, plan, communication, and interaction.

SELF-ASSESSMENT

Because faculty may be "unconsciously incompetent" in providing nursing advisement and help, self-assessment is a first step. According to Purnell (2008), one is unconsciously incompetent when one is not aware of cultural differences or when one unknowingly carries out actions that are not culturally congruent. Cultural blindness, cultural imposition, and culturally incongruent actions can cause cultural pain to others (Leininger & McFarland, 2002). The major aim of self-assessment is raising consciousness and self-awareness.

Here, self-assessment is a process in which the nurse educator systematically appraises various dimensions that can impact upon the achievement of culturally congruent advisement and helpfulness. A systematic assessment can be initiated using the dimensions described in Chapter 1, listed in Table 1.2, and illustrated in Figure 6.2. (A user-friendly Self-Assessment Tool-Academic (SAT-A) is available in the Cultural Competence Education Resource Toolkit [Jeffreys, 2010]). The realization that there are multidimensional variables influencing student–faculty interaction is overwhelming, yet these variables are essential to evaluate before developing a culturally congruent approach. In addition to raising consciousness and self-awareness, self-assessment can help identify areas of strengths and weaknesses and should be compared with students' own self-assessments and expectations.

Although the faculty member may be immersed within the "culture" of nursing education and be familiar with long-held nursing education CVB, it is important to be aware that unconscious and conscious CVB in nursing education and in one's own values and belief systems, many of which were developed long before entering the nursing culture, may influence practices, behaviors, and actions. For example, a nursing faculty member whose traditional cultural values favor direct eye contact for all communication and who views lack of eye contact suspiciously will need to be consciously aware of his or her underlying values and beliefs and aim to consciously avoid distrusting students based solely on this nonverbal cue.

Awareness of one's knowledge about different CVB, especially the CVB that most directly affect nursing student retention (through academic and psychological outcomes) must be explored (see Table 1.2). Although Table 1.2 presents a snapshot approach of selected CVB that may impact upon nursing student retention, it does allow for a quick comparison of different CVB. One benefit of this approach is that it evokes the awareness that there may be CVB in various cultures that the nurse educator is unaware of. The realization that one is not and cannot be "culturally competent" all of the time is often a powerful awakening. Becoming conscious of one's incompetence can be a humbling experience but frequently sparks a desire for obtaining cultural knowledge. Cultural awareness, desire, and knowledge are essential for the process of cultural competence (Campinha-Bacote, 2003).

Cultural knowledge is a thorough educational foundation about various CVB with the goal of comprehending and empathizing with others' perspectives. The nurse educator must assess one's cultural desire or motivation for engaging in the process of becoming culturally competent. Reflecting on the feelings one experiences and the actions taken when students' CVB are different from one's own CVB can further one's insight. Because the process of cultural competence is ongoing, nurse educators should examine their commitment toward achieving this goal. True commitment requires time, energy, persistence, extra effort to overcome obstacles, and willingness to learn from mistakes. Commitment is essential in achieving positive outcomes in student retention (Campbell & Davis, 1996).

Nurse educators must appraise the multidimensional factors influencing undergraduate nursing student achievement, retention, and success, or full understanding will not truly be achieved. Furthermore, they need to evaluate how CVB can influence persistence behaviors (Kuh &

Love, 2000). Nurse educators should reflect on the last time an updated review of the literature, workshop, or conference on student retention and success was completed. Again, appraisal of one's desire for updated knowledge and commitment in relation to other faculty responsibilities and available time should be critically determined.

Similarly, self-expectations of the advisor role and helpfulness toward students should be examined. Faculty often overlook the significant role that their attitudes and behaviors can have on student satisfaction and retention. (Bosher & Pharris, 2009; Lundquist, Spalding, & Landrum, 2002). Although the developmental advisement approach is strongly supported in the literature as offering the most benefits to enhance student academic and psychological growth and development, not all nursing faculty may value, support, or practice developmental advisement. In a developmental approach, student–faculty relationships encourage open communication, shared responsibility and power, caring, mentoring, total student development, self-direction, active help-seeking behaviors, and decision making. Developmental advisement is more focused on the "process" of learning whereas prescriptive advisement is grade-oriented, focused on the attainment of a prescribed product. Prescriptive advisement views the faculty advisor as the authority person who dispenses information and prescribes the measures needed for students to complete their curriculum requirements (Alexitch, 2002; Herndon, Kaiser, & Creamer, 1996).

Developmental advisement necessitates a commitment on the part of both faculty member and student; the advisor–advisee relationship changes over the educational process. Although the developmental approach is advocated in the NURS model, students may inwardly view faculty advisement and helpfulness differently. Not all students may value a developmental advisement approach. Often student perceptions and expectations about the faculty advisement role are different from that of the faculty (Baldwin & Wold, 1993; Gasper, 2009; Harrison, 2009; Lehna, Jackonen, & Wilson, 1996; Shultz, 1998; Trent, 1997; Winters, 1990). Additionally, expectations about "helpfulness" can be different than that of faculty (Bosher & Pharris, 2009; Poorman, Webb, & Mastorovich, 2002). The mismatch between student and faculty expectations and perceptions creates another barrier, whereby students can become disappointed and dissatisfied; poor psychological outcomes for the nursing program increase the risk for attrition. Consequently, faculty members should appraise their knowledge about student expectations and perceptions. Lack of knowledge or limited knowledge in this area identifies targets for further self-development. However, one must have the desire to obtain such knowledge and be committed to its pursuit amidst other faculty responsibilities. Finally, self-assessment should conclude with a listing of strengths, weaknesses, gaps in knowledge, goals, commitment, and priorities.

LITERATURE REVIEW

Next, a review of the nursing and higher education literature should be conducted. A review of the literature in psychology, anthropology, and sociology may also prove fruitful. Materials should be reviewed for gathering background information or updating previously gathered information about CVB, cultural competence, student retention, advisement, faculty helpfulness, help-seeking behaviors, and faculty–student interactions. Priority areas, weaknesses, or gaps in knowledge previously identified in the self-assessment can guide the review. Choice of a relevant conceptual framework can be instrumental to an organized review. For example, the NURS model can structure a systematic approach to the review and organization of retention literature. After gathering general background information, it may be appropriate to begin targeting specific student cultural groups, especially those with whom there is frequent interaction. The dimensions targeted in Chapter 1 (Table 1.2) and Figure 6.2 and can provide a guide for organizing specific information; however, it is vital to individually appraise each student and avoid stereotypical assumptions.

CONSULTATION AND COLLABORATION

Once sufficient background information has been reviewed and synthesized, collaboration with others should be initiated. Sufficient background knowledge is a precursor for successfully optimizing consultation and collaboration. The nurse educator will now have a mutually shared conceptual and empirical knowledge base with colleagues and experts that will promote deeper dialogue and added benefits. Consultation with experts in specific cultures, cultural competency, advisement, and student retention is helpful. Collaboration with colleagues (other nursing faculty) can help coordinate efforts and avoid unnecessary duplication. Consultation and collaboration can occur formally and informally via conferences, e-mail, Webinars, telephone, and meetings.

A major benefit of collaboration among faculty is that nurse educators can become aware of each other's expertise and interests. Other goals include learning from others, avoiding pitfalls, and gaining insight into special program-specific considerations. Still another plus is broadening information sources and soliciting conceptual and/or instrumental support from others.

STUDENT ASSESSMENT

The ability to gather relevant and valid cultural information is an essential component in the development of cultural competence (Campinha-Bacote, 2003). Moreover, a systematic appraisal of CVB is a precursor to determining the needs and priorities within a cultural context (Leininger, 1978). Promoting student self-assessment of CVB must be initiated in a positive supportive environment that embraces diversity. Students will need to feel comfortable exploring their own CVB in the context of the nursing educational setting and secondly will need to feel comfortable in sharing CVB with others, especially faculty. The literature suggests that students of different cultural backgrounds than faculty often feel isolated and reluctant to share differences for fear of reprimand, discrimination, or misunderstanding (Barbee & Gibson, 2001; Bessent, 1997; Bosher & Pharris, 2009; Campinha-Bacote, 1998b; Flinn, 2004; Kirkland, 1998; Kuh & Love, 2000; Labun, 2002; Manifold & Rambur, 2001; Tucker-Allen & Long, 1999; Villaruel, Canales, & Torres, 2001; Weaver, 2001; Yurkovich, 2001).

Encouraging students to explore their own CVB concerning such dimensions as listed in Table 1.2 will enhance awareness of cultural similarities and differences with peers, clients, and faculty. This awareness will aid in the development of cultural competence in professional settings with clients, peers, other health care professionals, and ancillary workers. Asking about students' expectations concerning faculty advisement and helpfulness in the classroom, clinical setting, college skills laboratory, and informal settings will publicize and emphasize the fact that faculty care and have the desire to help students. Students' perception that an instructor or advisor is asking about student needs is helpful in and of itself and creates a caring environment. Perceptions that faculty sincerely care about students and openly apologize for (cultural) mistakes is more important than flawless, superficial, and distant interactions with students.

Student assessment may be done formally through the use of survey tools; however, the development of valid and reliable survey tools that are free of cultural bias and social desirability response bias is a complicated and lengthy process (Jeffreys & Smodlaka, 1996). A previous review of literature may reveal already existing survey tools with adequate estimates of reliability and validity that can be used or adapted with permission. Use of a survey tool that has not been tested for validity and reliability not only provides questionable results but can impact adversely on student perceptions if items are offensive, misinterpreted, unclear, insulting, or culturally inappropriate. Such unwanted outcomes create dissatisfaction, added stress, and negatively influence retention.

Another formalized assessment approach may be using focus groups with select student groups (Yearwood, Brown, & Karlik, 2002). Dialogue with students, with a set of predetermined questions to guide the discussion and allow for comparison between student groups, will allow for unsolicited comments, solicited comments, and qualitative data that can add richness not achievable via a quantitative or close-ended survey questioning. Focus groups that are guided by peer mentors or faculty who are not in a teaching role may ease fear of penalty or adverse consequences. A systematic assessment can be initiated using the dimensions listed in Table 1.2. Student responses can then be compared with those of faculty.

In the classroom, clinical setting, or college laboratory, a simple technique may be to survey students anonymously on the first day. After an introduction, the instructor can express interest in meeting student needs through advisement and helpfulness and can ask students to write several ways that they believe the instructor can be helpful during the semester. It may also be beneficial to ask students to write anything that they experienced in the past that was not helpful or anything that they would perceive to be inappropriate or not helpful. This strategy can also be adapted to ask questions about faculty helpfulness in an informal setting.

Advisement and helpfulness should be developmental, that is, changing over time as student needs and expectations change, and so student assessment should be ongoing throughout the course and throughout the program at regularly scheduled intervals. For example, mid-semester, a classroom instructor may want to ask students to write comments again as before and compare with the group's previous responses. Over time, common trends or themes may emerge, especially in a particular clinical setting or classroom course component. A systematic program appraisal can provide an overview of successful strategies and outcomes (Padilla, 1999).

ANALYSIS

Insight into students' perceptions is important in meeting needs of adult learners (Knowles, 1984). A systematic analysis of students' self-assessment should identify realistic versus unrealistic expectations, areas of untapped or underutilized advisor role, trends among the students surveyed, group similarities, individual differences, and perceived student needs. A thorough and objective analysis to determine the gap between student and faculty expectations, perceptions of what is important, and level of cultural congruence should be estimated. Mismatches need priority attention. The analysis should list strengths and congruency as well as weaknesses, gaps, and incongruency. Analysis of findings may be enhanced through the review of relevant literature to explain findings, elaborate major points, and offer suggestions.

PLAN

Next, a written action plan is developed. Individual faculty can review student comments for areas of unrealistic or unclear expectations and then plan to address this in a group setting to clarify advisor and faculty role. Similarly, faculty can verbally and positively respond to realistic, clear, and important expectations in faculty–student interactions. Relevant issues reported in the literature and/or uncovered through consultation and collaboration should be incorporated. Another strategy may be to develop, distribute, and discuss an academic advising guide delineating responsibilities as an advisee and responsibilities of the advisor (Harrison, 2009). The advisor guidebook of the National Academic Advising Association (NACADA) can provide some foundational information generalizable to multidisciplinary college students (Roufs, 2007).

A plan for a faculty development workshop or series of workshops in enhancing culturally congruent advisement and helpfulness is central to promoting retention through positive psychological outcomes. Inadequate planning of effective advisement strategies appropriate for various students throughout the educational process supports the need for faculty development workshops (Bosher & Pharris, 2009; Braxton & Mundy, 2001; Gasper, 2009; Hammond, Davis, Hodges, & Warfield, 1997; Harrison, 2009; Hesser, Pond, Lewis, & Abbott, 1996; Kirkpatrick & Koldjeski, 1997; Labun, 2002; Nora, 2001; Rew, 1996; Sherrod & Harrison, 1994; Tucker-Allen & Long, 1999; Yoder, 2001). Nursing education goes beyond a single nurse educator. It is the whole nursing educational experience that impacts positively or negatively in the minds of students. One experience of cultural pain can do much to undermine the efforts of other faculty members who strongly advocate and consciously implement culturally congruent approaches.

The plan for faculty development should recognize that some faculty may fail to recognize the need for a workshop or may demonstrate reluctance to participate. Even if a workshop or series of workshops is mandatory, this does not necessarily mean that faculty will change values, beliefs, and traditions in favor of culturally congruent advisement and helpfulness. However, it is important to remember that all faculty members and students have CVB that may potentially be congruent or incongruent with each other and/or traditional nursing education values (Table 1.2). Both faculty and students may belong to multiple cultural groups, and the boundaries between cultural groups and affiliations is often unclear (Kuh & Love, 2000; Phinney, 1996). Therefore, formalized educational experiences concerning culture are necessary for all individuals, regardless of age, ethnicity, gender, sexual orientation, lifestyle, religion, socioeconomic status, or geographic location (Andrews, 1995; Jeffreys, 2000; Leininger, 1995b).

Table 6.2, Table 9.1, and Table 9.2 provide case examples contrasting culturally incongruent and culturally congruent student–faculty

Table 9.1 Examples of Culturally Incongruent and Culturally Congruent Advisement Approaches

ADVISEMENT SITUATION	CULTURALLY INCONGRUENT	CULTURALLY CONGRUENT
Shari arrives for academic course advisement accompanied by her husband. She states that she prefers having her husband with her. Shari's husband asks several questions concerning the nursing curriculum. Her CVB view decision making as a process involving her husband. Nonverbal communication cues (relaxed facial expression and relaxed body posture) suggest comfort with each other's presence during the advisement session.	Professor ignores the student's CVB and does not actively explore preferred advisement style. Professor imposes her own CVB by stating, "I will be glad to answer any questions that Shari has. Shari, if you want to be a professional nurse, you must learn to be assertive, speak for yourself, and make decisions on your own". *Result*: Shari and her husband experience cultural pain and feel embarrassed. Because they view the professor as an authority figure, they do not want to confront her. Instead, they remain quiet. Later, Shari and her husband decide that she should drop out of the nursing program.	Professor recognizes the importance of Shari's CVB. Professor states, "It is nice to see such strong family support. I hope that I will be able to answer your questions. If you would like to move your chairs into a more comfortable arrangement, please feel free to do so. I want to help you in the best way possible, so please let me know if something I say or do makes you uncomfortable or is unclear." *Result*: Shari and her husband feel that the professor genuinely cares about Shari holistically and is sincerely interested in accommodating their needs.

Table 9.1   Examples of Culturally Incongruent and Culturally Congruent
             Advisement Approaches (*continued*)

ADVISEMENT SITUATION	CULTURALLY INCONGRUENT	CULTURALLY CONGRUENT
Dana, a 25-year-old unmarried part-time student visits the nursing advisor for registration. She has her three small children with her. She expresses concern over getting daytime courses that coincide with the college childcare services. Her CVB place family responsibilities over all other responsibilities. Single parenting is not viewed negatively in her culture.	Professor holds traditional nursing values and beliefs as well as own CVB that are congruent with nursing CVB. Professor states, "When I went to school, we weren't concerned about things like that. None of us were married and none of us had children. School was the priority. Nursing is hard work and should be a priority." *Result*: Dana feels discouraged and experiences hurt, anger, and pain.	Professor acknowledges the importance of Dana's concerns, and compliments her beautiful children and her motivation to pursue her nursing degree. Professor offers to call the childcare guidance counselor to assist her with the childcare aspect. *Result*: Dana feels satisfied that the advisor respects and understands her values and beliefs.
Iris experiences a personal crisis during the last semester before graduation. The stress associated with the crisis situation interferes with her ability to complete assignments and tests successfully. Iris's CVB stigmatize psychological stress. Talking about one's personal feelings is taboo. Indirect verbal communication and periods of silence for reflection are the preferred communication patterns. Iris asks the advisor for help in improving her grades.	Professor values a direct approach that aims to encourage verbalization of feelings. Professor states, "You obviously are under a lot of emotional stress. I think you should talk about your feelings with me or a college counselor." *Result*: Iris experiences cultural pain and distress because her emotional stress is outwardly recognizable. She feels stigmatized and reluctant to talk about feelings. This results in negative psychological feelings associated with school.	Professor recognizes that students may view stress differently and that different advisement approaches may be needed. Professor states, "Last month I had a student whose grades dropped following a personal crisis. Sometimes students experience stress related to outside issues or events. Some students have benefited from speaking with a counselor about their feelings." (pause) *Result*: Iris does not feel stigmatized and is satisfied with the advisor's approach.

Table 9.2   Faculty Helpfulness beyond Class: Examples of Culturally
            Incongruent and Culturally Congruent Approaches

SITUATION	CULTURALLY INCONGRUENT	CULTURALLY CONGRUENT
Outside Maria is walking across the campus with her father and encounters her former nursing instructor. Maria's CVB place parents, elders, teachers, and nurses as highly respected individuals. Family and traditions are priorities; education is secondary. She formally introduces her father and instructor.	Professor values casual, informal interaction with students, thinking that this is helpful for all students. She states, "Oh, just call me Cathy. There's no need to be so formal." *Result*: Maria and her father experience cultural pain and embarrassment. Maria's father is concerned that Maria will abandon her traditional CVB. Maria feels pulled between her traditional CVB and pursuit of a nursing career.	Professor is comfortable with casual, informal interaction with students, yet respects alternative values. Professor does not attempt to impose her values, rather she graciously thanks Maria for the formal introduction and responds formally. *Result*: Maria and her father experience positive psychological outcomes (satisfaction).
Office Hours During office hours, several students asked the instructor's help for completing a written paper assignment. Pat does not understand how to complete a written paper assignment; however, his CVB are not congruent with self-initiated active help-seeking behaviors.	Professor holds CVB that value assertiveness, active help-seeking behaviors, and confrontation with authority. Professor states to her colleague, "I keep my office door open so students can stop by and ask for help. If students don't ask for help, they deserve the grade they get." *Result*: Pat still does not understand the assignment, fails the paper, resulting in poor academic outcomes and poor psychological outcomes.	Professor recognizes that help-seeking behaviors vary culturally and consciously makes an effort to follow up on students who do not seek help. Professor requests that Pat meet during office hours to discuss the written paper assignment, stating, "When students share their questions and feedback concerning papers and the class, it helps me a great deal. Could you please help me by stopping by to talk about the paper?" *Result*: Pat receives the necessary help needed and passes the assignment. Positive academic and psychological outcomes occur.

interactions and the resulting outcomes. These case examples can be incorporated into a plan to initiate discussion with faculty and students. Such dialogue may help promote inner reflection or self-awareness of one's CVB, cultural imposition, ethnocentric tendencies, and potential impact of cultural pain on nursing student retention. Using case examples can point out that despite the intent to help, one's actions may not always be helpful. In fact, they may be counterproductive, causing pain, conflict, dissatisfaction, and stress for the student. Planning communication strategies to convey faculty commitment and holistic caring about culturally diverse students is necessary to avoid misunderstandings and to enhance the quality of faculty–student interactions.

COMMUNICATION

Communicating that "culture matters" and that "students matter" requires an integrated, well-planned approach. Multimedia strategies to promote open communication, clarify misperceptions about the faculty advisor role, convey caring and helpfulness, and develop student–faculty partnerships in achieving cultural congruency should be proactive and ongoing. For example, communication can be initiated in new student orientations, on initial assignment to an advisor, on the first day of class/clinical via verbal, written, and other media format. Slides, PowerPoint presentations, videos, case examples, and other multimedia approaches can be used to supplement previous information and initiate discussions in large groups, small groups, or individual settings with students. The faculty advisor role, teacher's role, and student rights and responsibilities can be delineated and described in student newsletters, handout materials, student handbook, welcome letters to new students, course outlines, bulletin board postings, e-mail list serves, and Web pages. Messages that openly celebrate diversity encourage others to appreciate and embrace the diversity among students, faculty, clients, and society in general. Such messages permit the open sharing and exchange of cultural information that is a necessary precursor to mutually satisfying interactions with culturally different individuals.

INTERACTION

It is not sufficient for educators to have read about cultures, attended workshops, professed commitment to cultural competence, or surveyed students; faculty must take action and enter a new phase in the journey of achieving cultural competence. Campinha-Bacote (2003) calls this interaction phase "cultural encounter." Leininger (2002), however, defines cultural encounter as a situation in which someone meets or briefly interacts with a culturally different individual. Such a brief encounter fails to allow a deep understanding or an insight into the culture (Leininger, 2002a). In this book, cultural interaction refers to the ongoing, planned and unplanned situations in which faculty and students with various different CVB have shared experiences or interactions. The faculty member committed to the goal of developing cultural competence and providing culturally congruent advisement and helpfulness will make a concerted effort to actively initiate and engage in cultural interactions throughout the educational process and possibly beyond graduation and into the student's entry into the nursing profession.

Cultural interaction leads to a greater insight into the student's culture on the individual level. Interactions offer the opportunity to recognize the cultural variations that exist among individuals, families, and groups (Leininger, 2002). Through ongoing interactions, the discovery that cultural variations exist and impact differently on faculty–student interactions, persistence, and all dimensions of culture helps prevent stereotyping of individuals based on perceived cultural group affiliation. Cultural interaction fosters the exchange of CVB, thus facilitating personal growth, professional growth, and the development of cultural competence for educators and students. An initial interaction that values, appreciates, and embraces diversity will do much for encouraging the further exchange of information, values, beliefs, and ideas as well as promoting positive psychological outcomes (satisfaction and decreased stress) associated with the educational experience.

Entering a culturally different or unknown world can be intimidating or stressful, for fear of making a mistake or inadvertently doing something "wrong." Such fears are a barrier to initiating and engaging in substantive cultural interactions with students. Acknowledging ahead of time that mistakes may occur is important; however, learning from one's mistakes and moving forward is even more important. A "cultural mistake" can make one more consciously competent next time when encountering a similar or even different situation.

Cultural competency must never be taken for granted. One cannot really ever be totally culturally competent, but one can exert conscious effort into achieving cultural congruence. Insight can be enhanced by self-reflection and reflection-in-action (Schön, 1987). Reflection calls for ongoing self-assessment, updated knowledge, consultation, collaboration, student assessment, analysis, plan, communication, and cultural interactions.

Exhibit 9.1   Educator-In-Action Vignette

At a nursing faculty meeting, Professor Glass introduces the topic of "Culturally Congruent Faculty Advisement and Helpfulness" by sharing a personal experience. "I used to think of myself as being a helpful advisor to all students; however, this opinion changed recently. I realized that I made a cultural mistake with one of my students. This mistake set up obstacles for future communication and caused her obvious stress. I apologized immediately but later I always felt a gap was present. I realized that the increased number of new immigrant nursing students from diverse countries meant that I could not use the same approach with all students. I was also concerned that I may have offended others unintentionally. The next week in class, I asked students to reflect on their experiences with nursing faculty so far and anonymously write down helpful faculty actions, unhelpful faculty actions, student expectations about faculty advisement and helpfulness, and any cultural customs relevant to faculty–student interactions. Responses were amazing."

Professor Glass read several student comments that contrasted student perceptions, CVB, and student experiences with faculty.

1. "My advisor always stares right into my eyes during the registration advisement session. I get so uncomfortable that I feel as though I can't even speak."
2. "My advisor hardly ever looks me in the eye so I don't think she even sees me as a person."
3. "When nursing faculty greet me in the hall or library and offer to help me during office hours, it makes me feel like they care."
4. "My advisor was right behind me in the cafeteria line and didn't even acknowledge my greeting or say hello."
5. "When my advisor changed her office hours to Friday afternoons, she offered to set an alternate meeting time with me instead of making me change advisors. That made me feel as though she really cared about me and respected my religious beliefs."
6. "Thank you for asking about our (students') feelings, experiences, and concerns. Even if you do something other than what I expect, I will now feel as though you are trying to treat us as individuals and respect our cultural values and beliefs."

Other faculty members relate similar experiences and concerns about providing culturally congruent advisement and helpfulness. Faculty decide that the annual faculty development workshop topic will be "Culturally Congruent Advisement and Helpfulness: Strategies to Enhance Nursing Student Retention and Success." Subsequent plans are made to have a 2-day faculty retreat to critique the curriculum, recruitment and retention strategies, and advisement approaches for culturally sensitive approaches that embrace diverse cultures.

Several adjunct faculty members with full-time appointment at the HCI comment on the need for culturally congruent preceptor and supervisor roles to enhance nurse satisfaction and retention. The adjunct faculty members form a subcommittee to adapt the process of developing a culturally congruent approach to faculty advisement and helpfulness to the process of developing a culturally congruent approach to the preceptor and supervisor role. Plans to collaborate and cosponsor guest speakers between the school of nursing and several affiliating HCI hope to capitalize on pooled human and financial resources by creating proactive networks.

KEY POINT SUMMARY

- Faculty advisement and helpfulness is manifested through faculty actions such as encouraging realistic educational and career goals, promoting positive feelings of self-worth, verbalizing belief in the student's ability to succeed, listening to problems and concerns, expressing interest in academic progress, optimism, offering assistance, and presence.
- A culturally congruent approach to faculty advisement and helpfulness refers to those faculty actions that are tailored to fit with the student's CVB in order to promote, facilitate, or support meaningful, beneficial, and satisfying academic endeavors, career goals, and professional socialization.
- The process of developing cultural congruence and becoming "culturally competent" faculty advisors and helpful teachers includes self-assessment, literature review, consultation and collaboration, student assessment, analysis, plan, communication, and interaction.

C H A P T E R   1 0

Health Care Institutions: Inquiry, Action, and Innovation

Marianne R. Jeffreys, EdD, RN

Health care institutions (HCI) are in a unique position not only to encourage but also to expect ongoing cultural competence development and culturally congruent patient care (see Figure 10.1). Expectations must be partnered with structured, high-quality educational opportunities and incentives for enhancing cultural competence development that are motivated by true commitment for cultural competence rather than by accrediting agency mandates. Because cultural competence is defined as a multidimensional learning process that integrates transcultural skills in all three dimensions (cognitive, practical, and affective) and involves transcultural self-efficacy (confidence) as a major influencing factor, high-quality opportunities must be carefully planned and coordinated to integrate these components. The term "learning process" emphasizes that the cognitive, practical, and affective dimensions of transcultural self-efficacy (TSE) and transcultural skill development can change over time as a result of formalized education and other learning experiences.

Although informal interaction within the HCI can provide contact with other cultures that can have valuable and positive learning outcomes, especially if supplemented with appropriate formalized educational experiences, unguided interactions can unintentionally perpetuate stereotypes and misperceptions. One common misperception is that one member of a particular cultural group is the authority or example for all aspects of

243

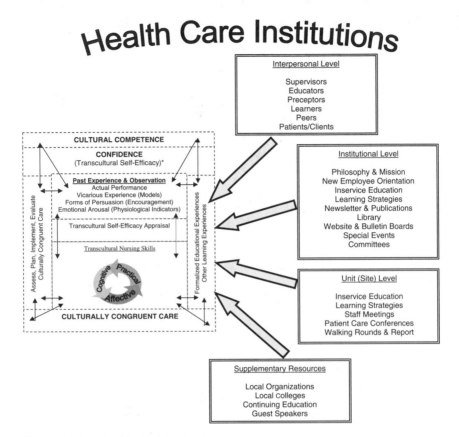

Figure 10.1 Health Care Institutions

the group's values, beliefs, and practices; hence, stereotyping may ensue. Another common misperception is that being a member of a minority group automatically makes one the authority on cultural competence for minority group(s) and on the process of promoting cultural competency development in others. Contrary to this unfounded belief, scholars support that all individuals, regardless of cultural background, need formalized preparation in transcultural nursing—at least on the generalist level (Andrews, 1995; Leininger, 1995b; Leininger & McFarland, 2002). Preparation on the generalist level emphasizes broad transcultural nursing principles, concepts, theories, and research study findings to care for clients of many different cultures (Leininger, 1989). Accrediting organizations have also addressed the need for formalized cultural competence education for all students, professionals, and/or staff members (AACN, 2008, 2009; AAMC, 2005; ADA, 2005, 2007; APA, 1994; APTA, 2008;

Gerstein et al., 2009; JCAHO, 2002; Lubinski & Matteliano, 2008; NASW, 2001, 2007, 2009; NLN, 2009; NLNAC, 2008a, 2008b, 2008c, 2008d, 2008e; Nochajski & Matteliano, 2008; Panzarella & Matteliano, 2008; Ponterotto et al., 2010; Suh, 2004).

Learners will be most motivated and interested in learning if immediate benefits to career goals and daily professional responsibilities are clearly evident and learning goals are realistic (Brookfield, 1986; Knowles, 1984) (see Figure 6.5). With increased globalization and the changing demographics and characteristics within and between cultural groups, it is unrealistic to expect that nurses will become specialists in caring for (or working with) all of the many different cultural groups that they may encounter. To become a specialist in one or more select cultural groups requires a series of specialized transcultural courses and concentrated fieldwork at the graduate level (Leininger, 1989; Leininger & McFarland, 2002). Although this type of formalized education occurs in an academic setting, the HCI has an important role in facilitating nurses' advanced degrees and/or advanced certifications. The HCI may provide incentives (flexible scheduling, promotions, released time, tuition reimbursement, forgivable loans, certified transcultural nurse certification fee and expenses) for nurses to become advanced practice nurses as transcultural nurse specialists. Transcultural nurse specialists will be valuable resources within the HCI and the surrounding cultural community.

It is realistic to expect that all nurses have the basic or generalist transcultural nursing skills needed to provide care for culturally diverse and different clients. It is also reasonable to expect nurses, who have been prepared as generalists, participate in ongoing educational programs designed to expand their learning with direct application to specific, targeted priority cultural groups in the surrounding communities. The advanced certificate program in cultural competence offers a unique, flexible, formalized graduate level *or* continuing education learning opportunity for nurses and other health professionals to expand their cultural competence education, develop cultural competence projects for implementation and evaluation in a variety of health care settings, and network with other health care professionals from near and far places (see Chapter 6) (Jeffreys, 2008). By providing incentives such as tuition reimbursement, professional recognition, and monetary bonuses for advanced certificates, degrees, and certifications, the HCI will actively create a climate in which culturally competent practice and innovations will flourish and grow.

Because few nurses have had formal preparation in transcultural nursing at entry into practice and because not all nurses will pursue higher education, the HCI assumes a great responsibility for assuring the public that nurses are prepared to provide culturally congruent care and that the care is appropriately rendered. Unfortunately, heightened patient acuity levels, the nursing shortage, poor nurse retention, inadequate staffing, rapidly changing culturally diverse patient populations, managed care, and limited resources create numerous, ongoing challenges for HCIs. First, patient care activities often must compete with educational programs. Second, providing ongoing education programs for nurses passing through a revolving door system of changing positions, units, agencies, and shifts presents obvious obstacles for synthesized learning connections that build upon previous learning. Third, the disheartened morale and dissatisfaction of many nurses drains valuable energy and motivation integral to learning. Finally, the number of nurses formally prepared in transcultural nursing, at the undergraduate or graduate level, who are actively employed in an HCI and who can adeptly develop their own and others' cultural competence is grossly inadequate. Although the AACN has now heightened attention on the inclusion of cultural competence throughout baccalaureate and graduate nursing education, most HCI nurses currently employed missed this accreditation mandate. Additionally, nurses prepared via diploma or associate degree programs (or foreign-educated) do not fall under AACN accreditation guidelines. Consequently, their exposure to formal (and informal) cultural competence education is not expected or standardized; therefore, it is questionable, unknown, and/or inconsistent.

Although the removal of obstacles and challenges is one obvious solution, it is beyond the scope of this book to tackle all of these issues. The author contends that offering strategies and incentives for ongoing cultural competence development (part of professional development) combined with tangible patient, personal, and professional outcomes will positively affect nurse's satisfaction and morale, thereby improving nurse retention and further enhancing patient care. Nurse educators, executives, and leaders in the HCIs are empowered to make a tremendous difference by promoting, facilitating, and evaluating cultural competence development. Each individual nurse, nurse educator, executive, or leader is empowered to make a positive difference; however, the greatest impact will be achieved through a coordinated, holistic group effort that thoughtfully weaves together relevant high-priority educational programs, unit-based initiatives, and supplementary resources.

Certain factors within the HCI may support cultural competence development, yet other factors may restrict its development. This chapter will propose some strategies for systematic inquiry into already existing facets of the HCI, while also suggesting strategies for developing new initiatives. This chapter aims to: (a) uncover, discover, and explore educational opportunities (within HCIs) for promoting cultural competency; (b) describe action-focused strategies for educational innovation; and (c) present ideas for evaluation (and reevaluation) of educational innovation implementation. Figures, tables, "Innovation in Cultural Competence" insert exhibits, and the "Educator-in-Action" vignette provide supplementary information to expand upon narrative text features. Major emphasis is placed on self-appraisal and determining educational priorities and goals.

SELF-ASSESSMENT

Similar to the process of cultural competency development in academia (Chapter 6), promoting cultural competency in the HCI requires considerable, sincere effort that must begin with self-assessment. Systematic self-assessment evaluates the various dimensions that can impact upon the educational process and on the achievement of educational outcomes (Jeffreys, 2004). Figure 10.2 depicts a systematic assessment within the HCI setting. Here, self-assessment refers to assessment of the individual staff nurse, nurse manager, nurse educator, nurse executive, administrator, and the organization. (Readers are encouraged to refer to Chapter 6 for an in depth discussion about self-assessment and Table 1.2 about dimensions of cultural values and beliefs. A user-friendly Self-Assessment Tool-Health Care Institutions (SAT-HCI) is available in the Cultural Competence Education Resource Toolkit [Jeffreys, 2010]. The SAT-HCI may be used individually and/or in groups; the SAT-HCI may be used alone or in conjunction with other toolkit items. (See instructions in Preface, page xix.) Finally, self-assessment should conclude with a listing of strengths, weaknesses, gaps in knowledge, goals, commitment, desire, motivation, and priorities.

As mentioned in Chapter 6, comprehensive understanding, skill, and desire are essential but not enough to effectively make a positive difference in cultural competence development. The author believes that resilient TSE (confidence) is the integral component necessary in the process of cultural competence development (of self and in others). TSE is the mediating factor that enhances persistence in cultural competence development despite obstacles, hardships, or stressors. Resilient TSE perceptions embrace lifelong learning in the quest to become "more" culturally competent and in the quest to assist others (learners and colleagues) to become more culturally competent.

Within the HCI there are many stressors or obstacles, therefore, it becomes increasingly important that individual staff nurses, nurse managers, nurse educators, nurse executives, administrators, and the organization develop and maintain resilience, motivation, commitment, and persistence for endeavors that foster cultural competence. It is proposed that individuals (and the organization) with resilient TSE perceptions

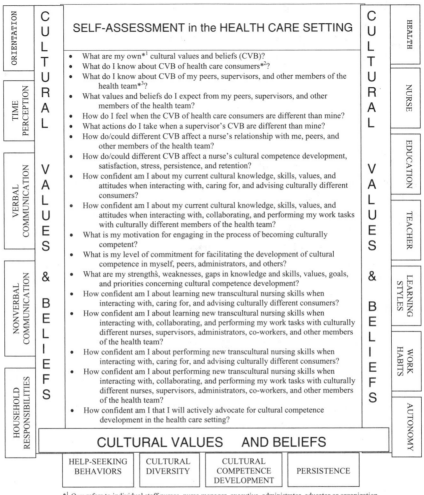

Figure 10.2   Self-Assessment in the Health Care Setting (Adapted from Jeffreys, 2004, p. 169)

persist in their endeavors to be active transcultural advocates or promoters of cultural competence in all dimensions of the HCI and professional practice. Figure 10.3 provides a guide for appraising values, beliefs, and actions and for determining whether or not one is an active role model in cultural competence development within the HCI or if there are factors restricting cultural competence development. (A user-friendly Active Promoter Assessment Tool-Health Care Institutions/Associations

Promoter	Values, Beliefs, and Actions	Promoter
Yes	Views cultural competence as important in own[1] life *and shares beliefs with others*[2,3]	No
Yes	Views cultural competence as important in staff's education, professional development, and future practice *and shares view with others*	No
Yes	Views own role to include active involvement in promoting cultural competence development among staff members *and shares view with others*	No
Yes	Routinely updates own knowledge and skills to enhance cultural competence *and shares relevant information with others*	No
Yes	Attends professional events concerning cultural competence development *and shares positive and relevant experiences with others*	No
Yes	Views professional event participation concerning cultural competence development as important in staff members' ongoing continuing education, professional development, and future practice *and shares view with others*	No
Yes	*Offers incentives to encourage staff members' participation in professional events*	No
Yes	Maintains professional partnerships focused on cultural competence development *and shares positive and relevant experiences with others*	No
Yes	Maintains membership(s) in professional organizations whose primary mission is cultural competence development *and shares positive and relevant experiences with others*	No
Yes	Views memberships in professional organizations/ associations (whose primary mission is cultural competence development) as important in staff's continuing education, professional development, and future practice *and shares view with others*	No
Yes	*Offers incentives to encourage other's participation in memberships in professional organizations/associations committed to cultural competence development*	No
Yes	Recognizes actual and potential barriers hindering the development of cultural competence *and initiates strategies to remove barriers*	No
Yes	*Implements strategies to encourage staff's development of cultural competence*	No
Yes	*Evaluates strategies implemented to encourage staff's development of cultural competence*	No

[1]*Own* refers to individual staff nurses, nurse manager, executive, administrator, educator or organization

[2]Active promoter/facilitator actions are indicated by italics

[3]*Other members of the health team* include professional and unlicensed health care providers

Figure 10.3 Self-Assessment: Active Promoter of Cultural Competence Development in the Health Care Institution

(APAT-HCIA) is available in the Cultural Competence Education Resource Toolkit [Jeffreys, 2010]. The APAT-HCIA may be used individually and/or in groups; the APAT-HCIA may be used alone or in conjunction with other toolkit items. (See instructions in Preface, Page xix.) It is proposed that the "actions taken to promote cultural competence development" is what makes one an active role model. Active role models influence cultural competence development in others by presenting opportunities for vicarious learning and via forms of persuasion (honest and judicious encouragement and feedback). By providing ongoing opportunities for high-quality mentoring, the HCI can enhance the power of modeling on self-efficacy appraisal and development of nurses at all levels within the HCI. The power of mentoring on nurses' professional development, satisfaction, quality of patient care, and retention has been well documented (Bosher & Pharris, 2009; Cavanaugh & Huse, 2004; Heller et al., 2004; Vance & Olson, 1998). E-mentoring is a strategy that can effectively connect nurses, mentors, and preceptors despite the barriers of distance, work schedules, and other responsibilities (Miller et al., 2008).

In addition, one needs to evaluate if the HCI is truly committed to the goal of cultural competence development and culturally congruent patient care for the right reasons. The right reasons mean guided by altruism, ethics, and patient advocacy rather than being motivated by accrediting body criteria that mandate evidence of cultural competence among employees and culturally competent health care among diverse client populations. This needs to be considered, because the relatively recent addition of cultural competence criteria by accrediting agencies correlate with many HCIs scrambling to produce evidence of cultural competence, especially when previously cultural competence was invisible, superficial, and/or unimportant. This applies for both minimum accreditation standards (standard accreditation) as well as for the more prestigious Magnet Status designation (Exhibit 10.1). One approach is to examine whether the HCI actively embraced cultural diversity and had cultural competence as a goal paired with opportunities for staff development prior to accrediting agencies' criteria mandating cultural competence. Actively embracing cultural diversity includes multiple, intensive strategies designed to recruit, retain, and encourage educational and career advancement among culturally diverse nurses, especially from groups underrepresented in nursing practice and nursing leadership. Tragically, cultural diversity within the nursing profession does not mirror the U. S. population; nurse leaders from underrepresented groups are even less visible (Burnes Bolton, 2004; Foley & Wurmser, 2004; Georges, 2004; Simpson, 2004; Swanson, 2004; Villarruel & Peragallo, 2004; Washington, Erickson, & Ditomassi, 2004). (The critical topic of enhancing cultural diversity within nursing is enormous; readers are referred to the current literature on nurse recruitment, retention, and professional advancement).

Exhibit 10.1   Overview of the Magnet Recognition Program® and Cultural Competence

Stephen R. Marrone, EdD, RN-BC, CTN-A
Deputy Nursing Director
Institute of Continuous Learning
State University of New York (SUNY)
SUNY Downstate Medical Center
Clinical Assistant Professor of Nursing
SUNY Downstate College of Nursing
Brooklyn, NY
Clinical Associate Professor of Nursing
Case Western Reserve University
Cleveland, OH
Adjunct Assistant Professor of Nursing Education
Teachers College Columbia University
New York, NY

The vision of the American Nurses Credentialing Center (ANCC), a subsidiary of the American Nurses Association (ANA), is that Magnet designated organizations will serve as the fount of knowledge and expertise for the delivery of nursing care in the global arena. To actualize this vision, the ANCC has articulated three principal goals of the Magnet Recognition Program® that include (1) promoting quality that supports professional nursing practice; (2) identifying excellence in the delivery of nursing services to consumers; and (3) disseminating nursing best practices (ANCC, 2009). Hence, the ANCC Magnet Recognition Program® was developed based on the ANA Nursing Administration: Scope and Standards of Practice (ANA, 2009) to recognize health care organizations that create and sustain a culture of nursing excellence and to serve as a venue for disseminating nursing best practices and strategies for the design of professional practice environments. Magnet designation is considered to be the highest recognition of nursing excellence globally (ANCC, 2008).

The Magnet Recognition Program® is based on findings of original research conducted in 1983 by the American Academy of Nursing (AAN) Task Force on Nursing Practice in Hospitals. The Task Force was commissioned to identify and describe the variables that created an environment that attracted and retained top nursing talent who promoted quality nursing care and outcomes (ANCC, 2009). These attributes of quality nursing practice are known as the 14 Forces of Magnetism. The 14 Forces of Magnetism include (1) quality of nursing leadership; (2) organizational structure; (3) management style;

(4) personnel policies and programs; (5) professional models of care; (6) quality of care; (7) quality improvement; (8) consultation and resources; (9) autonomy; (10) community and the health care organization; (11) nurses as teachers; (12) image of nursing; (13) interdisciplinary partnerships; and (14) professional development, and are incorporated throughout the Magnet Model.

The ANCC Magnet Model provides a framework for excellence in nursing practice and consists of five model components, namely, transformational leadership, structural empowerment, exemplary professional practice, new knowledge, innovations, and improvements, and empirical quality outcomes within an overarching framework of global issues in nursing and health care (ANCC, 2008). To achieve the Magnet designation, the ANCC utilizes a comprehensive and systematic approach to assess if the forces of magnetism are evident in the practice environment (ANCC, 2008). Successful organizations receive the Magnet designation for a period of 4 years and must redesignate every 4 years following a rigorous review of the professional practice environment.

In response to requests resulting from the changing demographics of health care consumers and providers, global trends in consumer and provider migration, the creation of international health care partnerships, the dissemination of new evidence, the use of technology, and the need for an international standard of nursing excellence, the ANCC Magnet Recognition Program® was expanded to recognize acute and long-term care organizations in the United States and abroad. As a result, cultural competency of health care practitioners in meeting the care needs of diverse and vulnerable patients, families and communities is a thread that is woven throughout the ANCC Magnet Model. Today, more that 300 health care organizations in the United States, Australia, and New Zealand have achieved the Magnet designation, the vast majority of which are located in the United States. There is a great international interest in the Magnet designation among the English-speaking countries of the world as well as in the Middle East where an expatriate health care workforce prevails.

Health care organizations that have been successful in achieving the Magnet designation and redesignation have well-designed and integrated cultural competency programs across the continuum of care and for all health care disciplines. Magnet designated organizations have developed, implemented, and evaluated comprehensive Diversity Models that enable them to provide evidence that describes how (1) respect for diversity is articulated in the organization and nursing mission, vision, values, strategies priorities, quality initiatives, and staff and patient satisfaction plans; (2) the organization and nursing addresses the health care needs of the community by establishing community partnerships and outreach programs; (3) the organization and nursing identifies and addresses disparities in the management of health care needs of diverse patient populations; and (4) nurses use resources to meet the unique and individual needs of patients and families (ANCC, 2008).

The oversight for Diversity Models is typically provided by a Chief Diversity Officer and/or a Transdisciplinary Diversity Council who have the requisite knowledge and experience in leading diversity initiatives. Diversity Models characteristically include (1) an organizational infrastructure (policies, procedures, strategic plan, performance criteria, and performance appraisal) that supports respect for and celebrates diversity and the minimization of health disparities; (2) the collection and analysis of demographic data by identifying the prevalent cultural, ethnic, linguistic, and spiritual groups represented among health care consumers and providers so as to design systems and processes to reduce health disparities related to culture and/or language; (3) collaboration among the diversity council, human resources, nursing retention and recruitment, and nursing and transdisciplinary councils to ensure an understanding of diversity issues within the organization; (4) establishing community partnerships with key cultural, ethnic, and spiritual leaders; (5) evidence-based initial and ongoing education and cultural competency assessment for practitioners, in general, and strategies to meet the culture care needs of the demographic characteristics of the service area; (6) cultural resources for practitioners at the point of care; (7) strategies to recruit, retain, and promote staff diversity representative of the service area at all levels of the organization; (8) language assistance (signage, interpretation services, and translation of critical documents (consents, patient education materials) in the key languages spoken by the groups represented among health care consumers; (9) culturally and linguistically sensitive grievance resolution procedures; (10) documentation systems that include an initial and ongoing patient cultural assessment and the integration and communication of assessment findings into the individualized transdisciplinary plan of care; and (11) evaluation of the impact and outcomes of the diversity model by benchmarking actual outcomes against established performance standards.

A major focus of the Magnet Recognition Program® is that organizations meet or exceed organizational, nursing, patient, and consumer outcomes when compared to national benchmarks. Outcomes such as overall patient satisfaction and satisfaction with nursing care, educational information, and pain management, and the impact of community outreach programs on community health and welfare are outcomes that may be influenced by the organization's commitment to the cultural competency of its practitioners. The successful achievement of Magnet Recognition is evidenced by creating and sustaining a "Magnet culture," a culture where a professional nursing practice environment, patient safety, quality patient outcomes, evidence-based practice, and transdisciplinary collaboration are woven into the fabric of the organizational infrastructure, thus providing consumers with the definitive standard of the quality of nursing care that they can be expected to receive.

A second approach is to consider "if the accrediting agency removed cultural competence from their evaluative criteria, would the HCI and its employees still allocate the same amount of time, money, and energy toward cultural competence development or would cultural competence be less valued?" These two major considerations are important because nurses exist within the organizational culture of the HCI and are greatly influenced by the opportunities, values, and expectations provided by the HCI (Neumann & Forsyth, 2008; Thorpe & Loo, 2003). Organizational cultures truly committed to cultural competence exert positive influence on nurses' values, commitment, satisfaction, and motivation (Leininger, 1994b). Furthermore, organizations that actively reach out to culturally diverse patients, nurses, and communities provide a wealth of opportunities and benefits to all. An important goal is to aim for optimal cultural competence, rather than merely "passing" accreditation criteria (i.e., the achievement of minimum standards). (See Chapter 1 and Preface.)

Motivation behind nurses' participation in cultural competence development inservices, continuing education, and/or workshops may not be ideal. For example, a nurse who attends a workshop because it is required for continued employment, salary increase, promotion, and/or transfer is extrinsically motivated by superficial or personal reasons, rather than intrinsically motivated by altruism, the desire for professional and personal growth and development, and improved patient care. Consequently, multidimensional learner characteristics will need to be evaluated before the design of any educational interventions. Typically, educators within the HCI are challenged with providing high-quality educational programs for nurses who represent cultural, educational, and career diversity (Bibb et al., 2003; Billings, 2004; Billings & Kowalski, 2008; Brathwaite, 2005; Collins, 2002; Harrington & Walker, 2004; Horsfall & Cleary, 2008; Mathews, 2003; Rashotte & Thomas, 2002; Schim et al., 2007). Developing strategies to shift extrinsic motivation to intrinsic motivation is one challenge for the HCI sincerely committed to developing cultural competence at high levels of excellence (optimal cultural competence). (See Chapter 12.) The author contends that cultural competence is unachievable unless individuals are intrinsically motivated; resilient TSE (confidence) will positively influence intrinsic motivation and persistence at cultural competence development of self and others.

EVALUATION IN THE HEALTH CARE INSTITUTION

Following the template for systematic evaluation in the academic setting (see Chapter 6), evaluation in the HCI begins with examining how visible (or invisible) cultural competency development is actively present: (a) overall within the institution; (b) specifically at the individual unit (site) level and; (c) via outside connections to supplementary resources. A systematic evaluative inquiry should also be guided by two additional questions: (1) To what degree is cultural competence an integral component within the HCI? and (2) How do all the cultural components fit together? (Figure 10.4) A thorough evaluation of what currently exists (Jeffreys Toolkit 2010, Item 16) serves as a valuable precursor to informed decisions, responsible actions, and new diagnostic-prescriptive innovations targeting staff development and improved patient care outcomes in the overall goal of achieving optimal cultural competence. The

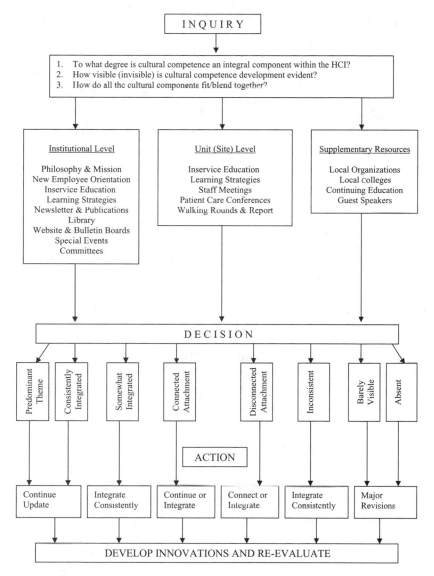

Figure 10.4 Systematic Inquiry for Decision, Action, and Innovation: Health Care Institutions (HCI)

following sections address major areas for inquiry, action, and innovation within the HCI.

Institution

Careful perusal of the HCI's philosophy, mission, and purpose may lend valuable insight into the HCI's worldview (perspective) on resources, resource allocation, profit goals, cultural diversity, cultural competence development, targeted patient populations and objectives, employee empowerment, nursing profession, decision making, and organizational priorities (Jeffreys Toolkit 2010, Item 16, Part 1). For example, a non-profit HCI, whose mission statement and philosophy attest to provide culturally congruent health care to culturally diverse individuals despite ability to pay, provides some beginning, favorable information concerning the desire to achieve cultural competence. However, without sufficient resources or strategies to (a) develop cultural competence of health care providers; (b) create culturally specific professional care actions; and/or (c) evaluate strategy outcomes, positive goal achievement is unlikely. Close inspection at the institutional level must also assess whether cultural competency development is emphasized substantially, equally, and symmetrically throughout the HCI beyond philosophy, mission, and purpose to such areas as new employee orientation, inservice education, learning strategies, newsletter and publications, library, Web site, bulletin boards, special events, and committees (see Chapters 11 and 12). Unfortunately, budget constraints, staffing shortage, and hospital restructuring has resulted in decreased HCI resources for new employee orientation, inservice education, and continuing education (Ellerton & Gregor, 2003 Pinkerton, 2004; Williams & Jones, 2004). Sample innovations particularly important to the development of cultural competence are presented in the Educator-in-Action Vignette and can also be used to guide inquiry. Several major areas will be described below.

New Employee Orientation

New employee orientation has the potential to initially introduce and reinforce the HCI's philosophy and purposes specifically concerning cultural competence development. Achievement of cultural competence must expand beyond meeting minimum levels of proficiency in clinical practice (product outcome view) to expecting ongoing efforts aimed at optimal cultural competence development in self and others (process view). Nurse educators at new employee orientations have the potential to make a tremendous difference by introducing, emphasizing, fostering, and nurturing cultural competence development throughout the new employee orientation (see Chapter 11). Emphasizing ongoing education as a professional commitment to lifelong learning has the potential to raise motivation for learning. By presenting learning goals and outcomes with long-term broader professional and personal benefits rather than as merely employer expectations, occupational tasks, or job requirements, the emphasis will be on professional expectations, standards, and excellence. Emphasis on autonomy, accountability, self-regulation, and ethics is consistent with professional standards and expectations (ANA, 2001, 2003, 2004) and can serve as intrinsic motivators (Kubsch et al., 2003). In contrast, mandatory workshops without connections to professionalism limit outcome results (Jones-Schenk & Yoder-Wise, 2002). Linking new employee learning with unit-specific examples and connections with other HCI resources and supplementary resources illustrates an easily accessible pathway to continue on the journey of cultural competence development paved by HCI's instrumental and philosophical support for cultural competence endeavors. For example, case study discussion and reflection transform passive classroom orientation into active, multidimensional, and synthesized learning (Rashotte & Thomas, 2002; Tomey, 2003; White, Amos, & Kouzekanani, 1999). Such multidimensional strategies should aim to optimize learning in the affective domain (Neumann & Forsyth, 2008). Supplementing learning with computer-assisted instructional programs, online continuing education programs, Web based programs, satellite TV programs, videotapes, and simulation programs are other innovative options discussed in the literature (Bibb et al., 2003 Carter & Rukholm, 2008; Harrington & Walker, 2004; JCAHCO, 2002; Mateo & McMyler, 2004; Matzo, et al., 2002; Pastuszak & Rodowicz, 2002; Piercy, 2004; Squires, 2002; Sweeney, et al., 2008).

As adult learners, new employees' motivation will be heightened with direct application and explicit ties to the unit (site) level (see Chapters 11 and 12). Partnering follow-up learning activities on the unit (site) level provides opportunities for applying general principles to specific patient situations. Assessing learner characteristics (including TSE perceptions) and pairing learners with experienced mentors who can serve as role models and offer encouragement will enhance cultural competence development. Self-efficacy perceptions will be greatly enhanced if models display effort and perform tasks successfully rather than models who complete the task effortlessly (Bandura, 1986; Schunk, 1987). Preparing preceptors adequately includes the use of techniques to enhance cultural competence learning, higher order-thinking (Davidson, 2009) and affective learning (Neumann & Forsyth, 2008).

Physiological indices such as manifestations of stress and anxiety also interfere with confidence and learning (Bandura, 1986). Typically, the stress of a new job, new orientation, and perhaps a new career (for graduate nurses) exist during orientations, thereby creating additional challenges. Although nurse residency programs or post-graduate training programs for new graduate nurses may present positive solutions, financial constraints and scarce human resources present grave limitations (JCAHCO, 2002). Sufficient supports for graduate nurses during the transitional process may include mentors, preceptors, prolonged general and unit-based orientation, review of reality shock phenomena and strategies for successful coping, positive professional socialization opportunities, and ongoing support beyond the orientation and probation period (Duchscher, 2004). Similarly, well-planned transitional interventions beginning with tailored orientation programs are strongly recommended for internationally recruited nurses (Sherman & Eggenberger, 2008; Zizzo & Xu, 2009) and inactive nurses returning to work (Hammer & Craig, 2008).

Unit (Site) Level

Although accountability for cultural competence development and culturally congruent health care delivery is a shared responsibility of individual staff nurses, nurse educators, and nurse managers, the nurse manager is ultimately responsible for holding staff accountable for developing and maintaining competencies (Mateo & McMyler, 2004). Delineating clear expectations and penalties for noncompliance, offering supportive strategies and rewards for developing competence, initiating corrective measures when necessary, and acknowledging positive achievements optimizes the achievement of successful outcomes and minimizes the risk of noncompliance (Mateo & McMyler, 2004). Again, emphasizing the importance of cultural competence development as a lifelong commitment to professional development and the enhancement of patient care reminds nurses of their individual responsibility to uphold professional standards. Thus, the shifted emphasis on individual professional accountability attempts to stimulate and nurture intrinsic motivation, thereby replacing the potentially, previously held, predominant influence of extrinsic motivators with true motivation and commitment (see Chapter 12).

Objectively appraising the daily routines, rituals, and activities specific within the unit (setting) and within the context of cultural competence and culturally congruent patient care as desirable outcomes requires time, expertise, and dedication. Table 10.1 presents select activities with cultural competence application common across a variety of settings. (Jeffreys 2010, Item 16). Because culturally congruent patient care begins with accurate, sensitive assessment of individual patient's cultural values, beliefs, practices, and behaviors, it is essential that the initial health history interview and physical examination incorporate cultural components visibly and substantially. First, inspection of the demographic

Table 10.1   Select Activities with Cultural Competence Application

Activity	Cultural Competence Application
Health History Interview	• Systematic cultural assessment is incorporated within the health history interview. • Interview form reflects key cultural assessment areas particularly relevant for setting or unit.
Physical Examination	• Physical examination assessments and documentation are adapted to meet cultural needs and biophysical differences • Physical examination form is free of cultural biases and includes physical assessment areas particularly relevant for setting or unit and for numerous different cultural groups
Change of Shift Report	Culture-specific care actions are discussed: • Preservation or maintenance • Accommodation or negotiation • Repatterning or restructuring
Patient Record	Culture-specific care actions are documented: • Preservation or maintenance • Accommodation or negotiation • Repatterning or restructuring
Patient Care Plan Patient Teaching Plan Patient Discharge Plan	Culture-specific care actions are planned, implemented, and evaluated: • Preservation or maintenance • Accommodation or negotiation • Repatterning or restructuring
Patient Care Conferences	• Topics focus on cultural competence development • Clinical topics include relevant case exemplars representing culturally diverse patients.
Walking Rounds	Incorporate culturally congruent approaches for introductions, communication, and physical examination
Staff Meetings	• Incorporate culturally appropriate strategies for cultural diverse staff • Address issues and topics to enhance cultural competence • Promote multicultural workplace harmony • Promote culturally congruent patient care • Include resources with cultural expertise as needed
Multidisciplinary Communication & Collaboration	Incorporate culturally congruent approaches for introductions, communication, and designing culture-specific care actions

(continued)

Table 10.1 Select Activities with Cultural Competence Application
(*continued*)

Activity	Cultural Competence Application
Unit-Based Inservice Education	• Topics focus on cultural competence development • Clinical topics include relevant case exemplars representing culturally diverse patients. • Utilize multidimensional teaching–learning strategies that incorporate cognitive, practical, affective dimensions, and transcultural self-efficacy • Relevant journal articles and other resources are available • Relevant information is posted on the staff bulletin board or in the communication book.
Patient Teaching Materials	Include literature and resources specific to consumers' ethnicity, religion, preferred language, socioeconomic status, geographic location, developmental level, educational level, and health needs.

form and health history interview (institution- or unit-specific) should be free of bias and reflect key cultural assessment areas particularly relevant for the setting or unit. For example, are patients (a) invited to self-identify with ethnic group affiliation(s) as an open-ended question; (b) asked to select one or more ethnic group affiliation options including an open-ended fill-in; (c) instructed to pick one category only; or (d) assigned a category by the admission nurse or physician? Examining whether health history forms include details about folk medicine practices, home remedies, spiritual rituals, and non-Western health practices should also appraise if questions are presented equally with questions about Western medicine, and whether questions are presented first, last, integrated, or as an afterthought. Subtle, culturally incongruent and insensitive messages may often be unintentional or unconsciously incompetent; however, they can hinder communication and assessment. Second, information forms are only meaningful if nurses (and other health professionals) have the appropriate knowledge, skills, values, and confidence to use them appropriately with culturally diverse patients and to document findings clearly.

It is important that assessment findings be translated into culturally specific and congruent plans of care; however, this activity must extend beyond mere written documentation. Active integration of culturally congruent patient care must extend throughout all unit- or setting-based activities such as change of shift report, walking rounds, patient care conferences, patient teaching, delegation of tasks, staff meetings, and multidisciplinary collaboration. Realistic and feasible opportunities for ongoing staff development and inservice education are enhanced through multidimensional teaching-learning innovations. Especially in times of limited financial and human resources, it is essential to determine priorities based on immediate needs, learner characteristics, and available resources (see Chapter 12).

PRIORITIZATION

Following transcultural generalist principles introduced or reintroduced at new employee orientation and reinforced through later inservices, subsequent educational opportunities for cultural competence development should be available, building on previous knowledge, skills, values, and confidence. Promoting cultural competence is a broad, massive topic to undertake, therefore determining priority focus areas will assist in the justification for allocation of limited resources (such as time, money, and expertise). The first question, What are the priority issues or focus areas? is subsequently followed by the second question, How can priority issues be determined? Although several approaches may be employed, this chapter will present a strategy comprising three main considerations: (1) target populations; (2) learner characteristics; and (3) educational resources. Table 10.2 presents sample questions to guide prioritization.

Determining target patient populations may be initiated throughout the HCI with specific focus on select units or be initiated at the unit-based level (see Chapter 12). The method of determining patient target areas should first begin by determining the presence of cultural groups present within the geographic region. Then, which groups use, do not use, or underutilize health care services should be determined, thereby contrasting actual patient profiles with potential patient profiles. Decisions can be further guided by considering national goals in eliminating health disparities as well as local issues. Justifiable and feasible rationale for the selected group must be defensible when considering learner characteristics and educational resources. In other words, target population selection should not be determined in isolation from other major considerations (see Educator-In-Action Vignette). Detailing an initial broad list of potential target patient populations demonstrates the existence of diverse cultural groups typically grouped together under broad demographic categories. If health care is to be truly culturally congruent, then culture care

Table 10.2   Sample Questions to Guide Prioritization

Sample Questions to Guide Prioritization

Target Populations
1. Which cultural groups are present in the geographic region and *USE* health care services?
2. Which cultural groups are present in the geographic region and *DO NOT USE or UNDER-UTILIZE* health care services?
3. Of the above groups, which ones should be targeted first?
4. Why? What is the underlying rationale?
   - Significant health problem
   - Largest cultural group
   - Newest cultural group
   - Victims of discrimination and bias
   - Marginalized group
   - Poorly understood group by health care personnel
   - Other
5. What are the specific desired goals for the targeted population(s)?

Learner Characteristics
1. What are learners' background, identity, values, and beliefs?

Profile Characteristics	*Affective Factors*
Age	Cultural values and beliefs
Ethnicity	Transcultural self-efficacy
Race	Motivation
Gender	
Socioeconomic	
Religion	
Primary (first) language	
Prior education	
Prior work experience	

2. What are learner strengths?
3. What are learner weaknesses?
4. What learning gaps are/may be present?
5. What biases are/may be present?
6. What prior *formalized* learning (related to culture) can provide a foundation for continued and ongoing learning?

Educational Resources
1. What learning opportunities for transcultural nursing exist(ed)?
2. What are the specific desired goals for the targeted population(s)?
3. What resources are currently available?
4. What resources are necessary to achieve goals of developing cultural competency for targeted population(s)?
5. What resources are most easily attainable?
6. Who can design, implement, and evaluate multidimensional strategies to maximize learning?

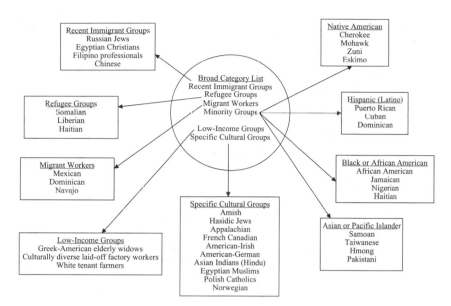

Figure 10.5 Determining Target Populations: Sample Broad Category List and Sample Detailed List

must be specific to specific cultural groups, necessitating differentiation within and between groups. Figure 10.5 presents a sample broad and detailed list.

A decision based on comprehensive assessment of patient populations, learner characteristics, and educational resources proposes realistic goals capitalizing on learner strengths and educational resources. Furthermore, creatively designing multidimensional teaching–learning strategies to enhance cultural competence development has the potential to bring learning to higher levels of synthesis and internalization and foster realistic self-efficacy appraisal and resilience. Ongoing inservice education or a series of transcultural workshops are two examples of education initiatives coordinated through staff development (see Exhibits 10.2–10.4; Figure 6.4). While this is important, fragmented educational components that are (or seem) disconnected from each other and from other activities within the HCI offer limited opportunities for cultural competence development. Coordinating the development of cognitive, practical, and affective learning requires much planning and interconnectedness. Connecting innovations in cultural competence development may be achieved through publicity, publications, special events, and committees and by developing a collaborative network of supplementary resources beyond the HCI. For example, if the systematic decision-making process results in the decision to target "Enhancing Cultural Competence in the Care of Recent Egyptian Immigrants," connecting innovations may be done by:

- Publicizing workshop series on bulletin boards, staff Web site or listserve, hospital Internet site, staff meeting announcement, flyer attached to paycheck, personal letter, flyers, personal communication between unit liaison nurse on each shift who will personally invite other staff nurses, hospital newsletter, and/or local newspaper and TV announcements.
- Purchasing, borrowing, organizing, and displaying relevant professional and consumer literature in HCI library.
- Offering traditional Egyptian food choices every Thursday for 2 months in the cafeteria, partnered with posters and handouts describing the food choices, cultural meaning of food, nutritional values, method of preparation, estimated cost per serving, dietary accommodations for patients on specific prescribed diets, and other relevant information. (Avoid planning activity during months with a large number of religious fast days.)
- Featured cultural expert who will be part of workshop series, continuing education program, consultation, and/or conference.
- Relevant journal article, brief article summary outline, appropriate referral resources, and pertinence to specific unit posted on staff bulletin boards on each unit.
- Agenda for the monthly institutional committee meeting for cultural competence development focuses on the designated topic.
- Collaboration and cosponsorship of conference focused on (or incorporating) selected topic with relevant Ethnic Nursing Organization, local chapter of Transcultural Nursing Society, or other professional organization.
- Creating an advisory board focused on the selected topic with related local organizations, universities, community groups, staff nurses, nurse educators, nurse executives, and other members of the multidisciplinary health care team.
- Quality assurance team develops comprehensive plan to evaluate educational innovations.

Supplementary Resources

For the HCI, utilization of selective supplementary resources outside the HCI has the potential to optimize cultural competence development. Examples of supplementary resources include local organizations, local colleges, continuing education programs, and guest speakers. Resources that embrace cultural diversity, by being culturally friendly and inclusive of culturally diverse and academically diverse health professionals and patients, create caring environments that foster feelings of integration, satisfaction, and cultural congruence with the nursing profession and educational institution. For example, the aforementioned supplementary resources outwardly display a celebration of diversity if respective brochures, posters, mentors, employees, workshops, invited guest speakers, events, meetings, and student participants appropriately represent a variety of cultural groups.

Appraising existing supplementary resources beyond their superficial appearance may uncover untapped areas necessitating further action, expansion, inclusiveness, and innovation. Similarly, discovery that supplementary resources do not exist suggests the need for immediate action and innovation. Several ideas are listed below:

- Develop collaborative partnerships with local college librarians
- Share new library resources for cultural competence development
- Revise HCI recruitment brochures to feature health care professionals of different age, gender, and cultural groups
- Advertise upcoming cultural events, holidays, and workshops on bulletin boards
- Host an international food festival
- Cosponsor a cultural workshop with STTI chapter and involve HCI employees as volunteers
- Sponsor nurses and other health professionals for participation in cultural nursing conference and/or elimination of health disparities conference
- Establish networks with local ethnic nursing organizations
- Host a local chapter meeting of the transcultural nursing society
- Raffle a membership in the Transcultural Nursing Society and local chapter
- Invite guest speakers from different cultural backgrounds to speak about cultural topics

EVALUATION

The most comprehensive education evaluation plan includes formative and summative components that are explicitly tied to the educational strategy's goal and purpose and are objectively measured. Formative evaluations assess the process of a strategy rather than outcomes and can be monitored as the strategy is implemented. Through systematic and ongoing formative evaluations, the documentation of specific activities and the identification of desired outcomes, anticipated strengths, as well as any difficulties, snags, weaknesses, and/or problems, will allow for diagnostic-prescriptive modifications based on learner's feedback obtained from consistent qualitative and quantitative data collection. Summative evaluations assess the achievement of desired learning outcomes or program outcomes and are monitored at the completion of the teaching strategy or educational program. Summative evaluations are strengthened via a multidimensional approach that includes cognitive, practical, and affective components using quantitative and qualitative data.

Every educational evaluation plan should include formative and evaluative components that are realistic, positively phrased, and provide valid, valuable feedback. Evaluation plans that are unrealistic and difficult to measure objectively should be avoided because data will be invalid, unreliable, and therefore useless. For example, a formative evaluation goal that states "All cultural competence workshop participants will rate all speakers as 'excellent'" does not allow for disparate responses that discriminate between different speakers' strengths. Disparate and discriminating responses are desirable to substantiate validity of responses or respondents' ability and willingness to think carefully about each item, differentiate between items, and select a thoughtful and honest response (Sudman & Bradburn, 1991). Modification of this goal as "The majority (or 80%) of cultural competence workshop participants will be satisfied with the overall program and individual program components as seen by at least 80% of workshop participants selecting a '4—satisfied' or '5—very satisfied' on the Workshop Evaluation Survey Tool (WEST)." Exhibit 10.2 presents an example of a formative evaluation plan, data collection, data analysis, and future implications. This example could be adapted to evaluate other cultural competence development initiatives within the institution, unit (setting) level, and supplementary (collaborative) resources (see also Exhibit 12.3).

Exhibit 10.2 Innovations in Cultural Competence Development: Formative Evaluation Plan, Implementation, and Implications

Goal: Staff nurses are satisfied with the Cultural Competence Development Series Workshops as seen by 80% of nurses selecting "4" (satisfied) or "5" (very satisfied) on the Workshop Evaluation Survey Tool (WEST).

- **What:** Satisfaction will be at least 80%
- **Who:** Among workshop participants (nurses)
- **Where:** Hospital workshop
- **When:** After completion of Workshop 1
- **How:** As measured by the WEST
- **Why:** Satisfaction level provides information for guiding future workshops, identifying areas of high, moderate, and low satisfaction. It is proposed that high levels of satisfaction will enhance cultural

competence educational learning, motivation, and transcultural self-efficacy.

Data Collection: WEST is administered after workshop 1 in a series of 5 planned "Enhance Your Cultural Competency" workshops given over the next 12 months.

Quantitative Data Analysis indicates:

- Overall satisfaction
- 87% of nurses selected "4" or "5" responses on the majority of WEST items
- 92% of nurses selected "4" or "5" responses on items concerning satisfaction with learning outcomes achieved within cognitive, practical, and affective domains.
- High satisfaction with speaker 1 and with the video
- Moderate satisfaction with guest speaker 2 and with the PowerPoint slides

Qualitative Data: Comments from respondents suggest that:

- Speaker 2 should wear a microphone and slides should be larger
- Workshops should be 15 minutes longer to allow for questions and to enhance learning
- Participants were unaware of the impact of own cultural values and beliefs on the care of culturally different patients.
- Workshop participants expressed appreciation with being asked for their feedback.

Empirically Based Interventions for Quality Improvement (some possibilities):

- Continue with workshop series
- Invite back speaker 1 and continue to show the video
- Invite back speaker 2 provided he/she uses a microphone and revises (enlarges) slides*
- Extend workshops 15 minutes to allow for questions and dialogue*
- Provide opportunity for nurses to discuss and share their raised awareness with each other*
- Continue to administer WEST after each workshop and modify or continue with educational strategies.
- Continue to emphasize importance of participants' feedback*

---

*Rationale for these interventions was provided by the solicitation of qualitative comments. Making decisions based solely on quantitative data is self-limiting. For example, based solely on the quantitative data in this scenario, speaker 2 might not have been invited back as a presenter despite expertise.

Within the HCI, summative evaluations may often target both measurable changes in the learner and changes in patient outcomes and cost outcomes. If changes are to be truly documented, it is extremely important that pretest measures are conducted before any strategy is implemented and that strategies are followed by appropriate posttest measures that permit valid and reliable data analyses. Without pre- and posttests, the influence of the intervention (independent variable) on the dependent variable(s) cannot be established. Although qualitative methodologies provide unique, valuable data that is usually otherwise unobtainable, the reality of current funding initiatives is that strong quantitative findings generally substantiate further funding for teaching and practice innovations. Qualitative data will add richness to the overall understanding of the phenomenon under investigation, thereby providing valuable information to guide future strategy interventions.

Constraints in HCI resources (money, staff, time, equipment) place increasing demands on conserving resources to those endeavors that have proved positive, desirable outcomes. "The return on investment in nursing will be reflected both in cost savings and in improvements in the safety and quality of care provided" (JCAHO, 2002, p. 17). It is therefore not only beneficial but it is essential to have patient outcome indicators that demonstrate tangible increases in HCI revenue, income, or access; decrease costs; or other positive outcomes. Such outcome measures necessitate quantitative methodology (Exhibit 10.3). Unfortunately, few studies have investigated the impact of cultural competence education on health outcomes, patient behavior change, satisfaction, or health care delivery (Fortier & Bishop, 2003), although the impact of culturally congruent patient care on clinical outcomes has been demonstrated (Majumdar et al., 2004; MSH, 2005). Measurable outcome indicators are needed (OMH, 2005). Cost savings can be demonstrated with increased nurse retention, increased staffing that eliminates the need for overtime or outside agency nurses, decreased staffing vacancies, and/or decreased absences that are specifically correlated with increased nurses' satisfaction following a sequence of workshops, special events, or other cultural competence initiatives. Evaluating changes in learners' TSE perceptions using the Transcultural Self-Efficacy Tool (TSET) presents a quantitative measure for evaluating changes within cognitive, practical, and affective dimensions (see Exhibit 10.4 and TSET Research Exhibit 10.1). TSET Multidisciplinary Healthcare Provider (TSET-MHP) version is adapted from TSET to measure and evaluate learners' confidence (TSE) for performing general transcultural skills among diverse client populations. Items are exactly the same as original TSET. Directions change "nurse" and "nursing" focus to "health care provider" focus, encompassing nursing and all other multidisciplinary health care provider groups. (TSET Research Exhibit 10.2 and Jeffreys 2010 Toolkit, Item 2).

Exhibit 10.3   Innovations in Cultural Competence Education: Summative Evaluation—Sample for Measuring Changes in Patient Outcomes (Access, Quality, & Cost)

Desired Outcome 1: Patient satisfaction among Mexican American patients at the diabetic outpatient clinic will increase following diabetic clinic RNs' completion of 5 "Cultural Competent Care for Mexican-Americans" workshops and as measured by the Patient Satisfaction Survey (PSS).

- **What:** Patient satisfaction will increase
- **Who:** Among Mexican American clients
- **Where:** At the diabetic clinic
- **When:** Following diabetic clinic RN's completion of 5 "Cultural Competent Care for Mexican-Americans" workshops
- **How:** *Measured by* the Patient Satisfaction Survey (PSS).
- **Why:** It is assumed that educational workshops specifically targeting culturally competent care for Mexican Americans within a specialty area (diabetic clinic) will result in the provision of more cultural competent care to Mexican Americans, thereby increasing patient satisfaction. Satisfaction is an indicator of enhanced quality of care.
- **Independent Variable:** Educational intervention (Cultural Competent Care for Mexican American workshops)
- **Dependent Variable:** Patient satisfaction

Independent Variable	Dependent Variable	Measurement Tool	Desired Outcomes
Workshops	Patient satisfaction	PSS	↑ satisfaction

Data Collection: Administer PSS to Mexican American patients at the diabetic clinic before the start of Workshop 1 and 1 month after Workshop 5. (Cross-sectional study design).

Data Analysis: Compare survey results.

- *Quantitative:*
  - Did PSS scores change in the expected direction?
  - What were patients most satisfied about?
  - What were patients least satisfied about?
  - Would patients refer others to use general hospital services?
- *Qualitative:* What comments and common themes emerged?

Results (select examples):

- *Quantitative:*
  - Statistically significant increases in PSS scores indicated a significant increase in overall patient satisfaction
  - Patients were most satisfied about the presence of bilingual personnel, variety of dietary samples specific for Mexican Americans as well as other samples that acknowledged the influence of acculturation and exposure to other multicultural foods available in the surrounding community.
  - Patients were least satisfied about the clinic hours and waiting times averaging approximately 40 minutes.
  - 78% of patients indicated that they would refer others to use general hospital services; this was an increase from last year's rate of 52%.

- *Qualitative:*
  - 90% of comments were positive, indicating satisfaction with various services within the clinic. In particular, patients noted the attentiveness, respect, and personalized attention of staff to cultural needs, especially the inclusion of family (as per patient's preference)
  - 10% of the comments indicated dissatisfaction related to clinic hours and waiting times. Several patients suggested hiring more staff to decrease waiting times and changing hours to coincide with the bus schedule.

Implications (some possibilities)

- Continue with cultural competence workshop series for newly hired employees
- Expand cultural competence workshop series to other specialty areas and units
- Expand cultural competence workshop series to target other cultural groups predominant in the area (as per prioritization guidelines suggested in Table 10.2 and Figure 10.5)
- Change clinic hours to coincide with the bus schedule
- Hire two more RNs and one more receptionist (bilingual preferred) for peak clinic hours
- Continue with a variety of dietary menus offered at the clinic
- Expand dietary menus in other areas and units to provide multiple options and personalize to patients' dietary preferences and uses

Desired Outcome 2: Hospitalization rates and ER usage among Mexican American diabetic clinic patients will decrease and regularly scheduled attendance at diabetic clinic appointments will increase following RN completion of Workshop 5 (increased access to primary preventive care, increased quality, decreased cost).

- **What:** Hospitalization rates and ER usage will decrease and regularly scheduled attendance at diabetic clinic appointments will increase
- **Who:** Among Mexican American diabetic clinic patients
- **Where:** Diabetic clinic
- **When:** Following RN completion of also as Workshop 5
- **How:** As measured by admission rates, ER usage rates, and clinic appointment attendance records
- **Why:** Increased access to primary preventive care (clinic appointment attendance records) will result in increased quality of care and decreased need for ER usage, thereby decreasing costs.
- **Independent Variable:** Educational intervention (Cultural Competent Care for Mexican American workshops)
- **Dependent Variable:** Hospitalization rates, ER usage, and regularly scheduled attendance at diabetic clinic appointments

Independent Variable	Dependent Variables	Measurement Tool	Desired Outcomes
Workshops	Hospitalization rates	Hospital records	↓ hospitalization rates
	ER usage		↓ ER usage
	Clinic attendance rates		↑ clinic attendance rates

Data Collection: Collect relevant data monthly for 3 months before initiating Workshop 1, monthly during Workshop series, and then monthly for 6 months after Workshop 5. (Also collect other data such as staffing trends, workshop series participants, and nurse retention to check for control, consistency, and/or extraneous variables.)

Data Analysis: Compare rates.

- What data trends occurred?
- What were the statistically significant results?
- Were there any threats to internal and external validity?

Results (select examples)

- Hospitalization rates decreased 14% (statistically significant)
- ER usage rates decreased 23% (statistically significant)
- Clinic attendance rates increased 47% (statistically significant)
- Low staffing during September (attributed to two nurses retiring, one nurse on maternity leave), and the hiring of per diem nurses (non-workshop participants) may have adversely influenced results

Interpretation (select examples)

- Positive changes were noted in the desired direction following the educational intervention (5 workshop series); however, some intervening variables (low staffing during September may have skewed the results, i.e., results may have been even more favorable)

Implications (some possibilities)

- Continue with data collection and compare results
- Continue to track staffing patterns for possible intervening variables
- Continue with workshop series for newly hired employees to the clinic area
- Expand workshop series to other targeted areas in the hospital and clinic settings with targeted cultural groups (based on prioritization determination)

Desired Outcome 3: Hospital annual revenue will increase 5% as seen by the increased number of new patients (using any hospital services) referred by Mexican American patients attending the diabetic clinic, by hearing about hospital's *Culturally Congruent Care for Mexican Americans* staff workshops, or by hearing about cultural sensitivity of nurses and as measured by annual revenue changes and New Patient Survey (NPS)

- **What:** Hospital annual revenue will increase 5%
- **Who:** New patients
- **Where:** Any hospital service
- **When:** Referred by Mexican American patients attending the diabetic clinic, by hearing about hospital's *Culturally Congruent Care for Mexican Americans* staff workshops, or by hearing about cultural sensitivity of nurses
- **How:** Measured by annual revenue changes and New Patient Survey (NPS)
- **Why:** Appraisal of costs associated with 5 workshop series in comparison with increased income generated as a result of referred clients pre-educational intervention and post-educational intervention will determine cost effectiveness. (gains versus losses).
- **Independent Variable:** Educational intervention (Cultural Competent Care for Mexican American workshops)
- **Dependent Variable:** Hospital revenue generated from new patients (using any hospital services) referred by Mexican American patients attending the diabetic clinic or by hearing about hospital's "Cultural Congruent Care for Mexican-Americans" staff workshops, or by hearing about cultural sensitivity of nurses.

Independent Variable	Dependent Variables	Measurement Tool	Desired Outcomes
Workshops	Hospital revenue	Annual revenue; NPS	↑ revenue (5%)

Data Collection: Ask new patients (using any hospital services) to complete New Patient Survey (NPS) (why they chose hospital)

- 3 months before initiating workshops and
- then monthly for 1 year after workshop 1

- *Data Analysis:* Calculate number of new patients and hospital revenue generated from new patients who chose hospital based on specified criteria.
- *Results:* (select sample)
  - Hospital revenue increased 3.89% from new patients who chose hospital based on specified criteria.
- *Implications* (select sample)
  - Continue to evaluate and track revenue changes based on specified criteria
  - Although hospital revenue did not increase to the desired outcome of 5%, hospital revenue increased 3.89%. This amount of increase was 73% greater than the amount invested in workshop design, implementation, and evaluation; therefore, workshops are not only cost-effective, but yield financially profitable results.

Desired Outcome 4: Hospital profits will exceed losses as seen by higher income generated from increased use of diabetic clinic services among Mexican Americans and decreased losses incurred from unpaid hospitalization costs resulting from managed care reimbursement guidelines.

- **What:** Hospital annual profits will exceed losses
- **Who:** Mexican American diabetics
- **Where:** Diabetic clinic services mostly as versus other hospital services
- **When:** In 1 year
- **How:** As measured by annual income and loss accounting records
- **Why:** Appraisal of costs associated with 5 workshop series in comparison with increased income generated as a result of referred clients pre-educational intervention and post-educational intervention will determine cost-effectiveness (gains versus losses).
- **Independent Variable:** Educational intervention (Cultural Competent Care for Mexican American workshops)
- **Dependent Variable:** Difference between hospital profits and losses (of specified criteria) or hospital income

Independent Variable	Dependent Variables	Measurement Tool	Desired Outcomes
Workshops	Revenue minus loss	Accounting records	↑ revenue, ↓ income loss

Data Collection: Collect respective data following method described in Desired Outcome 2.

Data Analysis: Analyze respective data following method described in Desired Outcome 2.

> **Exhibit 10.4**   Innovations in Cultural Competence Development:
> Summative Evaluation: Changes in Transcultural Self-Efficacy
> Perceptions with Implications
>
> *Goal:* After completion of the workshop series, workshop participants will
> have a *change* in transcultural self-efficacy (perceived confidence) for per-
> forming general transcultural nursing skills among diverse client populations
> as demonstrated by changes in subscale mean scores on the Transcultural
> Self-Efficacy Tool (TSET) in the anticipated direction from pretest to posttest.
> Specifically, low to moderate pretest scores will increase on posttest; supremely
> efficacious scores will decrease to moderate on posttest.
>
> - **What:** Transcultural self-efficacy perceptions will change
> - **Who:** Among workshop participants
> - **Where:** Hospital workshop series
> - **When:** After completion of the workshop series
> - **How:** as measured by the TSET.
> - **Why:** Transcultural self-efficacy is an integral component to cultural
>   competence education and is proposed to influence the provision of
>   cultural competent patient care; therefore, effectiveness of a cultural
>   competence education program can be measured via a comparison
>   of baseline TSE perceptions before the educational interventions and
>   after the educational intervention.
>
> | *Independent Variable* | *Dependent Variables* | *Measurement Tool* | *Desired Outcomes* |
> | --- | --- | --- | --- |
> | Workshops | TSE | TSET | Low or moderate TSE, → ↑
 Supremely efficacious→
 lower TSE to resilient |
>
> *Data Collection:* TSET is administered before "Enhance Your Cultural
> Competency" workshop 1 and after the last (fifth) workshop.
>
> *Data Analysis:*
> *Calculations on TSET pretest and TSET posttest*
>
> - Self-Efficacy Strength (SEST) scores (mean) were calculated for each
>   subscale.
> - It was an underlying assumption that no nurses in this setting would
>   select "1" or "2" responses on 20% or more of subscale responses;
>   therefore, Self-Efficacy Level (SEL) was not calculated.
> - Nurses were divided into low, medium, and high groups for each
>   subscale as per suggestions of the HCI statistician.
> - To determine items that nurses were most or least confident about in
>   each dimension, item means for the group were rank-ordered within
>   each subscale.

Comparative Tests:

- To detect significant differences between pretests and posttests on all calculations listed previously, *t* tests were performed.

Results: (Select examples)

- On both pretest and posttest, nurses were least confident with their knowledge and most confident about their values, attitudes, and beliefs concerning culturally different clients.
- Overall, nurses had statistically significant changes (increase) in SEST scores from pretest to posttest on the Cognitive and Practical Subscale.
- Statistically significant changes were not detected on the Affective Subscale although scores changed in the anticipated direction (increase).
- For each subscale, nurses in the "low" group on pretest demonstrated the greatest change in self-efficacy perceptions on the posttest.
- Demographic data indicated that the majority of nurses in the pretest "high" group on the Cognitive and Practical Subscale and who remained in the posttest "high" group for these two subscales had attended at least two conferences on cultural issues and/or completed a graduate course in Transcultural Nursing prior to the HCI workshop series.*

Limitations: Sample size, other potential threats to internal and/or external validity

Interpretation (select examples)

- When examining the results in relation to the underlying conceptual framework (Cultural Competence and Confidence Model), the results make sense conceptually.
- Statistically and practically significant changes occurred in anticipated directions (according to underlying conceptual framework and previous empirical results obtained using TSET). Therefore, the educational intervention made a measurable, significant difference in nurses' TSE perceptions.

Implications (some possibilities)

- Continue with cultural competence workshops and reevaluate.
- Expand cultural competence workshops to target other settings within the HCI and reevaluate with the TSET.
- Expand cultural competence workshops to target physicians and/or multidisciplinary professionals within the HCI and reevaluate using TSET physician and/or TSET-MHP format.
- Target future cultural competence workshops to address items that nurses were least confident about and reevaluate.

---

*This demonstrates the importance of relevant demographic data collection in interpreting results.

TSET Research Exhibit 10.1 Evaluating the Effects of Cultural Competency Training Using Self-Instruction Learning Packets

The Effects of Cultural Competency Training Using Self-Instruction on Obstetrical Nurses' Awareness, Knowledge, and Attitudes

Jeanette Velez, MA, CDP
Huron, a Cleveland Clinic Hospital
13951 Terrace R
East Cleveland, OH 44112

Research Report

Purpose: To measure the effect of cultural competency training using self-instruction on obstetrical nurses' awareness, knowledge, and attitudes.

Research Question: Is there a significant change in obstetrical nurses' awareness, knowledge, and attitudes (transcultural self-efficacy) after the completion of cultural competency training using self-instruction as measured by the TSET tool?

Study Design: Quasi-experimental

Sample:
    Size: 20
    Type of learner: Obstetrical nurses with an associate or baccalaureate degree working in an urban hospital.

TSET Data Collection
    Pretest: Data was collected at the beginning of the educational intervention
    Posttest: Data was collected at the completion of the educational intervention

Educational interventions/teaching–learning strategies: Self-Instruction-Learning-Packet (SILP) identical to a 7-hour training class on cultural competency designed by Dolgan (2001).

Data Analysis
Results: Nurses' transcultural self-efficacy (TSE) SEST scores changed significantly from pretest (pre-SILP) to posttest (completion of SILP) for nurses.

TSE SEST scores (n = 20)

	Mean	t-test	Significance
Overall TSET			
Pretest	197	−6.84	P<0.001
Posttest	236		
Cognitive Subscale			
Pretest	167	−7.59	P<0.001
Posttest	209		
Practical			
Pretest	180	−7.29	P<0.001
Posttest	226		
Affective			
Pretest	243	−5.63	P<0.001
Posttest	274		

SEL Scores were used for grouping into High, Medium, and Low:

Low: Select 1 or 2 responses on 80% or more items
High: Select 9 or 10 responses on 80% or more items
Medium: Select 3 through 8 responses on 80% items or
            does not fall into low or high groupings

Subscale	High	Medium	Low
Cognitive			
Pretest	1	19	0
Posttest	13	7	0
Practical			
Pretest	1	19	0
Posttest	10	10	0
Affective			
Pretest	10	10	0
Posttest	18	2	0

Discussion: There were no low scores reported in any subscale for either the pretest or posttest. The greatest percentage of pretest high scores occurred in the Affective subscale (50%) followed by the Cognitive and Practical at 5% each. The greatest percentage of posttest high scores occurred in the Affective subscale at 90% followed by Cognitive at 65% and Practical at 50%. The greatest increase in SEL scores occurred on the Cognitive and Practical subscales while the least change in scores was noted in the Affective subscale. There was no decrease in scores in any subscale between the pretest and posttest. The SEL scores for the Cognitive subscale exhibited the greatest percentage point improvement as a result of the SILP.

Program Evaluation
At the conclusion of the SILP training, participants were asked to complete a program evaluation. The evaluation measured knowledge, pre- and post-training, the level of satisfaction with the SILP, the percent of the average increase in knowledge and a question on the achievement of the course's objectives. Each item on the evaluation was rated on a four-point scale. Overall, nurses were satisfied with the SILP, a substantial increase in knowledge and skills was demonstrated, and all six course objectives were met.

The learning domains most affected in both Dolgan's 2001 study and Velez's 2005 study were the Cognitive and Practical realms.

Institutional Implications

1. The use of self-instruction learning packets may be as efficient as classroom instruction in training professional staff cultural competencies.
2. Continue using SILP
3. Continue collecting data using TSET

Dissemination of Results: Master's thesis; within institution

---

TSET Research Exhibit 10.2 Evaluating the Influence of an Educational Program among Nursing and Health Care Providers

Using the TSET to Measure the Influence of an Educational Program on Transcultural Self-Efficacy among Nursing and Health Care Providers

Stephen R. Marrone, EdD, RN-BC, CTN-A
Deputy Nursing Director
Institute of Continuous Learning
State University of New York
SUNY Downstate Medical Center / Health Science Center of Brooklyn
Clinical Assistant Professor of Nursing
SUNY Downstate College of Nursing
Brooklyn, New York

Purpose: The purpose of this study was to evaluate the influence of a cultural competence educational program on transcultural self-efficacy among nursing and health care providers.

Research Question: Is there a significant change in the perceived self-efficacy of nursing and health care providers after the completion of the cultural competence education program, as measured by the Transcultural Self-Efficacy Tool (TSET)?

Study Design: Quasi-experimental

Instrument: The TSET Multidisciplinary Healthcare Provider (TSET-MHP) version was used to measure the influence of the educational program on TSE among nursing and health care providers. Items are exactly the same as original TSET. Wording in the directions change the "nurse" and "nursing" focus to "health care provider" focus, encompassing nursing and all other multidisciplinary or transdisciplinary health care provider groups, faculty, and students.

TSET-MHP Data Collection

   Pretest: Data was collected at the beginning of the educational program
   Posttest: Data was collected online 8 weeks after the educational program

Educational Program Purpose

To provide nursing and transdisciplinary health care providers, faculty, and students with the requisite knowledge and skills for developing cultural competence.

Educational Objectives

The 8-hour educational program was designed to enable participants to:

   1. Integrate evidence-based best practices into the development of an organizational infrastructure and strategic plan that supports the provision of culturally competent health care;
   2. Design strategies that ensure the initial and ongoing cultural competency of transdisciplinary health care practitioners; and
   3. Formulate strategies for meeting the learning needs of diverse patients, families, students, and practitioners.

Setting

Brooklyn, New York, is one of the five boroughs that comprise New York City and is the most populous and second most diverse county in New York State. The State University of New York – SUNY Downstate Medical Center is the only academic medical center in Brooklyn. More than 2.6 million residents are served by SUNY Downstate.

Target Audience

The target audience included registered nurses and transdisciplinary health care practitioners at the point of care, advanced practice nurses, health care leaders and administrators, students and faculty of nursing and other health care disciplines.

Data Analyses Plan: Descriptive statistics; inferential statistics comparing pretest and posttest TSET-MHP subscale scores.

Preparation of a comprehensive summary report that substantially details yet succinctly highlights key findings via tables, figures, and/or bullet lists should be accompanied by easy-to-read descriptive text. A thorough, user-friendly evaluation that aims to include nurses (and multidisciplinary health care professionals) of varying levels of education and research expertise will enhance the application of the evaluation results and help prevent feelings of exclusion or being overwhelmed. The true potential of cultural competence development within the HCI can only be optimally realized when feelings of mutual respect, validation, inclusiveness, and group solidarity predominate, acknowledging the many important contributions each individual can make in promoting culturally congruent care. Creatively connecting the positive attributes and strengths of individuals within the HCI will maximize the institution's overall positive outcomes related to cultural competence educational strategies and innovations.

Exhibit 10.5   Educator-In-Action Vignette

During a staff meeting, several staff nurses verbalize feelings of inadequacy and lower confidence when caring for new groups of immigrant populations. The nurses represent diversity in age, gender, education, ethnicity, religion, race, and number of years in nursing.

Stella, the nurse manager, recognizes the need to promote cultural competence development for care of patients of diverse cultures; however, she recognizes the immediate priority to focus on select target groups, provide immediate feedback to these adult learners, and capitalize on learners' intrinsic motivation. Through guided questioning and dialogue, Stella assists the staff nurses to determine populations within the broad category of "recent immigrants" by detailing subcategories. Three major recent immigrant groups are identified: Russian Jews, Filipinos, and Dominicans.

To determine which group should be targeted first, Stella uses the sample questions to guide target population prioritization (see Table 10.2). By writing nurse's rationale, concerns, and goals on the chalkboard, nurses can easily visualize differences and similarities between the four groups. For example, although each group consisted of non-English speaking individuals, more Filipino clients were able to speak English than within the other groups. Of the three groups, Dominicans sought primary care less frequently, often first entering the hospital system with acute illness, advanced illnesses, or complications from chronic illnesses. As a result, poorer health outcomes and prolonged hospitalization within the constraints of managed care reimbursement also presented the HCI with financial losses.

Ed, the unit's professional development specialist (nurse educator), invites nurses to share learner characteristics by asking nurses to write down on an index card information about prior formalized learning (related to culture), including continuing education programs and academic courses. Nurses are invited to share any other concerns, interests, or information that they think may be helpful to assist in the decision and design of cultural competence development unit initiative. Here are some excerpts:

Maureen: "I graduated two years ago from a baccalaureate nursing program that had a required course in transcultural nursing. Culture care was integrated throughout my program and I had many guided opportunities in clinical with culturally diverse patients. During my senior semester break, I participated in a volunteer health service initiative with the university, providing care for indigent patients in the Dominican Republic. That experience made me realize that I have a lot to learn about cultures that are different than mine. Some of the other staff nurses expect me to be the expert on Dominicans, but I am not confident about my knowledge and communication skills.

Rosa: "Because I speak Spanish fluently, many of the other nurses automatically think I know everything about the Dominican culture and customs. Of course, I can translate information but sometimes I feel as though the patients and families are hesitant to trust me completely because I am not Dominican. It bothers me when my colleagues discount my concerns. One other nurse even said 'It's all the same—Puerto Rican, Dominican, Cuban—you all speak Spanish.' That really hurt my feelings."

Svetlana: "I am not confident about dealing with so many of the different cultures in the United States. Although I got my associate degree in nursing last June and am attending school part-time for my bachelor's degree, I still am overwhelmed by the differences from Russia where I spent 40 years of my life. I am proud to be a resource for the other nurses to help translate and provide quality care for the Russian patients."

Taylor: "I have attended several conferences on cultural competence presented by the State Nurses Association and the National Black Nurses Association. Next June I will be finished with my master's degree program. I think I would like to become an adjunct instructor at the university or a nurse educator within this institution, but I'm not sure. I feel it is important to have general background information about caring competently for cultures different than one's own. I would benefit from review of this necessary information first before focusing on any specific group."

Based on this information, Ed and Stella collaborate about learner strengths, weaknesses, learning gaps, biases, motivation, and confidence. Next, exploration of educational resources within the HCI reveals that an advanced practice nurse in the adult day hospital is also certified in transcultural nursing. Further exploration reveals that two nursing faculty members at a collaborating nearby university are actively involved in cultural competence research and teaching. Unfortunately, no one is a specialist within any of the three potential target populations; however, through professional associations and networks, an appropriate consultant/guest speaker could be selected.

Resource allocation (time, and honorarium for consultant) for cultural competence program development, implementation, and evaluation is approved at all executive levels within the HCI. Results from the pilot initiative will serve to guide future educational endeavors. Changes in learners, patient outcomes, satisfaction, nursing staffing patterns, and costs will be evaluated.

Based on the assessment of target populations, learner characteristics, and educational resources, Ed, Stella, and the unit staff mutually agree to focus on culturally congruent care for Dominican adults. This will occur only after introducing (or reviewing) general principles, skills, knowledge, concepts, and values concerning cultural competence (generalist approach).

Staff's survey results of preferred learning strategies support the use of the following innovative strategies:

- Fifteen-minute PowerPoint presentation reviewing general principles of cultural competence development
  - Presentation by nurse educator or certified transcultural nurse (CTN) on each shift (Week 1 and 2)
  - Posting of PowerPoint presentation on internal Web site
  - Slide handouts posted on unit bulletin boards
  - Bibliography list with select articles and books available on unit
- Three journal articles on cultural competence and assessment (general) (Week 2–4)
  - Posted on staff bulletin boards, internal Web site, and unit staff listserve
  - Bullet list outlining 10 key points of article posted on staff bulletin board
  - Bag lunch (breakfast or dinner) discussion

- Three journal articles or book chapters on culturally congruent care for Dominican Americans (Week 5–7)
  - (As above)
- Learning lunch with Guest Presenter/Consultant (Week 8)
  - Traditional Dominican foods prepared by Dominican American caterers
  - Cultural Learning Menu—1 paragraph description of food, meaning of food, etc.
  - Twenty-minute presentation
  - Fifteen-minute group discussion
  - Edited video clip of presentation, foods, and discussion (with permission) on internal Web site
- Weekly "tidbits and niblets" program (Williams & Jones, 2004) (Weeks 9–13)
  - Tiny bytes of cultural information, questions, and answers with references on index cards
  - Contact hours awarded for each tidbit completed
- Exploring Cultural Resource Links for Professional Education (Week 10)
  - Fifteen-minute presentation by librarian with appropriate expertise
  - Edited video clip and/or PowerPoint presentation on internal Web site
- Learning breakfast with Guest Presenter/Consultant (Week 11)
  - (As above with learning lunch, but different topic within the same cultural group)
- Exploring Cultural Resource Links for Patient Education (Week 12)
  - Fifteen-minute presentation by librarian with appropriate expertise
  - Edited video clip and/or PowerPoint presentation on internal Web site
- Learning dinner with Guest Presenter/Consultant (Week 13)
  - (As above with learning lunch, but different topic within the same cultural group)
- Panel discussion cosponsored by the HCI, nearby university, and two local nursing associations (Week 14)
- Staff meeting, discussion, and future plans (Week 15)

KEY POINT SUMMARY

- Within the health care institution (HCI), each individual nurse, nurse educator, executive, or leader is empowered to make a positive difference in cultural competence; however, the greatest impact will be achieved through a coordinated, holistic group effort that thoughtfully weaves together relevant high-priority educational programs, unit-based initiatives, and supplementary resources.

- Promoting cultural competency in the HCI requires considerable, sincere effort that must begin with self-assessment of the individual staff nurse, nurse manager, nurse educator, nurse executive, administrator, and organization.

- It is proposed that individuals (and the organization) with resilient TSE perceptions (confidence) persist in their endeavors to be active transcultural advocates or promoters of cultural competence in all dimensions of the HCI and professional practice.

- Selection of targeted priority areas should be based upon a comprehensive assessment of patient populations, learner characteristics, and educational resources.

- Close inspection at the institutional level must assess whether cultural competency development is emphasized substantially, equally, and symmetrically throughout the HCI beyond philosophy, mission, and purpose to such areas as new employee orientation, inservice education, learning strategies, newsletter and publications, library, Web site, bulletin boards, special events, and committees.

- Connecting innovations in cultural competence development may be achieved through publicity, publications, special events, and committees and by developing a collaborative network of supplementary resources beyond the HCI.

- Educational innovations should include a comprehensive formative and summative evaluation plan that is realistic, positively phrased, and measurable.

- Evaluating changes in learners' TSE perceptions using the TSET presents a quantitative measure for evaluating changes within cognitive, practical, and affective dimensions.

Case Exemplar: Linking Strategies—Spotlight on Employee Orientation Programs to Enhance Cultural Competence

Marianne R. Jeffreys, EdD, RN

Cynthia Karczewski, MS, RN

Although employee inservice programs can provide numerous ongoing opportunities for promoting cultural competence development, it is the employee orientation program (EOP) that can make the greatest impact. This is true for three reasons: (a) the main function of the orientation program is "education"; (b) the primary role of the employee is "learning" to apply old and new professional knowledge, skills, and attitudes in a new organizational culture and setting; and (c) the orientation program provides the foundation and framework for employees' work expectations and all future employee inservices. During the orientation, the expectations and values of the health care institution (HCI) are conveyed within the immediate context of the employment setting. HCIs that convey, expect, and support optimal cultural competence initially during the EOP set the standard at this high-quality level. If optimal cultural competence is highly valued by the HCI, employees will become enculturated into the organizational environment. Optimal cultural competence can also be supported by being criteria for annual evaluation, promotion, salary gain, and annual recognition. Conveying that minimal level performance is not looked upon favorably by the HCI motivates employees to continually seek to enhance cultural competence development, actively assess culture within the workplace, and implement decisive action plans to provide culturally competent patient care and facilitate multicultural workplace harmony.

The main purpose of this chapter is to describe a process of visibly integrating cultural competence throughout an existing EOP. Employee education is best facilitated through a collaborative partnership in cultural competence education and professional development between nurse educators, administrators, other professional nurses, and other health professionals. The ongoing, accessible opportunities for cultural competence education at the HCIs offer tremendous possibilities for optimal cultural competence. This is especially true if subsequent employee inservice programs build upon the foundations established via a well-planned EOP. For example, a well-planned EOP should: (a) substantively emphasize cultural competence throughout most content areas; (b) provide strategies and incentives for nurses to implement culture-specific care directly on their assigned unit or setting; and (c) intrinsically motivate nurses to actively engage in the ongoing quest for developing cultural competence in self and in others (see also Chapters 10 and 12).

Illustrative case exemplars, supplemented by detailed illustrations, will be threaded throughout the chapter, demonstrating easy application for a variety of unit-based or site-based settings. Evaluation of EOP components, including formative and summative evaluation strategies, will conclude the chapter.

EMPLOYEE ORIENTATION PROGRAM: INTEGRATING CULTURAL COMPETENCE

Visible and substantive integration of cultural competence in an existing EOP should be a systematic and well-planned process. This involves time, energy, money, commitment, collaborative partnerships, and a systematic plan. Figure 11.1 presents an eight-step process that can guide EOP revision. The two case exemplars (general hospital orientation and school nurse orientation) illustrate how this process can be adapted by other staff/employee nurse educators interested in developing diagnostic-prescriptive employee orientation programs for nurses and other licensed and unlicensed health care personnel. The EOP exemplars were designed for newly hired nurses within two different settings; however, the case

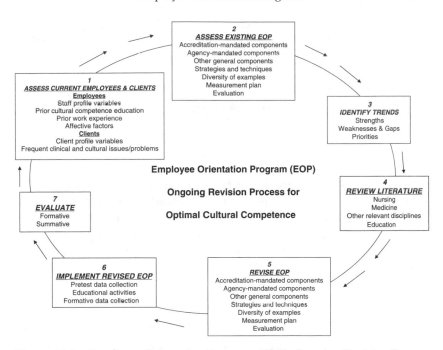

Figure 11.1 Employee Orientation Program (EOP): Ongoing Revision Process for Optimal Cultural Competence

exemplars have applicability for other health care personnel as well as other patient populations and settings.

The first step of the process involves three types of systematic assessments: (a) assess employee characteristics; (b) assess client characteristics; and (c) assess existing EOP. Assessment of the HCI is omitted here because it is assumed that the HCI interested in revising EOP to enhance cultural competence has already completed a detailed, systematic assessment (Chapter 10, Jeffreys Toolkit 2010, Items 11, 14, 16). Each beginning step will be described individually followed by a case exemplar that synthesizes assessment results.

Step 1—Assess Current Employees and Clients

Assess Employee Characteristics

An EOP should be designed for a specific employee population and have empirical support. The first step is to systematically assess both employee profile characteristics and affective factors. Profile characteristics include age, ethnicity, race, gender, socioeconomic background, religion, primary (first) language, educational background, prior cultural competence education, and prior work experience. Affective factors include cultural values and beliefs, transcultural self-efficacy (TSE), and motivation (see Chapters 1 and 10). Additionally, assessing the interaction of variables and for the presence or absence of multicultural workplace harmony or conflict is recommended (see Chapter 2).

Assess Client Characteristics

An EOP designed for specific, client examples reflective of patient populations and clinical problems will have most relevance to orientees and can have most benefit for patient populations by reducing health disparities among targeted populations. Assessment should include client profile variables, frequent clinical problems/issues, and frequent cultural problems/issues (see Chapter 10, Table 10.2).

Step 2—Assess Existing EOP

Although every HCI has some sort of EOP guided by accreditation-mandated and agency-mandated components, and most HCIs have at least the minimum level of cultural competence education mandated by accrediting agencies, too few HCIs actively advocate for optimal cultural competence. Assessment of the existing EOP for optimal cultural competence includes careful scrutiny of accreditation-mandated components, agency-mandated components, other general components, cultural competence components, strategies and techniques, diversity of examples, measurement plan, and evaluation. Obviously, mandated components must remain; however, they can be revised to be more reflective of cultural diversity and cultural competence education if needed. Other general components should be appraised for relevance in the overall orientation and benefit to employees, HCI, and clients as well as relevance to cultural competence development. Existing cultural competence education components should be evaluated for the placement within the EOP, connection to other components, depth, evidence-based content, appropriateness and relevance, and equality of emphasis in relation to other components. Examining the repertoire of teaching–learning strategies and techniques should take into account employee characteristics as well as the importance of learner-centered, reflective approaches with immediate relevance to the adult learner as recommended in the literature (Knowles, 1984; Brookfield, 1986). Three important questions are, To what extent are case examples representative of diverse patients, diverse employees, and diverse clinical issues? What types of examples are currently used? How do case examples develop or hinder cultural competence development in the workplace? Finally, assessment of the measurement plan and evaluation should be thoroughly reviewed, including any formative and summative evaluations of previous EOP.

Step 3—Identify Trends

Sifting through the above assessment results will assist in identifying data trends, showcasing strengths, uncovering weaknesses and gaps, and establishing priorities. In the school nurse case exemplar, the following assessment information supported the need for a revised EOP that emphasized and integrated cultural competence education:

1. Absence of prior cultural competence education program.
2. Increase in the cultural diversity of children, families, and communities.
3. Mismatch between the diversity of nurses, children, and parents.
4. Varying levels of motivation, interest, and commitment of nurses to cultural competence education.
5. Awareness that culture-specific care of clients (children and parents) could promote children's health, prevent illness, enhance clinical outcomes for existing health problems, and facilitate entry into the health care system.
6. Identification of actual and/or potential clinical problems directly and/or indirectly influenced by culturally incongruent versus culturally congruent care specific to the school setting.
7. Increase in multicultural workplace conflict, nurse dissatisfaction, high nurse transfer/attrition rates, complaints, and lawsuits.
8. The National Association of School Nurses identified the need to teach and learn about cultural competence and provide culture-specific care to diverse children (NASN, 2002).
9. Renewed administrative interest in cultural competence education throughout the local school system.

Step 4—Review Literature

A review of the nursing, medicine, and education literature as well as other relevant disciplines should be conducted. Materials should be reviewed for gathering background information about proposed clinical topics, culturally diverse patients and nurses, patient outcomes, cultural competence education strategies, evaluation methods, employee orientation/inservice and continuing education, and potential resources. Choice of a relevant conceptual framework can be valuable to provide structure and organization. For example, in the school nurse case exemplar, the Cultural Competence and Confidence (CCC) model and the measurement of transcultural self-efficacy perceptions provided the underlying framework for strategy design and evaluation. When reviewing literature concerning cultural competence education strategies, determining strategy strengths, limitations, and appropriateness of fit to the targeted population can help sort through various possibilities. Attention to the strategy's measurement and evaluation of outcomes is integral to determining selection and/or adaptation of strategies reported in the literature. One must be aware, however, that there is no panacea that one EOP will solve all problems and help prepare every nurse to become culturally competent. Realistically acknowledging that the EOP can be the foundational starting point for future employee cultural competence development is imperative.

Step 5—Revise EOP

When revising an EOP or any education inservice program, it is important to focus on the positive components that are already working effectively. Revising for the mere sake of doing something different without well-founded, empirical, and/or conceptual rationale is wasteful and counterproductive. Keeping what works and tying this into revisions will be most productive. For example, if an already existing case exemplar on the use of a professional interpreter for a non-English-speaking patient has had positive feedback from EOP participants and has met the desired educational outcomes, then this case exemplar should be retained (and continually reevaluated). Identifying what about the case exemplar captivated the audience can provide helpful guidelines to designing similar case exemplars for other topics. If time and other resources (money, expertise) permit, another teaching–learning strategy can be added to further develop cognitive, practical, and/or affective learning in the particular area. For example, adding on the 10-minute *Charades Communication Game* (Jeffreys, 1991), can be piloted.

Retaining accreditation-mandated and agency-mandated components is essential to maintaining accreditation and the operation of the particular agency. Finding creative, time- and cost-efficient ways of threading cultural competence, diversity, and multidimensional teaching–learning strategies throughout the EOP (with the intent of establishing a strong foundation for future employee inservices with integrated cultural competence) is challenging yet quite rewarding if successful. Determining what is successful (what works, what doesn't, and why) requires a thorough formative and summative measurement plan with timely evaluation of the results.

In the school nurse EOP, no formalized cultural competence education had been previously introduced; therefore, a formalized measurement plan and evaluation was also nonexistent. Consequently, the following revisions were proposed:

New School Nurse Orientation

The evidence-based, research-supported CCC model (Jeffreys, 2006) and valid, reliable corresponding questionnaire is proposed to guide the school nurse EOP, its implementation, and the evaluation of summative outcomes. The EOP includes self-assessment for each employee to determine one's own cultural values and beliefs as well as if the employee is an active promoter of cultural competence development in the workplace (Jeffreys 2010 Toolkit, Items 11, 14). The Transcultural Self-Efficacy Tool (TSET) will be given prior to the first class and again three months after orientation. It will be used to measure and evaluate participants' confidence for performing general transcultural nursing skills among diverse populations.

Next, the EOP will introduce and reinforce the Office of School Health's philosophy and purposes specifically concerning cultural competence development. The recent focus on cultural competence education by the National Association for School Nurses (2002) and the International Association of School Nurses will be highlighted. The emphasis will be on professional expectations, standards, and excellence as well as on autonomy and accountability. Ongoing education will be emphasized as a professional commitment to lifelong learning. New employees' motivation will be heightened with direct application in the school setting (Exhibit 11.1).

Exhibit 11.1   Enhancing Cultural Competence Development in School Nurses during the EOP: Purpose, Activity Components, Educational Objectives, and Content Exemplar

Title: An Introduction to Cultural Competence for School Nurses

Purpose: To introduce school nurses to concepts of cultural competence at the new employee orientation program

Main EOP Activity Overview: A series of three workshops lasting 45 minutes during new employee orientation utilizing the Cultural Competence and

---

Confidence Model (CCC) to develop cultural competence in newly hired school nurses. Direct application scenarios will demonstrate strategies for: (a) enhancing culturally congruent care of children, families, and communities and (b) multicultural workplace harmony

EOP Activity Components:

1. Administer the TSET and School Nurse Satisfaction Survey (SNSS)
2. Lecture/Discussion
3. Interactive PowerPoint and discussion
4. Use of world map to explore global migration
5. Case exemplars for direct application and analysis
6. Storytelling with reflection
7. Small group role play activities
8. Computer instruction on cultural competence resources
9. Generate open-ended questions related to how culturally competent school nurses can build positive parent and community partnerships and enhance child health
10. Generate open-ended questions related to how culturally competent school nurses can build positive staff relationships
11. Summary synthesis to guide school nurses for direct implementation of cultural competence strategies over the next 3 months prior to a follow-up seminar.

Future activity: In three months, regroup to discuss application of cultural competence in the school setting (multicultural employees, children, parents, and communities). Administer TSET and SNSS.

Educational Objectives	Brief Content Outline

Identify key terms, need, and concepts associated with cultural competence	1. Terms and Definitions
	  a. Culture
	  b. Cultural competence
	  c. Cultural confidence
	  d. Culturally congruent care
	  e. Transcultural nursing
	  f. Multicultural workplace harmony
	  g. Multicultural workplace conflict
	  h. Other
	2. Changing demographics
	3. Healthy People 2010
	4. Ethical and legal issues
	5. Conceptual models as resources
	  a. Leininger
	  b. Purnell
	  c. Jeffreys
	6. Relevance to school nurses

Educational Objectives	Brief Content Outline

Describe how school nurses can promote positive health outcomes through cultural competence using Pender's (2006) health promotion model. (Pender, et al., 2006)	A. Pender's (2006) Health Promotion Model: Brief overview of theoretical basis
	  1. Individual Characteristics and Experiences
	    a. Prior related behavior
	    b. Personal factors: biological, psychological, sociocultural
	  2. Behavior-Specific Cognitions and Affect
	    a. Perceived benefits and barriers to action
	    b. Perceived self-efficacy
	    c. Activity-related affect
	    d. Interpersonal influences (family, peers, and providers)
	    e. Situational influences
	  3. Behavioral Outcomes
	    a. Commitment to a plan of action
	    b. Immediate competing demands
	    c. Health-promoting behavior
	B. Cultural competence in the school nurse setting
	  1. Culturally incongruent case exemplars
	  2. Culturally congruent case exemplars
	  3. Internet-accessible cultural competence resources

Discuss how school nurses can promote multicultural workplace harmony through cultural COMPETENCE (Jeffreys, 2008)	Influence of cultural values on the multicultural workplace (Andrews & Boyle, 2008)
	  1. Cultural Values
	    a. Time orientation
	    b. Family obligations
	    c. Etiquette
	    d. Communication patterns
	    e. Space/distance
	    f. Touch
	    g. Meaning of work
	    h. Work ethic
	  2. Cultural COMPETENCE acronym for multicultural workplace (Jeffreys, 2008)
	  3. Preventing multicultural workplace conflict: case exemplars
	  4. Promoting multicultural workplace harmony: case exemplars

The specifics of the training include an introduction to the many cultures of the area residents. This will be done in a pictorial display, in chart and graph design, and in the use of a world map. Next, a 15-minute PowerPoint presentation introducing and defining general principles of cultural competence development will lead into prompting the participants to reflect back on their own cultural values and beliefs. As participants move through the EOP, cultural competence concepts will be woven into the expected provisions of care for local children, families, and communities. Additional computer training will help school nurses identity cultural competence resources that are readily available at one's fingertips and beyond.

In addition to the assumptions of the CCC model (Jeffreys, 2006; Chapter 3), several specific assumptions for the school nurse underlie the revised EOP:

1. Formalized cultural competence education initiated during the EOP will positively influence cognitive, practical, and affective learning about caring for and working with diverse cultures in the school setting and local communities.
2. Enhanced knowledge, skills, and attitudes about diverse populations will enhance the delivery of culturally competent care to school children, thereby better promoting children's health, preventing illness, improving clinical outcomes for existing health problems, and facilitating smooth entry into the health care system.
3. Enhanced knowledge, skills, and attitudes about diverse populations will better promote multicultural workplace harmony and prevent multicultural workplace conflicts.
4. A school workplace environment that actively embraces diversity in the workplace and offers strategies to improve school children's health and the relationships within and between local communities will lead to improved school nurse satisfaction, lower requested transfer rates, higher school nurse retention rates, and decreased complaints and lawsuits.
5. Increased school nurse satisfaction and retention within the assigned school will provide more continuity in care for children, thus enhancing health outcomes (e. g., less absence from school due to illness, less use of ER for nonemergency situations because of increased screening/intervention by school nurses).

Using school records and satisfaction questionnaire data, the above assumptions could be measured and evaluated by comparing data prior to and then later following the implementation of the revised school nurse EOP.

Newly Hired RN Hospital Orientation Program

To provide hospital-based examples for illustrative purposes, several areas for expansion will be described. For example, consider that an assessment of the current hospital EOP reveals limited mention of cultural considerations for pain assessment and management. Inclusion of pain assessment and pain management reflects recent accreditation-mandated guidelines based on research findings revealing that physicians and nurses commonly under-medicate patients for pain, thereby suggesting that more astute and routine assessments be conducted and more aggressive pain management strategies be implemented and evaluated. Despite research findings that identify differences in pain expression, genetic and ethnopharmacological differences in pharmacokinetics and pharmacodynamics between ethnic and/or racial groups, physicians and nurses continue to assess and treat pain based on a "one size fits all" approach. Revising the EOP on the accreditation-mandated (and ethically and legally mandated) topic of pain assessment and pain management to substantively include culture should provide essential cognitive knowledge, practical application (culturally competent interview and pain therapy/comfort skills), and affective components (value and appreciate the diverse expressions, meanings, and treatments of pain). Figure 11.2 presents a detailed health history form to incorporate various dimensions of culture within the general pain assessment following some background "holding" knowledge about the various meanings, expressions, and treatments of various types of pain.

To make this assessment immediately applicable in the clinical setting, adapting the questions or phrasing of questions to match the patient population is essential; following the general orientation with direct application through preceptors and mentors on the assigned clinical unit will assist nurses in the transition from the general to specific, immediate, and relevant situation, thus making it more meaningful moving from being "consciously integrated" within one's professional practice to "unconsciously integrated" within one's professional practice.

Although not an exhaustive or all-inclusive list, Table 11.1 also provides some additional examples for optimal cultural competence applicable for a variety of settings and applicable for both employees (personal relevance) and for patients (professional relevance). Presenting some simple case scenarios depicting culturally competent and culturally incompetent approaches that can be used as a discussion prompt within the EOP. Every topic within an existing EOP should be examined for cultural competence education opportunities. Because content validity experts affirmed that the TSET encompassed the content domain of transcultural nursing knowledge, skills, and attitudes appropriate in preparing a

COMFORT

General Patient Information

Patient Name _____ Age _____ Sex _____

Admitting Dx _____

Activity Level: _____ Diet _____

HISTORY (SUBJECTIVE DATA)

A) Location: _____ Internal _____ External _____

B) Duration: How long experiencing pain? _____

     Pain episode duration _____ Frequency _____

     Acute _____ Chronic _____

C) Intensity: no pain _____ mild _____ moderate _____ severe _____ worst pain _____

     Pain scale (0-10): _____

D) Quality: sharp _____ dull _____ diffuse _____shifting _____ burning _____

                      cramping _____ stinging _____ pinching _____ throbbing _____

                      shooting _____ sore _____ stabbing _____

E) Periodicity: continuous _____ intermittent _____ transient _____

Chronology: Changes in pain _____

Development/progression of pain _____

Aggravating factors _____

Alleviating factors _____

Associated factors _____

Analgesic Medication History

Name	Dose	Frequency	Last Dose	Pt's Understanding of Purpose

Past pain experiences _____

Previous methods for coping with pain _____

Effect of pain experience on: ADL_____

     lifestyle_____

     family role _____

     work role _____

     student role _____

Figure 11.2   Assessing Patient Comfort: A Culturally Competent Approach

Cultural Assessment – Interview

Ethnicity:_____Religion:_____

Gender Role:_____

Client's perceptions for the following:

A) Meaning of pain_____

B) Acceptable demonstrations of pain with:

    spouse_____children_____

    mother_____father_____

    others_____clergy_____

    nurse_____MD_____

C) Unacceptable demonstrations of pain with:

    spouse_____children_____

    mother_____father_____

    others_____clergy_____

    nurse_____MD_____

D) Acceptable measures to cope with pain_____

E) Unacceptable measures to cope with pain_____

F) Own role in pain relief_____

G) Family's role in pain relief_____

H) Nurse's role in pain relief_____

I) Physician's role in pain relief_____

J) Clergy's role in pain relief_____

K) Folk medicine practices_____

OBJECTIVE DATA

A) Behavioral (Voluntary) Responses

    guarding _____grimacing_____

    moaning_____crying_____

    refusal to move _____other_____

B) Physiologic (Involuntary) Responses

    Current T_____P_____R_____BP_____Baseline T_____P_____R_____BP_____

    vs during pain episode: T_____P_____R_____BP_____

    vs during peak action of analgesic: T_____P_____R_____BP_____

    Pupils dilated_____Pallor_____

    Muscle tension & rigidity_____

    Nausea_____Vomiting_____

    Fainting_____Unconsciousness_____

Figure 11.2 Assessing Patient Comfort: A Culturally Competent Approach (*continued*)

C) Affective (Psychologic) Responses

anorexia_____	depression_____
anxiety_____	fatigue_____
fear_____	withdrawal_____
restlessness_____	crying_____
anger_____	stoicism_____
hopelessness_____	powerlessness_____

D) Lab Data: Glucose: FBS_____ U/A_____ Fingerstick_____

Other:_____

Figure 11.2 Assessing Patient Comfort: A Culturally Competent Approach (*continued*)

generalist who must care for patients of many diverse cultures, the TSET could be used as a guide to current and additional topics within EOP.

Step 6—Implement Revised EOP

To facilitate smooth implementation, the program should be divided into various categories: pretest data collection, educational activities, and formative data collection. Each category should complement each other, receive adequate time and attention, be part of the overall program, and easily flow into the next category. For example, providing an environment conducive for pretest and formative data collection, verbally emphasizing the importance of completing the evaluations honestly and seriously, and allocating sufficient time for contemplative completion will convey institutional commitment to cultural competence education as well as add to the validity of findings that will guide future cultural competence educational programs. Learner-centered activities that thoughtfully provoke insights and application to the immediate workplace setting and individuals' career benefits are preferred over passive learning activities. A summary synthesis that ties together general principles of cultural competence with direct professional application will assist participants to incorporate cultural competence into all phases of the targeted topic (school nursing) (see Exhibit 11.1).

Step 7—Evaluate Revised EOP

As mentioned previously, a carefully orchestrated evaluation should be tied explicitly to the EOP measurement plan and should include both formative and summative components. Formative evaluations assess the process of a program rather than outcomes. Formative evaluations can be monitored as the program is implemented and can document specific

Table 11.1   Integrating Cultural Competence Components within EOP: Focus on Employee and Patient Needs

Topic	Organization	Employee	Patient	Sample Sites for Scenario Development & Discussion
Blood transfusion	Policy for refusing blood transfusions; patient documentation form Employee policy supporting religious freedom	Employees with religious beliefs against blood transfusion will delegate task to another appropriate person.	Patients who refuse blood transfusion will sign appropriate documentation form and receive alternate care as indicated. Risks to patient and prognosis information will be provided to patient.	OR RR Critical care units Medical oncology ER Labor and delivery
Pressure ulcer prevention and treatment	Policy for pressure ulcer prevention and treatment has written standards that address varying skin pigmentations. Photos depicting different stages and pigmentations accompany written standards. Varying CVB on skin care, physical examinations, etc. will be considered.	RN, physician, physician assistant, and other licensed personnel involved with skin assessment and care will assess pressure ulcer risk and treatment appropriate for patient's skin pigmentation and CVB.	Patient and/or significant other(s) will be informed of early signs and symptoms of pressure ulcer formation, strategies for prevention, wound healing, and treatment using terms, photos, and techniques consistent with patient's skin pigmentation and CVB.	Nursing home Rehabilitation unit Orthopedics Critical care units

(continued)

Table 11.1 Integrating Cultural Competence Components within EOP: Focus on Employee and Patient Needs (*continued*)

Topic	Organization	Employee	Patient	Sample Sites for Scenario Development & Discussion
HIPPA	Policy consistent with federal HIPPA guidelines. All employees undergo a mandatory training session on HIPPA, view an agency-created film incorporating all necessary HIPPA components with diverse employee and clinical examples	Information on the employee physical examination, subsequent employee health visits/treatment, and/or employee injury information will be assured of privacy under HIPPA	Patients who wish to include specific family members and/or significant other(s) in sharing of medical and other information will sign a standard agency form delineating who should be informed, what information should or should not be shared, and when.	Employee health Labor and delivery Medical-surgical unit Substance abuse Mental health clinic Nursery
Schedules	Policy to accommodate religious holidays, values, and beliefs into employee work schedule and patient care plan. Policy that employees working on inpatient settings work every other weekend.	Employees who cannot work complete weekends (Saturday–Sunday) due to religious reasons will work split weekends instead. Religious holidays whereby individuals cannot work will be accommodated in the work schedule.	Diagnostic procedures, surgery, & other appointments will be scheduled around patient's religious requirements. Any delay in scheduling that can potentially adversely affect health will be disclosed to the patient prior to decision.	Medical unit Surgical unit Outpatient mental health Pediatric unit ER

activities, identify difficulties, and allow for diagnostic-prescriptive modifications based on participants' feedback, using both quantitative and qualitative data (see Exhibit 10.2 and Exhibit 12.3).

Summative EOP evaluations should be monitored at a designated time period following the EOP. Aggregating and comparing data within and between EOP groups will be valuable in evaluating the achievement of educational and other outcomes. Collapsing several groups together to attain sufficient sample size for statistical comparison and relevance may be indicated. Because cultural competence education is a dynamic and multidimensional phenomenon, the success of any teaching strategy requires a multidimensional evaluation strategy. In the school nurse case exemplar, the EOP provides an action-oriented approach that combines cognitive, affective, and practical domains of learning. Because the TSET does not selectively target specific cultural groups and because it assesses cognitive, practical, and affective domains of learning, it is appropriate to use to develop a baseline of learners' needs, values, attitudes, and skills related to transcultural nursing and health care for school nurses caring for a wide variety of culturally diverse children. This is beneficial because the background information of school nurses encompasses various ages, languages, educational, work and cultural experiences. Within the measurement and evaluation plan, psychometric evaluation of the TSET will be conducted to provide further information about the tool's validity and reliability. Evaluation of TSE perceptions would gauge the effectiveness of the specific teaching interventions as well as assess changes in TSE perceptions over time. A new School Nurse Satisfaction Survey (SNSS) will need to be developed following recommended protocol for questionnaire development (Jeffreys & Smodlaka, 1996; Waltz, Strickland, & Lenz, 2005).

Following the preestablished plan for data collection and data analysis consistently and rigorously will help make the evaluation results more valid and reliable. This includes working diligently with previously established partners in the evaluation process such as the data collectors, director of institutional research, project assistant, and psychometric expert. Once the results are obtained and reviewed for statistical and practical significance, inferences from the data can guide future EOP activities, outcome measures, and desired outcomes. Ongoing assessment of employees and clients in conjunction with the EOP will help individualize EOP to help achieve optimal cultural competence.

KEY POINT SUMMARY

- A well-planned EOP should: (a) substantively emphasize cultural competence throughout most content areas; (b) provide strategies and incentives for nurses to implement culture-specific care directly on their assigned unit or setting; and (c) intrinsically motivate nurses to actively engage in the ongoing quest for developing cultural competence in self and in others.

- Visible and substantive integration of cultural competence into an existing EOP is presented as an eight-step process: assess current employees and clients, assess existing EOP, identify trends, review literature, outline ideas, revise EOP, implement revised EOP, and evaluate.
- Assessment of the existing EOP for optimal cultural competence includes careful scrutiny of accreditation-mandated components, agency-mandated components, other general components, cultural competence components, strategies and techniques, diversity of examples, measurement plan, and evaluation.
- The new school nurse orientation and hospital orientation case exemplars demonstrate easy application for a variety of hospital and other settings.
- Systematic EOP evaluation includes the assessment of formative and summative outcomes. Using the CCC model, summative evaluation includes the assessment of TSE using the Transcultural Self-Efficacy Tool as a pretest and posttest.

Case Exemplar: Linking Strategies—Spotlight on Employee Inservice Education to Enhance Cultural Competence

Marianne R. Jeffreys, EdD, RN

Patricia Bartley-Daniele, MSN, FNP-BC, CCRN, CNRN, CAPAN, CAPA

Karen Costello, BSN, RN, OCN

Providing culturally competent care is essential to a patient's well-being and recovery. Leininger (2002d) defines culturally competent nursing care as "the explicit use of culturally based care and health knowledge in sensitive, creative and meaningful ways to fit the general lifeways and needs of individuals or groups for beneficial and meaningful health and well-being or to face illness, disabilities or death" (p. 84). Examples of culturally competent care include "striving to overcome cultural, language and communication barriers; providing an environment in which patients from diverse cultural backgrounds feel comfortable discussing their cultural health beliefs and practices in the context of negotiating treatment options; and being familiar with and respectful of various traditional healing systems and beliefs" (U. S. Department of Health and Human Services Office of Minority Health, 2001, p. 8). In order to accomplish culturally competent care with culturally diverse patient populations and employees, the health care institution (HCI) must be truly committed to promoting and facilitating cultural competence development among all employees. Ongoing cultural competence education via employee inservices is an important mechanism toward achieving this goal.

This chapter describes a process of designing, implementing, and evaluating an employee inservice (EI) program to enhance cultural competence. EI education is best facilitated through a collaborative partnership in cultural competence education and professional development between nurse educators, other professional nurses, administrators, and other health professionals. The ongoing accessible opportunities for cultural competence education at the HCIs offer tremendous possibilities for optimal cultural competence. This is especially true if inservice programs build upon the foundations established via a well-planned employee orientation program that: (a) substantively emphasized cultural competence throughout all content areas; (b) provided strategies and incentives for nurses to implement culture-specific care directly on their assigned unit or setting; and (c) intrinsically motivated nurses to actively engage in the ongoing quest for developing cultural competence in themselves and in others. Extrinsic motivation refers to motivation that focuses on the goal-driven reasons, for example rewards or benefits earned when performing an activity (Lin, 2007). Intrinsic motivation indicates one's own pleasure and inherent satisfaction derived from a specific activity (Lin, 2007). Capitalizing upon both intrinsic and extrinsic motivators will optimize learning outcomes, transcultural self-efficacy (TSE), and the delivery of culturally specific patient care (see Chapter 10).

Two illustrative case exemplars from two different HCIs, supplemented by detailed illustrations, will be threaded throughout the chapter, demonstrating easy application for a variety of unit-based or site-based settings. Evaluation of EI components, including formative and summative evaluation strategies, will conclude the chapter.

EMPLOYEE INSERVICE: DESIGN, IMPLEMENTATION, AND EVALUATION

Employee inservice (EI) design, implementation, and evaluation should be a systematic and well-planned process. This involves time, energy, money, commitment, collaborative partnerships, and a systematic plan. Figure 12.1 presents an 11-step process that can guide EI development.

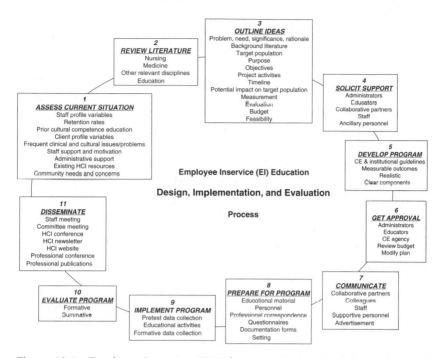

Figure 12.1 Employee Inservice (EI) Education: Design, Implementation, and Evaluation Process

The two case exemplars (perioperative nursing and bone marrow transplant [BMT] unit) illustrate how this process can be adapted by other staff/employee nurse educators interested in developing diagnostic-prescriptive employee inservice programs for nurses and other licensed and unlicensed health care personnel. The EI exemplars were designed for nurses already working in an HCI; however, the case exemplars have applicability for other health care personnel as well as other patient populations and settings. Additionally, the exemplars illustrate how the inservice can be implemented as a component of a larger, full-day inservice program (e. g., Nursing Educational Day) or as a separate, shorter, unit-based inservice.

The first phase of the process might appear to be "design," but there is really a predesign phase. This involves four steps: assessing the current situation, reviewing the literature, outlining ideas, and soliciting support. Each step will be described individually and within the context of the EI case exemplars.

Step 1—Assess Current Situation

An employee inservice program should be designed for a specific situation and have empirical support. The first step is to systematically assess the current situation, including staff profile variables, retention rates, prior exposure to formal and informal cultural competence education, client profile variables, frequent clinical and cultural issues/problems, staff support and motivation, administrative support, and the existing HCI resources (see Chapter 10).

In both of the EI case exemplars, the following assessment information supported the need for a unit-based/site-based cultural competence inservice program:

1. Absence of prior unit-based/site-based cultural competence education program
2. Increase in the cultural diversity of clients
3. Renewed administrative interest in cultural competence education throughout the HCI
4. Mismatch between the diversity of nurses and patient population
5. Varying levels of motivation, interest, and commitment of nurses to cultural competence education
6. Awareness that culture-specific care of patients could enhance patient clinical outcomes and prognoses
7. Identification of actual and/or potential clinical problems directly and/or indirectly influenced by culturally incongruent versus culturally congruent care specific to the unit/site

Step 2—Review Literature

Once the organizational climate seems favorable to supporting the educational endeavor, moving forward to conduct a systematic literature review is recommended. (In contrast, if the organizational climate is unfavorable or ambivalent, a systematic literature review documenting strong rationale for the educational endeavor is indicated.) A review of the nursing, medicine, other relevant disciplines, and education literature should be conducted. Materials should be reviewed for gathering background information about proposed clinical topics, culturally diverse patients, patient outcomes, cultural competence education strategies, evaluation methods, inservice and continuing education, and potential resources. Choice of a relevant conceptual framework can be valuable to provide structure and organization. For example, in the two case exemplars, the Cultural Competence and Confidence (CCC) model and the measurement of TSE perceptions provided the underlying framework for strategy design and evaluation. When reviewing literature concerning cultural competence education strategies, determining strategy strengths, limitations, and appropriateness of fit to the targeted population can help sort through various possibilities. Attention to the strategy's measurement and evaluation of outcomes is integral to determining selection and/or adaptation of strategies reported in the literature. One must be aware, however, that there is no panacea that one inservice program will solve all problems and help prepare every nurse to become culturally competent. Realistically weighing the possible benefits against the risk of doing nothing can help in the decision-making process. Realistically acknowledging that one cultural competence education inservice or continuing education program can be the starting point for future cultural competence development is important.

In the case exemplars, the inservice planners had previously compiled literature on cultural competence; however, an updated review of the nursing and health professions literature was necessary. Additionally, review of cultural competence education strategies, measurement and evaluation, psychology literature on motivation, and current clinical information on the specialized target areas were conducted systematically. Published journal articles and books were reviewed and organized into specific categories, expanding the current literature files and making future retrieval and updates easy.

Step 3—Outline Ideas

Beginning with a focused, manageable topic is a necessary, critical step. Attempting to collapse too much information, skills, and affective learning within a brief inservice will overwhelm the learner, dilute content, and result in superficial or minimal application in the actual clinical setting, thus defeating the intended purpose of achieving culturally congruent care and of promoting lifelong, ongoing cultural competence development among staff nurses. Planning a series of short inservices may meet the needs more appropriately and satisfactorily with nurses who are pulled in many directions on a busy unit and with other health care professionals who are pulled in many directions throughout the HCI.

Next, outline major areas and fill in details to expand the working outline. Major areas to include are:

- Problem, need, significance, and rationale
- Background literature
- Target population
- Purpose
- Objectives

- Project activities, timeline, and potential impact on target population
- Measurement and evaluation
- Budget
- Feasibility

In the case examplars, data from the preliminary appraisal of the HCI, unit, staff, and client profile (Step 1) strongly supported the need for a cultural competence inservice program. Furthermore, the background literature strongly documented the need for culture-specific care among perioperative patients and BMT patients. The broad goal was to enhance cultural competence among staff nurses. Exhibit 12.1 presents the purpose, target population, educational objectives, and activity components in an easy-to-read format. Brainstorming resulted in a list of possible activity and content components. Reviewing the list for feasibility eliminated some strategies. Finally, prioritizing the remaining components provided an outline of ideas that could be a starting point for soliciting support.

Exhibit 12.1 Title, Inservice/CE Purpose, Target Population, Educational Objectives, and Activity Components: Comparison of Two Case Exemplars

Title	
Enhancing cultural competence in patient teaching: Issues and examples for nurses working with diverse bone marrow transplant (BMT) patients	Perioperative nursing: Promoting cultural competence

Inservice/CE Purpose	
To enhance staff nurses' cultural competence in patient teaching among diverse BMT patients	To enhance perioperative nurses' cultural competence

Target Population	
BMT staff nurses at an HCI	Perioperative registered nurses at an HCI

Main Activity	
A 1.25-hour unit-based inservice targeting culturally competent patient teaching	3-hour hospital-based continuing education (CE) program with 25–30 perioperative RN participants

Educational Objectives

At the completion of the inservice, the learners will be able to:	1. Discuss the phases of perioperative nursing and its relationship to quality health care
1. Distinguish between different cultural competence terminologies	2. Describe key transcultural nursing concepts with direct application to perioperative nursing practice
2. Differentiate between culturally congruent and incongruent patient teaching.	3. Discuss the relevance of culturally competent perioperative nursing in the achievement of successful patient outcomes
3. Discuss areas of concern with providing culturally congruent teaching	4. Analyze the impact of CLAS standards and its effect on health literacy and culturally congruent perioperative nursing care
4. Incorporate cultural competence into patient teaching	5. Analyze the impact of medication reconciliation and culturally congruent nursing care
	6. Summarize strategies to promote culturally congruent perioperative nursing care

Activity Components

1. Administer the TSET	1. Administer the TSET
2. Lecture/discussion	2. Lecture/discussion
3. Interactive PowerPoint presentation/discussion	3. Interactive PowerPoint presentation/discussion
4. Short case scenarios about culturally congruent and incongruent patient teaching	4. Small group work analysis of clinical scenarios: Health literacy, medication, reconciliation, ambulatory patient discharge
5. Reflection	5. Reflection
6. Generate open conversation among staff nurses using probing questions about their concern and/or ideas regarding their provision of culturally congruent teaching with diverse patients	6. Group leader summary of clinical scenarios' themes
7. Dialogue and brainstorming on "How to incorporate cultural competence into patient teaching on the unit"	7. Guided synthesis summary to incorporate cultural competence into all phases of the perioperative process

Step 4—Solicit Support

Although soliciting support can seem time-consuming, the benefits of having conceptual and instrumental support commitments are invaluable and help build alliances and partnerships. Although both are important here, soliciting significant amount of instrumental support commitments is an essential precursor to preparing an EI program proposal.

While this step may seem similar to the assessment of support in Step 1, it has many important differences. First, this step builds on the collaborative relationship initiated in Step 1 that should then evolve (or be nurtured) into a collaborative partnership. A collaborative partnership can have varying degrees of direct or indirect supportive involvement but all could be potentially critical to the approval of an EI program and ultimately its success.

At this point of more formalized commitment to specific tasks, the anticipated timeline for the tasks should be mentioned. This gives more structure and organization. For instance, if the timeline is not realistic, it can be adjusted now before writing it in the proposal and setting one up for failure later in the implementation and evaluation phases. Before preparing a proposal, it is important to tease out what strategies are feasible and realistic and what would be more problematic. In this way, the presence or absence of support will result in a modified list of possible strategy components. Instrumental support cannot occur without conceptual support; however, conceptual support without instrumental support greatly limits the possibilities of EP success. Evaluating staff support for various components is crucial before entering the design phase (program preparation and approval).

The following examples are applicable to the EI:

- General objective of inservice (enhancing cultural competence) is approved by director of nursing education, clinical nurse educator, and nurse manager.
- Date and time for the inservice is negotiated and approved by director of nursing education, clinical nurse educator, and nurse manager.
- Several staff nurses agree to participate in the inservice and encourage their colleagues to participate
- Nurse manager agrees to make announcements to encourage staff participation
- Administrators commit to support release time for inservice planner/educator
- HCI statistician agrees to actively assist with questionnaire processing and data analysis
- Administrators agree to allocate funds for the CE application form, healthy snacks, and photocopying

Step 5—Develop Program

In the case exemplars, the broad goal (enhancement of cultural competence) listed in the outline of ideas (Step 3) needed to be explicated to fit with the terminology and format used in the CE application guidelines.

Table 12.1 Enhancing Cultural Competence in Patient Teaching: Issues and
Examples for Nurses Working with Diverse Bone Marrow
Transplant (BMT) Patients: Educational Objectives and Brief
Content Outline

Educational Objectives	Brief Content Outline
1. Distinguish between different cultural competence terminologies	Introduction to cultural competence terminology (a) Culture (b) Cultural competence (c) Culturally congruent care (d) Transcultural self efficacy

2. Differentiate between culturally congruent and incongruent patient teaching	1. Patient teaching
	(a) Culturally congruent
	  • Case scenario
	  • Case scenario
	(b) Culturally incongruent
	  • Case scenario
	  • Case scenario
	2. Nursing implications

3. Discuss areas of concern with providing culturally congruent patient teaching	1. Concern of nurses (a) Nurses' feelings (b) Nurses' concerns (c) Areas of improvement 2. How to effectively address the areas of concern
4. Incorporate cultural competence into patient teaching	1. Strategies for incorporation (a) Cultural assessment (b) Communication (c) Plan (d) Implementation (e) Evaluation 2. Patient teaching resources (a) Telephone medical interpreter services (b) Patient information in various languages (c) Hospital-based interpreter services 3. Other suggestions from nurses

The initial draft focused on the development of educational objectives,
activity components, and content outline (Exhibit 12.1, Tables 12.1 and
12.2). Next, the draft was expanded to develop budget, measurement,
and evaluation components (Exhibits 12.2 and 12.3). Program development also aimed to be realistic and clear with measurable outcomes.
The initial draft was then modified to facilitate learner-centered, unit- or
setting-specific components within the specified time frame and budget
proposed.

Using CE and institution-specific guidelines and terminology as well
as theoretical and empirical support from the literature, the evaluation
plan included formative and summative evaluation measures. Although

Table 12.2 Perioperative Nursing: Promoting Cultural Competence—
Educational Objectives and Brief Content Outline

Educational Objectives	Brief Content Outline

1. Discuss the phases of perioperative nursing and its relationship to quality health care	1. Perioperative nursing phases
	  (a) Preadmission
	  (b) Preoperative
	  (c) Intraoperative
	  (d) Postoperative
	  (e) Discharge
	2. Perioperative nursing quality indicators
	  (a) Efficient use of resources
	  (b) Regulatory requirements
	    • Healthy People 2010
	    • Joint Commission
	    • ANCC (Magnet)
	    • Office of Minority Health: National Standards for Culturally Linguistic and Appropriate Services (CLAS)
	    • American Society of Perianesthesia Nurses
	    • Reimbursement

2. Describe key transcultural nursing concepts with direct application to perioperative nursing practice	1. Transcultural nursing concepts
	  (a) Culture, values, and beliefs of patients, family, community, and health care professionals
	  (b) Process of Cultural Competence in the Delivery of Health Care Services (Campinha-Bacote)
	    • Awareness
	    • Skill
	    • Knowledge
	    • Encounters
	    • Desire
	  (c) Relationship between culturally congruent care and transcultural self-efficacy (Jeffreys)
	    • Cognitive
	    • Practical
	    • Affective

3. Discuss the relevance of culturally competent perioperative nursing in the achievement of successful patient outcomes	Components of culturally congruent perioperative nursing care:
	  (a) Hand-off communication
	  (b) Medication reconciliation
	  (c) CLAS standards
	  (d) Informed consent
	  (e) Patient advocacy

Table 12.2 Perioperative Nursing: Promoting Cultural Competence—
Educational Objectives and Brief Content Outline (*continued*)

Educational Objectives	Brief Content Outline
4. Analyze the impact of CLAS standards and its effect on health literacy and culturally congruent perioperative nursing care	Health literacy and culturally congruent versus culturally incongruent perioperative nursing care scenarios a) Preadmission b) Preoperative c) Intraoperative d) Postoperative e) Discharge
5. Analyze the impact of medication reconciliation and culturally congruent nursing care	Ambulatory patient discharge and culturally congruent nursing care a) Health teaching b) Health literacy c) Hand-off communication d) Medication reconciliation e) Follow-up
6. Summarize strategies to promote culturally congruent perioperative nursing care	Culturally competent perioperative nursing care scenarios analyses a) CLAS and health literacy scenario b) Ambulatory patient discharge scenario

the CE guidelines focused primarily on quantitative results documenting the perceived achievement of objectives, presenter's expertise, and appropriateness of teaching strategies, the measurement of nurse's TSE perceptions were written into the evaluation plan. The justification for this inclusion was based on empirical evidence and the underlying conceptual model. As an added incentive for nurses' completion of the TSET pretest and posttest, the perioperative inservice plan offered an opportunity for TSET participants to win a Basic Life Support inservice voucher during a witnessed raffle.

Exhibit 12.2 Sample Budget

Budget
The project's budget allocation and justification are detailed below:

Description:	Justification/Rationale:	Amount:
1. Release time for staff nurse with Advanced Certificate in Cultural Competence	Develop, implement, plan, and evaluate project	In-kind ($36/hr × 40hrs = $1440)

Description:	Justification/Rationale:	Amount:
2. Media Personnel	Assist with media set-up	In-kind ($28/hr × 4hrs = $112)
3. Paper Supplies	Handouts & TSET	(In-kind + $75)
4. Secretarial Support	Generate handouts & TSET	$10/hr × 3hrs = $30
5. Advertising	Flyers & word of mouth	In-kind ($50)
6. Conference Room	Location for inservice	In-kind ($500)
7. Beverages & Snacks	Nutrition for the inservice	$150
8. Data Processing TSET and Demographic Questionnaire	Analyze changes among the BMT staff nurses' TSE perceptions.	In-kind ($36/hr × 8hrs = $288)
		Total = $2770.00 In-kind Total = $2590.00 Budget Needed = $255

Exhibit 12.3   Sample Educational Activity (Formative) Evaluation: Perioperative Nursing: Enhancing Cultural Competence

Part I Instructions: *Please complete the following statement by circling the one number that describes your rating. The rating scale ranges from 1 to 4, where 1 = poor; 2 = fair; 3 = good; and 4 = excellent.*

	Poor	Fair	Good	Excellent
1. To what extent did the objectives relate to the overall purpose?				
(a) Discuss the phases of perioperative nursing and its relationship to quality health care	1	2	3	4
(b) Describe key transcultural nursing concepts with direct application to perioperative nursing practice	1	2	3	4
(c) Discuss the relevance of culturally competent perioperative nursing in the achievement of successful patient outcomes	1	2	3	4

	Poor	Fair	Good	Excellent
1. To what extent did the objectives relate to the overall purpose?				
(d) Analyze the impact of CLAS standards and its effect on health literacy and culturally congruent perioperative nursing care	1	2	3	4
(e) Analyze the impact of medication reconciliation and culturally congruent nursing care	1	2	3	4
(f) Summarize strategies to promote culturally congruent perioperative nursing care	1	2	3	4
2. To what extent have you achieved the objectives of this session?				
(a) Discuss the phases of perioperative nursing and its relationship to quality health care	1	2	3	4
(b) Describe key transcultural nursing concepts with direct application to perioperative nursing practice	1	2	3	4
(c) Discuss the relevance of culturally competent perioperative nursing in the achievement of successful patient outcomes	1	2	3	4
(d) Analyze the impact of CLAS standards and its effect on health literacy and culturally congruent perioperative nursing care	1	2	3	4
(e) Analyze the impact of medication reconciliation and culturally congruent nursing care	1	2	3	4
(f) Summarize strategies to promote culturally congruent perioperative nursing care	1	2	3	4
3. Rate the expertise of the presenter:	1	2	3	4
4. To what extent were the teaching strategies appropriate?	1	2	3	4
5. Overall, the program was. . .	1	2	3	4
6. Was this program fair, balanced, and free of commercial bias?	Yes	No		

Part II

1. Describe three ways that you will incorporate cultural competence into your role as a perioperative nurse:
2. Were the clinical scenarios helpful in relating cultural competence into the clinical setting? Explain.
3. What suggestions do you have for future continuing educational offerings that would meet the needs of culturally diverse patients and staff?

Other Comments:

_____

_____

_____

_____

_____

Thank you.

Several tasks should receive priority, because they involve a series of steps, are time-consuming, and involve several people and/or committees; the interrelated tasks include IRB approval, demographic questionnaire development, and questionnaire permission. Actually, questionnaire development and permission is necessary prior to requesting IRB approval, therefore these two received the highest prioritization. To request permission for TSET use, the EI planners/educators wrote typewritten, signed letters on letterhead stationery to the TSET author (Jeffreys, 2004) and current copyright holder/publisher (Springer Publishing Company). (See sample permission letter, Jeffreys Toolkit 2010, Item 19.) Requests to adapt or use items from the Demographic Data Sheet-Nurses (Jeffreys Toolkit 2010, Item 9) were also submitted as necessary, because this was prior to the availability of the Jeffreys Cultural Competence Education Toolkit (2010) and the permission stipulations specified for educational or institutional purchases. (See permission guidelines contained in Jeffreys Toolkit 2010 coversheet and in Preface page xix.)

When adapting or developing demographic questionnaires, review by peers with expertise in content, psychometrics, and organizational culture is recommended. The suggestions presented in Chapter 5 concerning demographic data collection and analyses offer a valuable guide in determining what should be included. For peer evaluators, a cover letter explaining some background information and purpose of the demographic questionnaire, requested due date, a self-addressed stamped envelope, and an instruction sheet for rating items should accompany the questionnaire. The ratings and comments of the reviewers provide the basis for revisions. Review by a psychometric expert should support that the demographic data questions are in a format that can easily be scanned, interpreted, and analyzed using a statistical program. Chapter 5 presents valuable guidelines on interpreting data and avoiding pitfalls in the data collection and analyses process.

Several EI program revisions resulted in a final EI program proposal that was submitted in a timely fashion according to the IRB and other administrative procedures at the respective HCIs.

Step 6—Get Approval

Final *official* approval from administrators, educators, and the CE agency are necessary to proceed. When a program is approved, it is important to review the budgetary allocations for specific categories and check if there are any restrictions or added guidelines. Additionally, IRB stipulations and recommendations concerning data collection, processing, and analyses must be considered. Budgetary and time constraints as well as IRB stipulations may require some modifications from the original proposed program. These modifications should be finalized before entering the next phase of preimplementation. The preimplementation phase acknowledges that there are two essential steps that need to be done before program implementation: communication and preparation. For the EI, no major changes from the original EI program proposal were noted.

Step 7—Communicate

Once the EI program is approved and the budgetary plan modifications are finalized, the inservice planner/educator should communicate that approval has been received. The important questions to consider are with whom to communicate, what needs to be communicated, and how to communicate. Essentially, what must be communicated is that approval was received and how this will involve the other collaborative partner(s).

Collaborative partners or those individuals who committed time, expertise, service, or some other instrumental support toward the proposed EI program should be contacted personally. A telephone contact followed by a written memo or copy of the CE and/or HCI administrator approval letter and the EI program proposal may be indicated depending on the type of partnership required and level of involvement. Memos that communicate the necessary details serve as reinforcement to the verbal communication.

A copy of the CE approval letter should be forwarded to the administration as per HCI protocol. A copy should also be forwarded to all unit-based administrators and the institution-wide nursing education department. Announcements made at staff, committee, and other pertinent meetings can be made both verbally and in the form of a written memo or information sheet. Postings on bulletin boards, newsletter and electronic announcements, and mailings will help advertise and market the program.

In the case exemplars, colorful and captivating flyers succinctly highlighted major program components including time, place, purpose, target audience, objectives, and participant benefits. In the perioperative case exemplar, announcement of CE approval from the state nurses association was forwarded to the appropriate administrators and other collaborative partners by the inservice planner/educator. Scheduled meetings with nurse educators, nurse managers, and other collaborative partners endeavored to build on the communication, commitments, and partnerships established previously in Steps 1 and 4.

Step 8—Prepare for Program

Allocating a sufficient amount of time for program preparation is important. Making a list of what needs to be done, by whom, and the needed date of completion can help prioritize program preparation components. Preparation may include creating or obtaining educational materials and documentation forms, selection and orientation of personnel, duplicating materials (questionnaires, flyers, educational handouts), and arranging the physical setting.

In the case exemplars, a timeline was originally submitted with the EI program proposal which this served as a valuable guide (Exhibit 12.4).

Exhibit 12.4   Timeline for Perioperative Nursing: Promoting Cultural Competence Employee Inservice Program

Timeline

March

1. Collaborate with HCI Director of Nursing Education
2. Collaborate with HCI clinical nursing educator (surgical service)
3. Distribute and collect Quality and Culture Quiz to all registered nurses
4. Develop educational inservice "Perioperative Nursing: Enhancing Cultural Competence" program purpose and objectives
5. Identify budget, feasibility, and timeline

April

1. Complete analysis of Quality and Culture Quiz with Cultural Committee
2. Obtain permission from Dr. Jeffreys and Springer Publishing Company for use of TSET
3. Apply for IRB approval for administration of TSET
4. Utilize Demographic Data for collection with TSET for registered nurses
5. Revise lesson plan and objectives
6. Meet with Perioperative Nursing Educational Day Planning Committee
7. Develop program schedule and confirm all presenters' topics.
8. Submit final continuing education form to state nurses' association
9. Revise budget, feasibility, and timeline.
10. Complete IRB requirements and online training related to research.

May

1. Incorporate Quality and Culture Quiz findings into identification of educational needs
2. Develop PowerPoint presentation handout
3. Confirm date and place of presentation
4. Request healthy snacks from HCI catering service
5. Follow-up on IRB approval for administration of TSET

June

1. Update literature review related to perioperative nursing, cultural competence, and health literacy.
2. Submit PowerPoint handouts, attendance, and evaluation tool for duplication
3. Obtain/Finalize IRB approval for administration of TSET

July–August

1. Advertise Perioperative Nursing fall program in Nursing education electronic newsletter
2. Advertise program on central and unit-based bulletin boards
3. Develop registration list

September

1. Meet with Periopertive Nursing planning committee for final confirmation and coordination with other education offerings
2. Review registration list
3. Coordinate handout packet preparation

October

1. Distribute TSET at beginning of continuing education program
2. Presentation of Perioperative Nursing: Achieving Cultural Competence as part of the Perioperative Nursing educational day
3. Distribute TSET at the end of the continuing education program

November–December

1. Analysis of TSET, continuing education evaluation, and demographic data using scanning software (or hand data entry) and SPSS
2. Prepare research report and PowerPoint presentation

January

1. Presentation of TSET findings and continuing education program evaluation results to the Director of Nursing Education and the Cultural Committee
2. Disseminate findings to Dr. Marianne Jeffreys and grant funding agencies.
3. Perform witnessed raffle for BLS voucher for TSET participants and announce winner in nursing education electronic newsletter
4. Meet with the Director of Nursing Education for planning of future cultural competence continuing education programs throughout the HCI

Spring of Next Year

1. Present poster of Perioperative Nursing: Enhancing Cultural Competence program and TSET findings at the annual HCI Nursing Research Day
2. Submit abstract to upcoming local, national, and/or international conferences
3. Prepare manuscript for submission to refereed journal

Step 9—Implement Program

A well-developed and detailed EI program proposal accompanied by an itemized timeline can serve as the guide for program implementation (Exhibit 12.4). To facilitate smooth implementation, the program should be divided into various categories: pretest data collection, educational activities, and formative data collection. Each category of the program should complement each other, receive adequate time and attention, be part of the overall program, and easily flow into the next category. For example, providing an environment conducive for pretest and formative data collection, verbally emphasizing the importance of completing the evaluations honestly and seriously, and allocating sufficient time for contemplative completion will convey institutional commitment to cultural competence education as well as add to the validity of findings that will guide future cultural competence educational programs. Learner-centered activities that thoughtfully provoke insights and application to the immediate workplace setting and individual's career benefits are preferred over passive learning activities. A summary synthesis that ties together general principles of cultural competence with direct professional application will assist participants to incorporate cultural competence into all phases of the targeted topic (patient teaching on the BMT unit or perioperative process) (Exhibit 12.1).

Step 10—Evaluation

As mentioned previously, a carefully orchestrated evaluation should be tied explicitly to the EI program proposal's measurement plan and should include both formative and summative components. Formative evaluations assess the process of a program rather than outcomes. Formative evaluations can be monitored as the program is implemented and can document specific activities, identify difficulties, and allow for diagnostic-prescriptive modifications based on participants' feedback, using both quantitative and qualitative data (Exhibit 12.3).

Summative evaluations should be monitored at the conclusion of a series of cultural competence education inservice programs or at a designated time period following a single EI program. Aggregating and comparing data within and between EI groups will be valuable in evaluating the achievement of educational and other outcomes. Collapsing several groups together to attain sufficient sample size for statistical comparison and relevance may be indicated. Because cultural competence education is a dynamic and multidimensional phenomenon, the success of any teaching strategy requires a multidimensional evaluation strategy. In the two case exemplars, the EI provides an action-oriented approach that combines cognitive, affective, and practical domains of learning. The inservice planners/educators noted that "The Cultural Competence and Confidence model (CCC) integrates these concepts that explain, describe, influence, and/or predict the phenomenon of learning (developing) cultural competence"(Jeffreys, 2006, p. 25). Cultural competence educational opportunities influence learners' confidence (transcultural self-efficacy) and ability to practice culturally sensitive nursing care. Within each of the HCI, cultural competence continuing education would become part of an integrated plan to provide culturally congruent care, enhance nursing professional development, and facilitate culturally sensitive health outcomes. The evaluation of transcultural self efficacy (TSE) perceptions would help assess learning, educational strategies, and contribute to transcultural nursing education and research. Following the preestablished plan for data collection and data analysis consistently and rigorously will help make the evaluation results more valid and reliable. This includes working diligently with previously established partners in the evaluation process such as the data collectors, director of institutional research, project assistant, and psychometric expert. Once the results are obtained and reviewed for statistical and practical significance, inferences from the data can guide future EI program activities, outcome measures, and desired outcomes. Additionally, comparing results from administering the TSET posttest immediately after a single cultural competence EI with results from delayed administration (6 months post educational intervention) and/or following a series of cultural competence workshops will yield new information.

Step 11—Disseminate

Professional development and the advancement of a profession relies on the active, ongoing dissemination of empirical findings that substantiate existing information, add to the depth and breadth of professional knowledge, and challenge professionals to explore new dimensions. Dissemination of quantitative and qualitative findings and outcomes or benefits from the EI should be conducted on an internal as well as external level. Sharing information internally via staff meetings, committee meetings, HCI newsletter, HCI Web site, or HCI conferences should be routinely incorporated with the EI process. Dissemination via discipline-specific and multidisciplinary professional conferences and publications shares valuable information on a broader level. Dissemination outside the HCI encourages conservation of limited human and financial resources typical of many HCIs as well as promotes the pooling of resources created by networking and sharing empirically supported cultural competence EI programs, rather than spending exorbitant amounts of time and energy continually recreating from scratch programs that may or may not work. Timely dissemination of conceptual, process, and empirical aspects of the EI program is highly recommended. In the case exemplars, a dissemination plan has been proposed (Exhibit 12.4)

KEY POINT SUMMARY

- Ongoing, accessible opportunities for cultural competence education at the HCI offer tremendous possibilities for optimal cultural competence, especially if inservice programs build upon the foundations established via a well-planned employee orientation program that: (a) substantively emphasized cultural competence throughout all content areas; (b) provided strategies and incentives for nurses to implement culture-specific care directly on their assigned unit or setting; and (c) intrinsically motivated nurses to actively engage in the ongoing quest for developing cultural competence in self and in others.

- The 11-step EI process includes: assess current situation, review literature, outline ideas, solicit support, develop program, get approval, communicate, prepare for program, implement program, evaluate program, and disseminate.
- The perioperative nursing and bone marrow transplant patient teaching case exemplars illustrate each step individually, describe EI activity components, and demonstrate easy application for a variety of unit-based or site-based settings
- Using the CCC model, summative evaluation includes the assessment of TSE using the Transcultural Self-Efficacy Tool (TSET) as a pretest and posttest.

CHAPTER 13

Professional Associations

Marianne R. Jeffreys, EdD, RN

Professional associations (see Figure 13.1) provide unique opportunities for professional socialization, networking, skill enhancement, knowledge expansion, and professional attitude development (Betts & Cherry, 2002; Joel & Kelly, 2002). Because professional associations possess a potentially powerful and extensive ability to network together diverse and talented groups of professionals beyond a single health care institution (HCI) or academic setting, they can exert tremendous influence on promoting, disseminating, and advancing cultural competence development. Collectively and individually, professional associations, leaders, and members are challenged to take definitive actions that prioritize and enhance cultural competence development. Although each member is empowered to make a positive difference, the greatest impact will be achieved through a coordinated, holistic group effort that purposely interconnects all dimensions of the association—which will no doubt reflect well on the association far beyond its membership. Such actions necessitate empirically and conceptually supported inquiries, actions, and innovations motivated by true commitment for optimal cultural competence that is expressed substantially in the philosophy and mission, structure, events, activities, and networks of the association.

Despite the type of professional association (broad purpose association, specialty practice association, or special interest association), all professional associations can potentially make a real difference in developing culturally competent nurses and other health professionals: to enhance quality of care among culturally diverse patients. Certain factors within the professional association may support cultural competence

Professional Associations

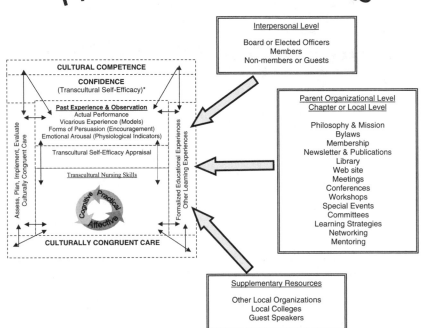

Figure 13.1   Professional Associations

development; yet other factors may restrict its development. This chapter highlights strategies for (a) identifying educational opportunities (within professional associations) for promoting cultural competency; (b) recognizing and overcoming barriers and challenges; and (c) developing action-focused strategies for educational innovation. The following section addresses key features for inquiry, action, and educational innovation within the professional association.

SELF-ASSESSMENT

Similar to the process of cultural competency development in academia (Chapter 6) and the HCI (Chapter 10), promoting cultural competency in the professional association requires considerable sincere effort that must begin with self-assessment. Systematic self-assessment evaluates the various dimensions that can impact upon the educational process and on the achievement of educational outcomes (Jeffreys, 2004). Figure 13.2 depicts a systematic assessment within the professional association. Here,

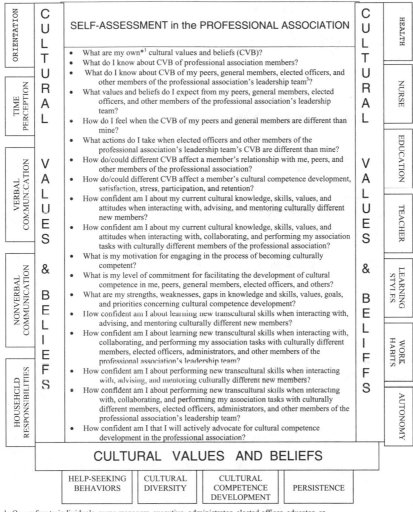

Figure 13.2 Self-assessment in the professional association (Adapted from Jeffreys, 2004, p. 169)

self-assessment refers to assessment of the individual member, elected officers, administrators, and the organization/association. (Readers are encouraged to refer to Chapter 6 for an in-depth discussion about self-assessment and Table 1.2 about dimensions of cultural values and beliefs. A user-friendly Self-Assessment Tool-Professional Associations (SAT-PA) is available in the Cultural Competence Education Resource Toolkit [Jeffreys, 2010]. The SAT-PA may be used individually and/or in groups;

the SAT-PA may be used alone or in conjunction with other toolkit items. (See Preface, page xix.) Finally, self-assessment should conclude with a listing of strengths, weaknesses, gaps in knowledge, goals, commitment, desire, motivation, and priorities.

As mentioned in Chapter 6, a comprehensive understanding, skill, and desire are essential but not enough to effectively make a positive difference in cultural competence development. The author believes that resilient transcultural self-efficacy (confidence) is a critical and integral component in the process of cultural competence development (of self and in others). Transcultural self-efficacy (TSE) is the mediating factor that enhances persistence in cultural competence development despite obstacles, hardships, or stressors. Resilient TSE perceptions embrace lifelong learning in the quest to become "more" culturally competent and in the quest to assist others (learners and colleagues) to become more culturally competent.

Within the PA there are many challenges and obstacles, therefore it becomes increasingly important that individual members, elected officers, administrators, and the organization develop and maintain resilience, motivation, commitment, and persistence for endeavors that foster optimal cultural competence. It is proposed that individuals (and the organization) with resilient TSE perceptions persist in their endeavors to be active transcultural advocates or promoters of cultural competence in all dimensions of the PA and professional practice. Exhibit 13.1 provides a guide for appraising values, beliefs, and actions and for determining whether or not one is an active role model in cultural competence development within the PA or if there are factors restricting cultural competence development. (A user-friendly Active Promoter Assessment Tool-Health Care Institutions/Associations (APAT-HCIA) is available in the Cultural Competence Education Resource Toolkit [Jeffreys, 2010]. The APAT-HCIA may be used individually and/or in groups; the APAT-HCIA may be used alone or in conjunction with other toolkit items. (See Preface, page xix for use within health care institutional and professional association settings). It is proposed that the "actions taken to promote cultural competence development" is what makes one an active role model. Active role models influence cultural competence development in others by presenting opportunities for actual and vicarious learning and via forms of persuasion (honest and judicious encouragement and feedback). By providing ongoing opportunities for high-quality mentoring, professional associations can enhance the power of modeling on self-efficacy appraisal and professional development at all levels within the PA. The power of mentoring on nurses' professional development and satisfaction has been well documented (Bosher & Pharris, 2009; Cavanaugh & Huse, 2004; Heller et al., 2004; Vance & Olson, 1998).

Exhibit 13.1 Self-Assessment: Active Promoter of Cultural Competence Development in the Professional Association

Promoter	Values, Beliefs, and Actions	Promoter
Yes	Views cultural competence as important in own[1] life *and shares beliefs with others*[2]	No
Yes	Views cultural competence as important in members' education, professional development, and future practice *and shares view with others*	No
Yes	Views own role to include active involvement in promoting cultural competence development among members *and shares view with others*	No
Yes	Routinely updates own knowledge and skills to enhance cultural competence *and shares relevant information with others*	No
Yes	Attends professional events concerning cultural competence development *and shares positive and relevant experiences with others*	No
Yes	Views professional event participation concerning cultural competence development as important in members' ongoing continuing education, professional development, and future practice *and shares view with others*	No
Yes	*Offers incentives to encourage members' participation in professional events*	No
Yes	Maintains professional partnerships focused on cultural competence development *and shares positive and relevant experiences with others*	No
Yes	Maintains membership(s) in professional organizations whose primary mission is cultural competence development *and shares positive and relevant experiences with others*	No
Yes	Views memberships in professional organizations/ associations (whose primary mission is cultural competence development) as important in members's continuing education, professional development, and future practice *and shares view with others*	No
Yes	*Offers incentives to encourage others' participation in memberships in professional organizations/associations committed to cultural competence development*	No
Yes	Recognizes actual and potential barriers hindering the development of cultural competence *and initiates strategies to remove barriers*	No
Yes	*Implements strategies to encourage members' development of cultural competence*	No
Yes	*Evaluates strategies implemented to encourage members' development of cultural competence*	No

[1] *Own* refers to individual members, elected officers, or association
[2] Active promoter/facilitator actions are indicated by italics

In addition, one needs to evaluate if the PA is truly committed to the goal of cultural competence development, cultural diversity within the profession, and culturally congruent patient care. One approach is to examine whether the PA actively embraced cultural diversity, cultural competence education, and recruitment of diverse members as priority goals partnered with strategic implementation plans prior to the relatively recent, popular attention to cultural diversity. Actively embracing cultural diversity includes multiple, intensive strategies designed to recruit, retain, and encourage educational and career advancement among culturally diverse nurses, especially from groups underrepresented in nursing practice and nursing leadership. Tragically, cultural diversity within the nursing profession does not mirror the U. S. population; nurse leaders from underrepresented groups are even less visible (Burnes Bolton, 2004; Foley & Wurmser, 2004; Georges, 2004; Simpson, 2004; Swanson, 2004; Villarruel & Peragallo, 2004; Washington, Erickson, & Ditomassi, 2004). (The critical topic of enhancing cultural diversity within nursing is enormous; readers are referred to the current literature on nurse recruitment, retention, and professional advancement).

Sincere, active commitment of members' individual and collective participation in cultural competence development and culturally diverse membership initiatives should be continually challenged to reach optimal levels. Settling for the status quo within a professional association is unacceptable—striving to reach outside the box (comfort zone) to evoke positive change within a PA takes constant energy and effective, visionary leadership. The author contends that cultural competence is unachievable unless individuals and groups of individuals (via memberships and participation in professional associations) are intrinsically motivated. Resilient TSE (confidence) will positively influence intrinsic motivation and persistence at cultural competence development of self and others. Resilient confidence in the power of professional associations and dynamic group action will move the achievement of optimal cultural competence forward.

EVALUATION IN THE PROFESSIONAL ASSOCIATION

Consistent with the evaluation of educational opportunities for cultural competence development in academic and health care settings, it is equally necessary to closely examine how visible (or invisible) cultural competency development is in the professional association. Certainly, examining interpersonal characteristics, the parent association and affiliated chapters, and supplementary resources in this regard requires courage, commitment, time, energy, and a systematic plan. An evaluative inquiry can be guided by two additional questions: (a) To what degree is cultural competence an integral component? and (b) How do all the dimensions of the association fit together to support cultural competence development? (See Figure 13.3) A thorough evaluation of what currently exists (Jeffreys Toolkit 2010, Item 17) serves as a valuable precursor to informed

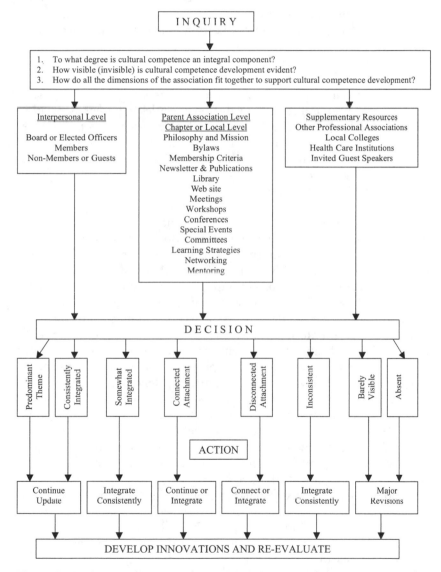

Figure 13.3 Systematic Inquiry for Decision, Action, and Innovation in Professional Associations

decisions, responsible actions, and new diagnostic-prescriptive innovations targeting members' development and the overall goal of achieving optimal cultural competence.

A detailed critique of the association's philosophy and mission, bylaws, membership, newsletter and publications, library, Web site, meetings, workshops, conferences, special events, committees, learning strategies, networking, and mentoring is an ambitious endeavor requiring much diligence, humility, honesty, and dedication. It may be a startling realization that a professional association is not as involved in optimal cultural competence development as it could be (or should be). Systematic evaluation helps identify association strengths, weaknesses, inconsistencies, and gaps related to cultural competency development. Guided and purposeful reflective self-appraisal at an individual member level, parent association level, and/or chapter level will provide valuable insight and perspective. On close scrutiny, threads of culture and cultural competency should be equally and substantially evident throughout the association's structure, activities, and resources.

Examination must differentiate between superficial and substantial evidence. For example, a professional association may sponsor a workshop on "Health Promotion and African-American Populations in Urban Communities," appearing to meet an association mission statement that states, "disseminate information to promote health among culturally diverse populations." Yet, the workshop may not actually promote cultural competence development if the multidimensional cultural values and beliefs (CVB) of a clearly defined cultural group are never thoroughly explored (see Table 13.1) As a second example, mission statements that incorporate such phrases as "cultural competence," "cultural diversity," and "culturally congruent care" may appear to value cultural competence. However, without the implementation of any actions and innovations that actively enhance cultural competence development, such mission statements are meaningless, misleading, and even harmful (see Table 13.2). Associations are challenged to effectively integrate cultural competence throughout all aspects of the association to provide long-lasting learning and desirable outcomes among culturally diverse professionals and beyond the immediate membership population. Because culturally diverse individuals have diverse learning needs, strengths, values, and beliefs, offering different types of multidimensional active learning activities will be most beneficial (Brookfield, 1986; Gaffney, 2000; Horsfall & Cleary, 2008; Kelly, 1997; Williams & Calvillo, 2002; Yoder, 2001). (Various learning strategies are discussed in Chapter 6).

A close scrutiny of association brochures, membership applications, newsletters, journals, other publications, library, and Web site should assess whether cultural competency development is emphasized

Table 13.1 Going beyond Topic and Title: Searching for Substantive Evidence of Cultural Competence

Topic/Title	Poor Example	Better Example
Prostate cancer (PC) screening practices among African American (AA) middle-aged men	(1) Focuses on disease process and reported statistics of PC screening practices among AA men (2) Mortality rates correlated with late screening practices (3) Includes recent immigrants and/or refugees from Haiti, Trinidad, Jamaica, Barbados, Nigeria, Kenya, South Africa as well as descendents of American slaves.	(1) Introductory focus on cultural beliefs, values, and practices associated with health promotion and illness prevention (2) Specific focus on CVB, and practices associated with prostate screening among AA.
Culture and sensitivity for wound care: New innovations in clinical practice	Focuses on the diagnostic procedure of obtaining a wound culture, providing wound care, evaluating culture and sensitivity (C&S) results, administering appropriate anti-infective medications, and evaluating healing.	Presents an overview of wound healing; variation in skin pigmentation, healing, and scarring; compares and contrasts beliefs, traditional healing practices, non-Western modalities for wound healing; stigmas and values associated with different types of wounds; and suggests implications for nursing practice using a culturally sensitive approach
A culturally congruent diet for Hispanic patients with diabetes	(1) Presents national statistics for incidence, complications, and mortality associated with diabetes contrasting "Hispanic" category with patients who identify as "white, non-Hispanic." (2) Presents Hispanics as one cultural group. (3) No discussion of cultural meanings and beliefs associated with different types of food. (4) Only presents Mexican foods (e. g., tamales, enchiladas, and tacos) as appropriate substitutions on food pyramid. (5) No discussion of culturally preferred teaching–learning styles	(1) Statistics presented. (2) Limitations associated with broad categorization of all Hispanics as a homogenous group discussed. (3) Presents a table contrasting several different subgroups within Hispanic category, listing common foods, uses, methods of preparation, nutritional value, and meaning associated with food. (4) Discusses "hot and cold" theory common to most Hispanic groups. (5) Case study illustrates cultural pain and distress experienced by a Puerto Rican patient with diabetes who is given a bilingual patient booklet entitled "Diabetic Diets for Mexican-Americans" and a second booklet discussing steps to becoming an American citizen.

Table 13.2 Outcome Responses to Professional Association's Components

Area	Positive Outcome (Promoting Optimal Cultural Competence)	Negative Outcome (Barriers to Cultural Competence)
Mission and philosophy	"I noticed that the professional association's mission and philosophy listed cultural competence development throughout the document. It made me feel like it was an important component and that my cultural values and beliefs (CVB) would be respected."	"I noticed that the PA's mission and philosophy listed cultural competence development as part of a bullet list, including it last. In contrast, other themes were much more predominant throughout the document. I felt like the PA was not really sincere in its mission toward cultural competence and diversity. I am looking for a PA that will help me develop my cultural competence and respect me as a unique individual. I do not feel this PA will meet my needs."
Newsletter	"I was really pleasantly surprised to see an article in the clinical specialty association's newsletter that discussed subtle racism in the workplace. It enlightened me that I am actually carrying out actions with some of my coworkers that are culturally insensitive. I was really pleased to see that the newsletter has a regularly featured column devoted to cultural issues particularly relevant to this clinical specialty but also applicable across many specialties."	"I can't believe the clinical specialty association's newsletter presented the inclusion of cultural considerations within nursing as a *new* idea. And, I can't believe the newsletter gave credit to this new idea to a nurse within the PA who has never even conducted any research on any subject. When I wrote a letter to the editor and sent a list of current and classic transcultural nursing references, her response was 'Thank you for your letter. Due to space limitations, we cannot publish your materials. We will file your reference list in our editorial file.'"
Membership brochure	"As a new graduate nurse on a tight budget, I was so pleased to see reduced rates and a mentoring program for new graduate nurses. I also noticed that the mentoring program offered the option to pair new graduates with a member of a similar ethnic or racial background, gender, or area of interest. Because I went to a nursing school where almost 95% of the students were my age, gender, religion, ethnic, and racial background, I had never thought about groups who were different than me and what their experience might be like entering a predominantly white, female,	"As a soon-to-be graduate nurse, I was motivated by my senior instructor to join the state nurses' association and become part of a professional association that could really make a positive difference in health care for this state. With the NCLEX examination soon approaching, I also needed to envision myself as a nurse—as part of an important profession. When I looked at the membership brochure photos, I couldn't find one person that looked like me. If 27% of my state's general population and 10% of the state's

(continued)

	nursing profession. It gave me something to think about and made me realize I have much to learn. I was thinking about requesting a mentor who was different from me so I could learn about a different experience and become more culturally knowledgeable with my patients and coworkers."	registered nurse population identifies with my racial group, why don't I see a relatively comparative proportion of photos of nurses and patients representing my group? I felt very discouraged and even questioned if I could really make it in the nursing profession."
Web site	"When perusing the PA Web site, I noticed a Web site heading for the 'Association strategies to enhance diversity within the profession.' As a member of an underrepresented group, I was thrilled. Then I clicked on the heading and was brought to a page that said, 'Under construction.' Three months later, I went back to the page and it was comprehensively updated along with other features and announcements on the PA Web site had been updated."	"When perusing the PA Web site, I noticed a Web site heading for the 'Association strategies to enhance diversity within the profession.' As a member of an underrepresented group, I was thrilled. Then I clicked on the heading and was brought to a page that said, 'Under construction.' Three months later, I went back to the page and nothing had changed, although other features and announcements on the PA Web site had been updated."
Conference	"Usually at the end of a conference, I am so totally tired that I can't even focus anymore. But the panel of speakers at the very end of the conference really tied together many aspects of the overall clinical conference by presenting application to select cultural groups. I liked that the panel represented a culturally diverse group of men and women in the profession who worked in academia and clinical areas but were also active members within my PA. I also liked that they first presented a brief overview of select literature and research on their group and then identified when they presented their own personal opinion. The separation between scholarliness, application, and opinions was important for my learning to develop my own cultural competence."	"How could the PA present such an incompetent group of panel speakers on 'Meeting the needs of culturally diverse patients'? The 3 speakers represented one of the several federal census categories—but where was my group?—I have a culture too. It would have been OK to just focus on 3 groups for this particular workshop (and then take general information to apply to other groups and/or have different groups represented in the future, but that should have been explained in the beginning). The speakers had no knowledge of the scholarly and clinical work done already with these groups; yet they presented their personal views as the views of all members within that category. The culturally diverse students I brought to the conference even expressed their concern about this."

Table 13.2   Outcome Responses to Professional Association's Components (*continued*)

Area	Positive Outcome (Promoting Optimal Cultural Competence)	Negative Outcome (Barriers to Cultural Competence)
Journal	*Ronnie:* "I haven't read the journal of the clinical specialty association in a few years. The research articles generally compared and contrasted new medications, procedures, or treatments for patients with a particular disease. Then, I picked up the journal the other day and was surprised to find two articles that compared and contrasted effectiveness of a medication and a treatment regimen between two distinct cultural groups usually collapsed under a cultural label comprising many cultural groups. I then checked the published purpose of the journal and was pleased to see that a revised purpose included presenting clinical specialty research to help eliminate health disparities and recognize culturally diverse populations." *Terry:* "I'm not really into all that cultural stuff. I'm a real clinical nurse. I didn't think the articles had relevance to me, but because I deal with these clinical issues, I decided to read them. I realized that sometimes when some of my patients had idiosyncratic reactions to drugs, I suspected that they did not accurately follow the prescribed regimen when their response was normal for them based on ethnopharmacological evidence that I was unaware of. Now, I am glad the journal will publish more articles like this so I can become a better clinical nurse. That's important to me."	*Kay:* "I can't believe that the peer reviewers of this journal focused on culture rejected our manuscript." *Jay:* "Yes, some of the comments the reviewer's wrote are even more unbelievable. We did the literature search and discovered a cultural topic and group not discussed in the nursing literature that demanded attention. We clearly presented the scholarly literature from other disciplines that substantiated its significance. One reviewer even wrote that this cultural group does not need attention when there are other groups more important." *Kay:* "Well, I was very angry and thought about not renewing my membership next year. But, after thinking about it some more, I realized that it was even more important to become active within the organization to broaden the thinking outside the traditional comfort zone of the majority members of the PA." *Jay:* "Yes, I feel the same way. It's great that our manuscript was accepted for publication in a multidisciplinary journal focused on culture. By the reviewers' comments, it was obvious they were not only scholars but open-minded and willing to think outside the box."

Meetings	"This PA is truly committed to an inclusive environment that embraces cultural diversity. During the membership meeting, the president chaired the meeting and demonstrated respect and gave equal attention to all diverse members and opinions."	"This PA is superficially committed to an inclusive environment and does not embrace diversity. During the membership meeting, the president chaired the meeting and demonstrated different degrees of respect and attention to members who were similar to her in age, education, and racial background. Oppositional views were quickly dismissed without listening to supporting rationale."
Special Events	"The PA special events committee met to plan an awards dinner. One of the members brought up that the proposed date was on a religious fast day. Although approximately 5% of the membership represented that religious group, the committee felt that all members should feel they could attend. The date was then changed to another date that would not conflict with any religious or ethnic holidays, fasts, requirements, or events. It was good to see the committee's decision process documented in the PA minutes so that all members could become more culturally aware and see that the PA was committed to inclusiveness."	"The PA special events committee met to plan an awards dinner. One of the members brought up that the proposed date was on a religious fast day. Another member said that the awards dinner had always been on the third Wednesday of that month, and approximately 5% of the membership represented that religious group and usually never attended the dinner, so therefore the date did not need to be changed. The date was not changed. This discussion was not documented in the minutes; however, the committee member who recognized the date as a potential conflict verbally discussed the meeting with me and other PA members informally."

substantially, equally, and symmetrically in all dimensions (see Table 13.2). Using the general questions depicted in Figure 13.3 and Jeffreys Toolkit 2010, Item 17, associations can conduct a systematic inquiry, make a decision, choose an action, and then develop innovations. For example, if the consensus of the association's board members decide that cultural issues are "barely visible" in the association newsletter and Web site, the action chosen should be to make major revisions, develop innovations, and reevaluate within a specified time period. Collaboration with other association members and outside experts will be essential to the overall goals and process. As a second example, an association's program development committee may decide that the annual program topics last year presented cultural competence as an "add-on" or "disconnected attachment." Thereafter, the chosen action will be to connect together with a common theme and closing address during the next annual program and reevaluate. A documentation log to document cultural competence plans, actions, and evaluations can help PAs on target with achieving goals for optimal cultural competence (Jeffreys Toolkit 2010, Item 20).

Certain factors will enhance the ability to conduct an intensive critique. These include psychological factors, practical factors, and expertise factors. Ideally, all conditions should be favorable for a critique to be most successful and valid. Psychological factors include: intrinsic motivation, extrinsic motivation, commitment, willingness to make changes, open-mindedness, satisfaction, minimal stress, positive group dynamics, and perceived benefits. Practical factors include time, location and setting, workload, financial resources, board and membership support, bylaws, secretarial support, technical resources, facilities, and energy. Expertise factors include the level of expertise (educational preparation and actual task experience) in evaluation, professional associations, group process, concept mapping, cultural competence development, teaching and learning cultural competence, teaching and learning process, adult learners, culturally diverse members, and learner characteristics.

BARRIERS

Unfortunately, there is a tragic decline in the number of professional association members who have time to serve as volunteers (Shinn, 1998). Furthermore, the number of members with the necessary expertise to conduct a thorough evaluation, propose changes, initiate actions, and implement innovations is sparse. Association leaders will need to recruit, guide, and mentor others in this evaluative process. Undoubtedly, strong, effective leadership is vital to the success of any professional association and its endeavors to facilitate cultural competence development. A major task for professional association leaders is to mentor others as leaders, especially reaching out to nurses who have been traditionally underrepresented in nursing (Bolton, 2004; Georges, 2004; Keltner, Kelley, & Smith, 2004; Thompson, 2004; Villarruel & Peragallo, 2004). Appraisal of the association's membership profile in relation to the general population of nurses, neighboring communities, elected leaders within the professional association, and criteria for membership will provide helpful information to guide the association's membership recruitment, retention, and mentoring initiatives. For example, a local chapter of an association whose main mission centers on cultural competence, located in a culturally diverse urban community, should have culturally diverse members representative of the population of nurses and should have culturally diverse qualified elected leaders. (Although recruitment and retention of professional association members is an important issue, it is beyond the scope of this book to address this here. Readers are referred to other sources in the literature.)

Another barrier is the devaluing of professional association participation in contrast to other activities. For example, when making tenure and promotion decisions, multidisciplinary committees at universities value a journal publication over service to an association. This is consistent with an individualistic worldview that places the emphasis on individual achievement and accomplishments over group achievements and successes. Although nursing faculty members are expected to belong to professional associations, funding to support memberships, conference fees, and travel is severely limited or virtually nonexistent, especially in public institutions. Similarly, a nurse who agrees to work 4 hours of overtime will receive more positive tacit, indirect, and direct feedback and support from supervisors and colleagues than a nurse who declines to work overtime to attend a professional meeting for 4 hours. Again, the short-term perspective is myopic; it does not examine the long-term benefits that would result from supportive professional development activities such as increased satisfaction and nurse retention. Professional associations today face different challenges than academia and HCIs in finding effective ways of promoting cultural competence development. The level of involvement is confounded by the shortage of nurses and nursing faculty. For example, nursing associations are competing with nurse dissatisfaction in the workplace, fatigue, stress, and time. Nursing associations are also competing with heavy faculty workloads exacerbated by increased nursing student enrollment; lack of sufficient, qualified faculty; and decreased university funds.

Other serious obstacles include the increased proliferation of professional associations, limited numbers of members and resources, duplication of efforts, competition for membership, and high-energy demands in a rapidly changing multicultural society (Shinn, 1998; Skaggs & DeVries, 1998). The question arises whether the proliferation of associations has fragmented professional unity and depleted the dynamic energy required to maintain routine activities and invigorate new ideas, explore new directions, stimulate positive change, create new vision, and spark needed innovations within the association and the profession. Furthermore, mandatory membership in a professional association through workplace unions may unintentionally shift focus on to salary, benefits, and workplace conditions rather than on strategies for advancing the science and scholarship of nursing. The challenge is to invigorate, motivate, and involve nurses who initially joined an association because of a unionized workplace to appreciate, value, support, and contribute efforts to advance the nursing profession and optimal cultural competence development.

ACTIONS AND INNOVATIONS

Pacquiao (2004) urged collaboration between associations and agencies in order to capitalize and pool together strengths and expertise, resources to achieve more positive outcomes (success), and avoid duplication of efforts. The idea of joint memberships in professional associations is one option to maximize an association's economic and human resource potential (Shinn, 1998). Often, professional associations have similar missions and attract similar potential members. For example, national ethnic nursing organizations, the Transcultural Nursing Society (international), local chapters of the previous associations, and other similar professional associations share an interest in cultural issues and health care. It takes constant energy to recruit and keep members in any one association and prevent the recycling of the same members as elected officers and/or task force committee members.

Similarly, local chapters of Sigma Theta Tau, broad professional associations, specialty associations, alumni associations, colleges, and HCIs may also plan events focused on cultural competence development, thus creating further challenges. More cosponsorship of professional events, meetings, and conferences through the ongoing collaborative network development as well as less (unintentional) competition between activities will have a more positive effect on participation, energy, fees, attendance, quality, and willingness to volunteer. How successful will any conference be if multiple conferences, which generally draw a wide audience of nurses, are held in the same city within a few months of each other and/or feature overlapping topics, speakers, and/or agenda? (In such a case, justification to attend more than one conference will be challenging; see Educator-In-Action Exhibit 13.2). Sites of conferences and traveling expenses, time, energy, work release, and distance are important considerations. Examining the existence of supplementary resources available to associations locally, nationally, and internationally is a necessary first step in widely disseminating high-quality educational programs to enhance cultural competence development. Innovative use of technology can serve to build community within and between professional associations. Examples include teleconferencing (audioconferencing and videoconferencing), webcasting, chat rooms, online discussion boards, and electronic meeting rooms (Zalon, 2008). The severe nursing shortage further underscores the need to pool resources and share responsibilities within and between associations.

Cultural competence workshops for individuals who realize that cultural competence development is an ongoing, lifelong commitment and who routinely participate in educational pursuits and/or are actively engaged in activities aimed at advancing cultural competence in self and in others serve a valuable purpose. However, these workshops do not reach individuals who are unaware, inefficacious, supremely efficacious, and/or uninterested in cultural competence development. Another challenge is for individuals active within associations that prioritize cultural issues to leave their "comfort zone" and venture into new associations less zealous in cultural competence development. Sharing cultural perspectives at meetings, presenting a PowerPoint presentation or poster presentation concerning culture relevant to the audience, joining committees, and suggesting cosponsorships are some innovations that can be done individually or in groups.

Committees, networking, and mentoring within and between professional associations have a great potential to enhance cultural competence and confidence. (see Exhibit 13.2). As mentioned in Chapters 6 and 10, comprehensive understanding, skill, and desire are essential but not enough to effectively make a positive difference in cultural competence development. The author believes that resilient TSE (confidence) is the integral component necessary in the process of cultural competence development (of self and in others). TSE is the mediating factor that enhances persistence in cultural competence development despite obstacles, hardships, or stressors. Resilient TSE perceptions embrace lifelong learning in the quest to become "more" culturally competent and in the quest to assist others (learners) to become more culturally competent. Professional associations have the potential to develop and nurture resilient TSE perceptions in their members through appropriate educational programs, role modeling, encouragement, and mentoring.

Exhibit 13.2   Educator-In-Action Vignette

Consider the two scenarios below and their potential impact on achieving optimal cultural competence:

Scenario 1

Several nurses belonging to the same Nursing Alumni Association engage in an e-mail discussion about upcoming professional conferences. Some excerpts are included below:

April: "Next week, on April 15, there is an all-day conference on 'Meeting Health Care Needs of Diverse Communities" at Community Hospital in Urban City, sponsored by the Local Nurses Association. The keynote speaker is Dr. Popular. Are you interested in attending? The conference fee is $60 including lunch and five CEs."

Mae: "If I knew ahead of time, I would have requested the day off. Unfortunately, we only get two conference days a year. I am on a committee at my Ethnic Nurses' Association. We are planning a cultural conference for May 7. It will be held at the Lodge two streets from Community Hospital. Dr. Popular is also the keynote speaker."

June: "That's interesting. Why didn't I know this before? The rest of the faculty in conjunction with our school's Sigma Theta Tau chapter is sponsoring "Cultural Awareness Day" on June 15. It will be an all-day symposium in which area nurses involved in projects related to cultural issues will be invited to conduct an oral or poster presentation. We have not decided on a keynote speaker yet, however, Dr. Popular is on the list of potential contacts. I am on the planning committee and also have responsibilities as chapter Vice President. There are so few volunteers that the planning tasks are overwhelming."

Julie: "Any of those conferences and events sounds interesting and I'd like to go. Did you know that the National Association conference theme is focused on culture and health? It is going to be held in Urban City in July so I can't afford to fly out twice to the same place in such a short time. The budgetary constraints at Public University make it impossible to request funds unless a faculty member is presenting orally at a larger conference. Fortunately, my abstract was accepted. I would have liked to share my study results at any of your association conferences."

Augustino: "Well, I am now hesitant to mention that the regional research alliance has also selected the theme of culture and health. We sent out a call-for-abstracts in March but only received four by the deadline. The conference is scheduled for August 1–2 in Suburban Town, only 20 minutes outside of Urban City. I am chairperson of the conference planning committee and can't persuade members to join the other three people on the committee. We already put a nonrefundable deposit on the State University's auditorium."

April: "As secretary of State University's Nursing Alumni Association, I am aware that the annual September alumni and student event at State University has invited Dr. Popular to speak about culture and health. It hasn't been officially announced yet. I don't even know if I can attend the event because my clinical specialty nurses association is having their annual program on the same day in the West Section of Urban City. There should be more discussion about culture and cultural competence within that association."

Conference Results: Each of the associations' conference events is minimally attended. Interested nurses are forced to choose which conference to attend. Active association members on the planning committee are exhausted from conference tasks. The thought of planning a future event is overwhelming. Although the majority of the association conferences "break even" between expenses and income generated, two of the associations lose money and only one makes a small profit. The poor attendance discourages potential new members from joining associations.

Scenario 2

Several nurses belonging to the same Nursing Alumni Association engage in an e-mail discussion about mutual collaboration, coordination, and cosponsorship of conference events, themes, speakers, and topics to avoid duplication, discourage competition for membership and attendance, promote common professional goals, pool human and financial resources, share responsibilities, and enhance the achievement of conference outcomes. Some excerpts are included:

April: Why don't we work together and plan a joint one-day conference focused on cultural competence? Local hospitals, universities, and professional associations are interested in this topic. By working together, we can share human and financial resources, attract a larger and more diverse audience, promote active networking between individuals and groups who might not ordinarily meet, and produce a high-quality conference for diverse groups.

Mae: That's an excellent idea. Let's make it a broad theme to attract a broader audience and plan a year in advance to attract key speakers with busy schedules, solicit abstracts for poster presentations, and permit people to "save the date." Of course, we will submit for CEs.

June: What about a conference theme called "Striving for Optimal Cultural Competence in the Changing Health Care Environment: Issues for Health Professionals, Educators, and Researchers"? That covers almost everyone. We can be sure to have a key speaker with expertise in each one of the major areas (health care setting, academia, research).

April: Let's take a vote. (everyone votes) Well, it's unanimous. Let's talk about the date.

Julie: Well, we should first avoid conflicts with other conferences locally, regionally, nationally, and internationally to avoid competition for the audience and presenters. We also need to avoid holidays. I have the nursing Web site calendar here. It looks like October 9 of next year might be good. It will give us 13 months to plan.

Augustino: That also coincides with the opening of State University's new 800-seat auditorium and conference center in September, opening in Urban City. Perhaps we can see if the university will donate the space and cosponsor the conference.

June: At a recent nursing faculty meeting, our chairperson asked us to think about sponsoring an event at the new facility that would network alumni, nurses from surrounding clinical agencies, full-time faculty, adjunct faculty, and students. I think faculty would be receptive of our idea.

April: I am on the cultural diversity committee at Community Hospital in Urban City. We were also seeking to plan an event. Many nursing graduates of State University are employed here. There is a natural link between Community Hospital and State University.

Augustino: The regional research alliance usually hosts a fall conference, usually in Suburban City. I am on the conference planning committee. We were discussing the possibility of expanding our membership campaign by changing the site to a more diverse and easily accessible site, such as Urban City. We have $1000 set aside for a keynote speaker. Perhaps we could donate the honorarium and another organization could pay for transportation expenses.

June: State University has a major name hotel right on the campus. We generally put up guest speakers there and pay for their meals in the hotel restaurant. It is still a cost, but considerably more economical. We could also ask State University's Sigma Theta Tau chapter to cosponsor with us and donate some toward expenses. Private University's chapter sometimes cosponsors events with us. We could also invite them. Of course, we will also need volunteers for several committees.

Julie: Three of us also locally belong to three different ethnic nursing associations and three different clinical specialty groups. We should also solicit support from them.

Results

The five nurses brainstorm, refine beginning ideas, and solicit support from the professional associations and agencies where they have affiliations. As a result, several organizations work together to plan, cosponsor, and conduct a well-attended, high-quality conference: State University, Sigma Theta Tau chapters from State and Private University, Regional Research Alliance, Community Hospital, two ethnic nursing associations, one clinical specialty group, Nursing Alumni Association, and Suburban Women's Clinic.

KEY POINT SUMMARY

- Professional associations possess a potentially powerful and extensive ability to network together diverse and talented groups of professionals beyond a single HCI or academic setting; therefore, professional associations can exert tremendous influence on promoting, disseminating, and advancing optimal cultural competence development.
- A systematic evaluation of the association's philosophy and mission, bylaws, membership, newsletter and publications, library, Web site, meetings, workshops, conferences, special events, committees, learning strategies, networking, and mentoring helps identify association strengths, weaknesses, inconsistencies, and gaps related to cultural competency development.
- Barriers to optimally enhancing cultural competence development through professional associations include the increased proliferation of professional associations, limited numbers of members and resources, devaluing of professional association activities, duplication of efforts, competition for membership, and high-energy demands in a rapidly changing multicultural society.
- Committees, networking, and mentoring within and between professional associations have a great potential to enhance cultural competence and confidence.

CHAPTER 14

New Priorities: Challenges and Future Directions

Marianne R. Jeffreys, EdD, RN

Currently, the process of cultural growth and change (cultural evolution) is strongly influenced by rapid growth in worldwide migration and changes in demographic patterns, marking a new and challenging era for health professionals. More than ever before, health professionals will be expected to provide culturally congruent care to many diverse "culturally different" patients and families. This new era demands a focused, committed, and transformational change that prioritizes optimal cultural competence development through innovative actions guided by systematic inquiry, empirical findings, and conceptual models. This new era necessitates optimism, resilient confidence, and a visionary plan with a prioritized focus.

A first priority is to comprehensively understand the process of becoming culturally competent, recognizing that optimal cultural competence is a multidimensional lifelong learning process rather than a final product. Limited research focused on understanding this "learning" uncovers the need to more fully understand the complex process before jumping ahead and implementing randomized and disconnected teaching interventions. Learning is more than an accumulation of cognitive, practical, and affective skills; learning, persistence for learning, motivation, and skill performance are strongly influenced by psychological factors. Gaining insight into the learner's perceptions will be an essential component to identifying learner's strengths, weaknesses, gaps, and needs.

In this book, the Cultural Competence and Confidence (CCC) Model was presented as an organizing framework for examining and understanding the multidimensional factors involved in the process of learning cultural competence. TSE (transcultural self-efficacy, meaning the perceived confidence for learning and performing transcultural skills among culturally different patients) is a major influencing factor. The model emphasizes that the cognitive, practical, and affective dimensions of TSE and transcultural skill development can change over time as a result of formalized educational and other learning experiences. In addition, the Transcultural Self-Efficacy Tool (TSET) was proposed as a valid and reliable tool for measuring and evaluating changes in TSE perceptions within the cognitive, practical, and affective domains. The CCC model offers a theoretical perspective on the process of cultural competence; however, the model is tentative and will require modification with new empirical data. Through the use of the TSET and the new Cultural Competence Clinical Evaluation Tool (CCCET), researchers can further appraise the underlying assumptions and relationships proposed in the model.

A second priority is to creatively design, implement, evaluate, and modify empirically supported teaching–learning strategies that effectively weave together the main threads of professional life (academia, health care institutions [HCIs], and professional associations) into a resilient fabric that can effectively meet changing climates and unforeseen challenges of the future. Part III of this book suggests strategies for inquiry, action, and innovation within each aspect of professional life; however, educational research remains grossly inadequate in evaluating learner needs and outcomes. The TSET was proposed as a tool for assisting educators in identifying inefficacious learners (at risk for avoiding transcultural skills), identifying supremely efficacious learners (at risk for inadequate preparation and performance of transcultural skills), and developing diagnostic-prescriptive teaching interventions; ongoing research with the TSET and CCCET will expand psychometric knowledge and practical application.

The chapter suggests some empirical directions for further inquiry, based on the major areas highlighted in this book. The suggestions are not meant to be exhaustive but are offered with the intent to stimulate new ideas and invite health professionals to explore new paths in the winding journey toward developing optimal cultural competence in self and in others.

FUTURE DIRECTIONS

Theoretical Framework

More studies using constructs, assumptions, and relationships from the CCC model should be conducted across a wide range of settings and health disciplines. Several underlying assumptions about the model have already been supported empirically (Jeffreys, 2000) and have been presented in Chapter 4 using the TSET. Studies in progress using the TSET and the new CCCET will provide data to substantiate or modify the CCC model. Quantitative and qualitative studies should be carried out using different groups of students and health professionals to compare similarities and differences based on gender, age, professional experience, ethnicity, race, religion, geographic region, and other demographic variables.

Qualitative Studies

Qualitative studies will add to nursing knowledge by exploring such topics as the:

- "Lived experience" of learners' changing transcultural perceptions.
- Perceived influence of select educational experiences on transcultural skills in the cognitive, practical, and affective dimensions.
- Perceived influence of changes in confidence levels and the impact on culturally congruent care, learning, and/or professional satisfaction.
- "Lived experience" of promoting, facilitating, and nurturing transcultural learning and self-efficacy in academia, HCIs, or professional associations.

Quantitative Studies

Future longitudinal, cross-sectional, or quasi-experimental studies (using the TSET exclusively or in combination with the CCCET) may help evaluate the effectiveness of select, sequential, integrated, or combined teaching interventions on outcome performances such as culture care competencies, knowledge, skills, patient satisfaction, positive patient outcomes, and confidence. The TSET has been used to:

- Identify transcultural skills perceived as more difficult or stressful by learners
- Identify at-risk learners (inefficacious or supremely efficacious/ overconfident)
- Develop a composite of learner needs, values, attitudes, and skills concerning transcultural nursing
- Evaluate the effectiveness of teaching interventions
- Assess changes in self-efficacy perceptions over time

The replication of quantitative studies using the TSET will add depth to the existing knowledge base; addition of CCCET, CSAT-DD, and other assessment tools will expand empirical knowledge. Evidence-based educational innovations and ongoing research, guided by empirically and conceptually supported literature, can effectively guide the transformation necessary to prepare culturally competent health professionals who exceed minimum standards striving for and/or achieving optimal cultural competence. Several current quantitative studies target nursing faculty who participate in workshops to enhance cultural competence throughout the curriculum. Such studies must also aim to reach beyond the minimal integration of cultural competence toward the optimal integration of cultural competence. Researchers should carefully consider which quantitative design and which quantitative measures are most suited for their study purpose and population, especially because funding agencies frequently stipulate the evaluation of outcomes using valid and reliable quantitative measures.

Psychometric Studies

The TSET demonstrated adequate reliability and validity consistently across several studies. Findings supported that the TSET assesses the multidimensional nature of TSE, yet also differentiates between cognitive, practical, and affective learning dimensions. Ongoing psychometric tests of reliability and validity should be incorporated into every study using the TSET, because reliability and validity is not an inherent property of the instrument but only an estimate that may vary among different samples.

Similarly, various scoring and grouping methods proposed in this book (Chapter 4 and Jeffreys Toolkit 2010) require ongoing testing with various sample populations. Although the TSET was originally designed for undergraduate nursing students and psychometric properties have been explored with several samples of undergraduate nursing students and nurses in a variety of settings, the instrument has also been requested for use and/or adaptation for use with nurses, graduate nursing students, physicians, and other health professionals in various countries. Comparison of psychometric properties across varied samples and settings will lend new insight into the possible uses and/or limitations surrounding the instrument. Additionally, the new TSET-MHP provides an opportunity to measure TSE before and after cultural competence education (workshops, conferences, or other strategies) involving multidisciplinary groups. Furthermore, detailed evaluation of adapted and/or translated versions of the instrument will need to be conducted. As new statistical procedures are developed, psychometric studies using these new techniques should be routinely conducted, expanding the repertoire of psychometric tests and results by which researchers can evaluate research findings generated by the TSET.

Replication

Multiple replication of studies are necessary to assess the reliability of a given construct (Braxton, 2000). Replication with similar and different study samples and settings will add depth to the growing body of knowledge concerning cultural competence and confidence. Developing a program of research that builds upon previous findings will enhance understanding about the complex process of cultural competence. Reaching out to other researchers interested in similar studies will permit wider replication among more diverse samples, further expanding knowledge beyond geographic boundaries and settings.

Collaboration and Partnerships

Collaboration between researchers prior to study design and during all phases of the research process will help decrease threats to internal and external validity as well as to promote new ideas and collaborative projects. Developing partnerships between researchers in academia, HCIs, and professional associations will provide the opportunity to connect the wide spectrum of professional activities and roles within a common goal of developing optimal cultural competence and providing culturally congruent care for all culturally diverse patients. In addition, connections within and between disciplines in the United States and beyond will provide another mechanism for reaching out and achieving a broader synthesis for advocating optimal cultural competence beyond the borders often imposed by discipline separation.

Dissemination

Wide dissemination of research findings using the TSET, CCCET, CSAT-DD, CCC model, and other assessment tools discussed in this book (and found in Jeffreys 2010 Toolkit) should be a consistent and strategically planned component of the research process rather than an inconsistent or haphazard occurrence. Using the research report template (Jeffreys 2010 Toolkit Item 21) and the examples provided in the TSET Research Exhibits throughout the book, researchers can document key information that can easily be retrieved by others seeking to conduct cultural competence education research, implement evidence-based cultural competence education strategies, and/or synthesize the state of research thus far. Unfortunately, some research results are hidden in dissertations, master's theses, obscure journals, institution reports, and grant evaluation reports that rarely (or never) have the opportunity to surface beyond a small reader audience. Even more obscure are the research results that are only shared at a conference, workshop, or meeting and are not publicized or retrievable beyond the single presentation. In order for dissemination to be a consistent and strategically planned component of the research process, dissemination plans should be clearly identified and include submitting a manuscript for publication in a peer-reviewed journal (see Chapter 12). Publication in a peer-reviewed journal will permit indexing and easy retrieval by readers. Researchers who are new to the publication process should seek mentors who can provide guidance, constructive criticism, and encouragement. If nursing education scholarship is to advance amidst the critical nursing faculty shortage, experienced authors and researchers must be willing to mentor others.

CONCLUSION

Societal needs, ethical guidelines, legal issues, and professional goals declare the need to view optimal cultural competence development as a real priority. Such a view necessitates a conscious, committed, and transformational change in current professional practice, education, and research. Individually, every health professional is empowered to positively contribute to this transformational change through an active role in ongoing professional self-development. As active partners, health professionals can continually seek to understand the process of developing optimal cultural competence in self and in others, mentor colleagues, integrate research findings into education and practice, question the status quo, uncover new directions for cultural competence research, implement new innovations, and be open to new ideas. Chapter discussions, corresponding diagrams, and toolkit items explored the steps essential for optimal cultural competence development: self-assessment, active promotion, systematic inquiry, decisive action, innovation, measurement, and evaluation—steps that can continue to guide the ongoing quest for developing optimal cultural competence in self and in others. Within purposeful professional partnerships, health professionals will not be alone in the endeavor to promote cultural competence; they will exercise resilience and persist despite challenges and obstacles. Such resilient energy will be maximized through an ongoing open, caring environment that embraces diversity within and between health professions as well as appreciates diversity within and between patients, families, and communities.

Shaping such an environment amidst managed care, the nursing shortage, faculty shortages, financial constraints, and intergroup and intragroup conflicts presents numerous challenges; however, positive change is possible. Through diligence and coordinated group efforts, the goals of culturally congruent care and multicultural workplace harmony

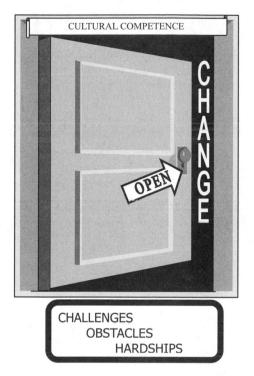

Figure 14.1 Stepping over challenges: Opening the door to change

may be achieved. The first step is to step over challenges and open the door to change (Figure 14.1). Whatever inquiries, actions, and innovations are done (or not done) today will influence the future. Let's join together and make a positive difference through ongoing inquiry, action, and innovation.

KEY POINT SUMMARY

- The new era in health care demands a focused, committed, and transformational change that prioritizes optimal cultural competence development.
- A first priority is to comprehensively understand the process of becoming culturally competent, recognizing that optimal cultural competence is a multidimensional lifelong learning process rather than a final product.
- Steps essential for optimal cultural competence development include: self-assessment, active promotion, systematic inquiry, decisive action, innovation, measurement, and evaluation.

- A second priority is to creatively design, evaluate, and modify empirically supported teaching–learning strategies that effectively weave together the main threads of professional life (academia, HCIs, and professional associations) into a resilient fabric that can effectively meet changing climates and unforeseen challenges of the future.
- The CCC model can guide future directions for inquiry, action, and innovation.
- Based on the major areas highlighted in this book, directions for research include:
  - Theoretical framework
  - Qualitative studies
  - Quantitative studies
  - Psychometric studies
  - Replication
  - Collaboration and partnerships
  - Dissemination

References

Abrums, M.E., & Leppa, C. (2001). Beyond cultural competence: Teaching about race, gender, class, and sexual orientation. *Journal of Nursing Education, 40*(6), 270–275.

Adams, C.E., Murdock, J.E., Valiga, T.M., McGinnis, S., & Wolfertz, J.R. (2002). *Trends in Registered Nurse Education Programs: A comparison across three points in time—1994; 1999; 2004*. Retrieved April 2, 2003, from http:// nln.org/aboutnln/nursetrends .htm.

Alexitch, L.R. (2002). The role of help-seeking attitudes and tendencies in students' preferences for academic advising. *Journal of College Student Development, 43*(1), 5–19.

Alien, D. (1990). *The curriculum revolution: Radical revisioning of nursing education. Journal of Nursing Education, 29*, 312–317.

American Association of Colleges of Nursing. (2009). *Establishing a culturally competent master's and doctorally prepared nursing workforce*. Washington, DC: Author.

American Association of Colleges of Nursing. (2008). *Cultural competency in baccalaureate nursing education*. Washington, DC: Author.

American Dental Association. (2005). *Access to care*. Chicago, IL: Author.

American Dental Association. (2007). *Accreditation standards for advanced general dentistry education programs in dentistry*. Chicago, IL: Author.

American Nurses Association. (1998a). *Position statement on cultural diversity in nursing practice*. Retrieved January 30, 2005, from http://nursingworld.org/readingroom/position/ethics/etcldv.htm.

American Nurses Association. (1998b). *Position statement on discrimination and racism in health care*. Retrieved January 30, 2005, from http://nursingworld.org/readingroom/position/ethics/etdisrac.htm.

American Nurses Association. (2001). *Code for nurses with interpretive statements.* Washington, DC: Author.

American Nurses Association. (2003). *Nursing's social policy statement* (2nd ed.). Washington, DC: Author.

American Nurses Association. (2004). *Nursing: Scope and standards of practice.* Washington, DC: Author.

American Nurses Association. (2009). *Nursing administration: Scope and standards of practice* (3rd ed.). Silver Spring, MD: American Nurses Association.

American Nurses Credentialing Center. (2009). *ANCC magnet recognition program.* Retrieved June 22, 2009, from http://nursecredentialing.org/Magnet.aspx.

American Nurses Credentialing Center. (2008). *Application manual: Magnet recognition program.* Silver Spring, MD: American Nurses Credentialing Center.

American Psychiatric Association (1994); *Diagnostic and statistical manual of mental disorders* (4th ed). Washington, DC: Author.

American Physical Therapy Association (2008). *Blueprint for teaching cultural competence in physical therapy education,* Author.

Anderson, K.L. (2004). Teaching cultural competence using an exemplar for literary journalism. *Journal of Nursing Education, 43*(6), 253–259.

Andrews, M.M. (1992). Cultural perspectives on nursing in the 21st century. *Journal of Professional Nursing, 8* (1), 7–15.

Andrews, M. (1995). Transcultural nursing: Transforming the curriculum. *Journal of Transcultural Nursing, 6*(2), 4–9.

Andrews, M.M., & Boyle, J.S. (2008). *Transcultural concepts in nursing care.* (5th ed.). Philadelphia: Lippincott Williams & Wilkins.

Andrews, M., Burr, J., & Janetos, D.H. (2004). Searching electronically for information on transcultural nursing and health subjects. *Journal of Transcultural Nursing, 15*(3), 242–247.

Antonio, A.L. (2001). Diversity and the influence of friendship groups in college. *Review of Higher Education, 25*(1), 63–89.

Association of American Medical Colleges (2005). *Cultural competence education.* Washington, DC: Author.

Baldwin, D. (1999). Community-based experiences and cultural competence. *Journal of Nursing Education, 38*(5), 195–196.

Baldwin, D., & Wold, J. (1993). Students from disadvantaged backgrounds: Satisfaction with a mentor-protégé relationship. *Journal of Nursing Education, 32,* 225–226.

Bandura, A. (1977). Self-efficacy: Toward a unifying theory of behavioral change. *Psychological Review, 84*(2), 191–215.

Bandura, A. (1982). Self-efficacy mechanism in human agency. *American Psychologist, 37*(2), 122–145.

Bandura, A. (1986). *Social foundations of thought and action: A social cognitive theory.* Englewood Cliffs, NJ: Prentice-Hall.

Bandura, A. (1989). Regulation of cognitive processes through perceived self-efficacy. *Developmental Psychology, 25*(5), 729–735.

Bandura, A. (1995). On rectifying conceptual ecumenism. In J.E. Maddux (Ed.), *Self-efficacy, adaptation, and adjustment: Theory, research, and application.* (pp. 347–375). New York: Plenum.

Bandura, A. (1996a). Reflections on human agency. In J. Georgas, M. Manthouli, E. Besevegis, & A. Kokkevi (Eds.), *Contemporary psychology in Europe: Theory, research, and applications (proceedings of the 1Vth European Congress of Psychology).* (pp. 194–210). Seattle, WA: Hogrefe & Huber.

Bandura, A. (1996b). Regulation of cognitive processes through perceived self-efficacy. In Jennings, G-H. (Ed.), *Passages Beyond the Gate: A Jungian Approach to Understanding the Nature of American Psychology at the Dawn of the New Millenium.* Needham Heights, MA: Simon & Schuster Custom Publishing, pp. 96–107.

Bandura, A. (1997). *Self-efficacy: The exercise of control.* New York: W. H. Freeman.

Bandura, A., & Schunk, D.H. (1981). Cultivating competence, self-efficacy and intrinsic interest through proximal self-motivation. *Journal of Personality and Social Psychology, 41,* 586–598.

Barbee, E.L., & Gibson, S.E. (2001). Our dismal progress: The recruitment of non-whites into nursing. *Journal of Nursing Education, 40*(6), 243–245.

Bartz, B., Bowles, M., & Underwood, J.R. (1993). Student experiences in transcultural nursing. *Journal of Nursing Education, 32*(5), 233–234.

Bellack, J.P. (2009). Integrating diversity. *Journal of Nursing Education, 48*(9), 475–476.

Bernal, H., & Froman, R. (1987). The confidence of community health nurses in caring for ethnically diverse populations. *Image: Journal of Nursing Scholarship, 19,* 201–203.

Berry, J.M., West, R.L., & Dennehey, D.M. (1989). Reliability and validity of memory self-efficacy questionnaire. *Developmental Psychology, 25,* 701–713.

Bessent, H. (1997). *Strategies for recruitment, retention, and graduation of minority nurses in colleges of nursing.* Washington, DC: American Nurses Publishing.

Betts, V.T. & Cherry, B. (2002). Health policy and politics. In Cherry & Jacob (Eds.), *Contemporary nursing: Issues, trends, and management,* (2nd Edition). Philadelphia, PA: Mosby, 219–235.

Bevis, E., & Murray, J. (1990). The essence of the curriculum revolution: Emancipatory teaching. *Journal of Nursing Education, 29,* 326–331.

Beyer, B. (1987). *Practical strategies for the teaching of thinking.* Boston, MA: Allyn & Bacon.

Bibb, S.C., Malebranche, M., Crowell, D., Altman, C., Lyon, S., Carlson, A., Miller, S., Miller, T., & Rybarczyk, J. (2003). Professional development needs of registered nurses practicing at a military community hospital. *Journal of Continuing Education in Nursing, 34*(1), 39–45.

Bilinski, H. (2002). The mentored journal. *Nurse Educator, 27*(1), 37–41.

Billings, D. (2004). Teaching learners from varied generations. *Journal of Continuing Education in Nursing, 35*(3), 104–105.

Billings, D., & Kowalski, K. (2004). Teaching learners from varied generations. *Journal of Continuing Education in Nursing, 35*(2), 104–105.

Billings, D., & Kowalski, K. (2008). Inclusive teaching. *Journal of Continuing Education in Nursing, 39*(7), 296–297.

Billings, D.M., & Kowalski, K. (2009). Nurses working with librarians. *Journal of Continuing Education in Nursing, 40*(1), 16–17.

Bloom, B.S., Enlgehart, M.D., Furst, E.J., Hill, W.H., & Krathwohl, D.R. (1956). *Taxonomy of educational objectives: Handbook I, cognitive domain.* New York: McKay.

Bolan, C.M. (2003). Incorporating the experiential learning theory into the instructional design of online courses. *Nurse Educator, 28*(1), 10–14.

Bolton, L.B., Giger, J.N., & Georges, C.A. (2004). Structural and racial barriers to health care. In, Fitzpatrick, L. (Ed.), *Annual review of nursing research, Vol. 22*, pp. 39–58.

Bosher, S.D., & Pharris, M.D. (2009). *Transforming nursing education: The culturally inclusive environment.* New York: Springer.

Botstein, L. (2008). Higher education and public school in twenty-first century America. *Thought and Action, 24*, 101–110.

Boyce, B.A.B., & Winne, M.D. (2000). Developing an evaluation tool for instructional software programs. *Nurse Educator, 25*(3), 145–148.

Brady, D., Wellborn-Brown, P., Smith, D., Giddens, J., Harris, J., Wright, M., & Nichols, R. (2008). Staying afloat: Surviving curriculum change. *Nurse Educator, 33*(5), 198–201.

Brathwaite, A.E.C. (2005). Evaluation of a cultural competence course. *Journal of Transcultural Nursig, 16*(4), 361–369.

Braxton, J.M. (Ed.), (2000). *Reworking the student departure puzzle.* Nashville, TN: Vanderbilt University Press.

Braxton, J.M., & Mundy, M.E. (2001). Powerful institutional levers to reduce college student departure. *Journal of College Student Retention: Research, Theory, & Practice, 3*(1), 91–118.

Brookfield, S.D. (1986). *Understanding and facilitating adult learning.* San Francisco, CA: Jossey-Bass.

Brookfield, S. (1987). *Developing critical thinkers.* San Francisco, CA: Jossey-Bass.

Brown, S.D., Lent, R.W., & Larkin, K.C. (1989). Self-efficacy as a moderator of scholastic aptitude: Academic performance relationships. *Journal of Vocational Behavior, 35*(1), 64–75.

Burchard, E.G., Avila, P.C., Nazario, S., Casal, J., Torres, A., Rodriguez-Santana, J.R., et al. (2004). Lower bronchodilator responsiveness in Puerto Rican than in Mexican subjects with asthma. *American Journal of Respiratory Critical Care Medicine, 169*, 386–392.

Burnes Bolton, L. (2004). Cultural diversity in leadership. *Nursing Administration Quarterly, 28*(3), 163–164.

Burr, P.L.; Burr, R.M.; & Novak, L.F. (1999). Student retention is more complicated than merely keeping the students you have today: Toward a "seamless retention theory." *Journal of College Student Retention, 1*(3), 239–253.

Callister, L.C., Khalaf, I., & Keller, D. (2000). Cross-cultural comparison of the concerns of beginning baccalaureate nursing students. *Nurse Educator, 25*(6), 267–271.

Cameron-Traub, E. (2002). Western ethical, moral, and legal dimensions within the culture care theory. In: Leininger, M. & McFarland, M. (Eds.), *Transcultural nursing: Concepts, theories, research, and practice* (pp. 169–177), New York: McGraw-Hill.

Campbell, A.R., & Davis, S.M. (1996). Faculty commitment: Retaining minority nursing students in majority institutions. *Journal of Nursing Education, 35*(7), 298–303.

Campbell-Heider, N., Rejman, K.P., Austin-Ketch, T., Sackett, K., Feeley, T.H., & Wilk, N.C. (2006). Measuring cultural competence in a family nurse practitioner curriculum. *Journal of Multicultural Nursing and Health, 12*(3), 24–34.

Campinha-Bacote, J. (1998a). *The Process of Cultural Competence in the Delivery of Healthcare Services: A Culturally Competent Model of Care* (3rd ed.). Cincinnati, OH: Transcultural C.A.R.E. Associates.

Campinha-Bacote, J. (1998b). Cultural diversity in nursing education: Issues and concerns. *Journal of Nursing Education, 37*(1), 3–4.

Campinha-Bacote, J. (1999). A model and instrument for addressing cultural competence in health care. *Journal of Nursing Education, 38*, 203–207.

Campinha-Bacote, J. (2003). *The process of cultural competence in the delivery of healthcare services: A culturally competent model of care* (4th ed.). Cincinnati, OH: Transcultural C.A.R.E. Associates.

Candela, L., Michael, S.R., & Mitchell, S. (2003). Ethical debates: Enhancing critical thinking in nursing students. *Nurse Educator, 28*(1), 37–39.

Candela, L., Dalley, K., & Benzel-Lindley, J. (2006). A case for learning-centered curricula. *Journal of Nursing Education, 45*, 59–68.

Carmines, E., & Zeller, R.A. (1979). *Reliability and validity assessment.* Newbury Park, CA: Sage.

Carter, L.M., & Rukholm, E. (2008). A study of critical thinking, teacher–student interaction, and discipline-specific writing in an online educational setting for registered nurses. *The Journal of Continuing Education in Nursing, 39*(3), 133–138.

Cavanaugh, D.A., & Huse, A.L. (2004). Surviving the nursing shortage: Developing a nursing orientation program to prepare and retain intensive care unit nurses. *Journal of Continuing Education in Nursing, 35*(6), 251–256.

Cervone, D. (1989). Effects of envisioning future activities on self-efficacy judgments and motivation: An availability heuristic interpretation. *Cognitive Therapy and Research, 13*(3), 247–260.

Chang, M.K. (1995). Bridging the cultural gap. *Urologic Nursing, 15*(14), 123–126.

Chartrand, J.M. (1990). A causal analysis to predict the personal and academic adjustment of nontradtional students. *Journal of Counseling Psychology, 37*(1), 65–73.

Chinn, P. (1990). GOSSIP: A transformative art for nursing education. *Journal of Nursing Education, 29,* 317–321.

Choudhry, S., Ung, N., Avila, P.C., Ziv, E., Nazario, S., Casal, J., et al. (2005). Pharmacogenetic differences in response to albuterol between Puerto Ricans and Mexicans with asthma. *American Journal of Respiratory Critical Care Medicine, 171,* 563–570.

Christiaens, G., & Baldwin, J.H. (2002). Use of dyadic role-playing to increase student participation. *Nurse Educator, 27*(6), 251–254.

Christianson, L., Tiene, D., & Luft, P. (2002). Web-based teaching in undergraduate nursing programs. *Journal of Nursing Education, 27*(6), 276–282.

Ciesielka, D. (2008). Using a wiki to meet graduate nursing education competencies in collaboration and community health. *Journal of Nursing Education, 47*(10), 473–476.

Colling, J. & Wilson, T. (1998). Short-term reciprocal international academic exchange program. *Journal of Nursing Education, 37*(1), 34–36.

Collins, J.M. (2002). Reflections on the changing learning needs of nurses: A challenge for nursing continuing educators. *Journal of Continuing Education in Nursing, 33*(2), 74–77.

Comrey, A.L. (1973). *A first course in factor analysis.* New York: Academic Press.

Constantine, M.G., & Watt, S.K. (2002). Cultural congruity, womanist identity attitudes, and life satisfaction among African American college women attending historically black and predominantly white institutions. *Journal of College Student Development, 43*(2), 184–193.

Constantine, M.G., Robinson, J.S., Wilton, L., & Caldwell, L.D. (2002). Collective self-esteem and perceived social support as predictors of cultural congruity among black and Latino college students. *Journal of College Student Development, 43*(3), 307–316.

Costello, A.B., & Osborne, J.W. (2005). Best practices in exploratory factor analysis: four recommendations for getting the most from your analysis. *Practical Assessment Research & Evaluation, 10*(7). Retrieved January 24, 2010, from http://pareonline.net/genpare.asp?wh = 4 = costello

Courage, M.M., & Godbey, K.L. (1992). Student retention: Policies and services to enhance persistence to graduation. *Nurse Educator, 17*(2), 29–32.

Cowan, D.T., & Norman, I. (2006). Cultural competence in nursing: New meanings. *Journal of Transcultural Nursing, 17*(1), 82–88.

Cowen, K.J., & Tesh, A.S. (2002). Effects of gaming on nursing students' knowledge of pediatric cardiovascular dysfunction. *Journal of Nursing Education, 41*(11), 507–509.

Critchley, K.A., Richardson, E., Aarts, C., Campbell, B., Hemmingway, A., Koskinen, L., Mitchell, M.P., & Nordstrom, P. (2009). Student experiences with an international public health exchange project. *Nurse Educator, 34*(2), 69–74.

Crow, K. (1993). Multiculturalism and pluralistic thought in nursing education: Native American world view and the nursing academic world view. *Journal of Nursing Education, 32*(5), 198–204.

Cummings, P.H. (1998). Nursing in Barbados: A fourth-year elective practice experience for nursing students and registered nurses. *Journal of Nursing Education, 37*(1), 42–44.

Daniel, G.R. (1992). Beyond black and white: The new multiracial consciousness. In M.P.P. Root (Ed.), *Racially mixed people in America* (333–341). Newbury Park, CA: Sage.

Davidhizar, R., Dowd, S.B., & Giger, J.N. (1998). Educating the culturally diverse healthcare student. *Nurse Educator, 23*(2), 38–42.

Davidhizar, R. & Giger, J.N. (2001). Teaching culture within the nursing curriculum using the Giger-Davidhizar model of transcultural nursing assessment. *Journal of Nursing Education, 40*(6), 282–288.

Davidhizar, R., & Lonser, G. (2003). Storytelling as a teaching technique. *Nurse Educator, 28*, 217–221.

Davidson, J.E. (2009). Preceptor use of classroom assessment techniques to stimulate higher-order thinking in the clinical setting. *The Journal of Continuing Education in Nursing, 40*(3), 139–143.

Davidson, P.M., Meleis, A., Daly, J., & Douglas, M. (2003). Globalisation as we enter the 21st century: Reflections and directions for nursing education, science, research and clinical practice. *Contemporary Nurse, 15*(3), 162–174.

Dearman, C.N. (2003). Using clinical scenarios in nursing education. In M. Oermann & K. Heinrich (Eds.), *Annual Review of Nursing Education, Vol. I*, New York: Springer, 341–355.

De Chesnay, M., Anderson, B. A. (2008). *Caring for the vulnerable: Perspectives in nursing theory, practice, and research.* Boston: Jones and Bartlett.

Delgado, C., & Mack, B. (2002). A peer-reviewed program for senior proficiencies. *Nurse Educator, 27*(5), 212–213.

Department of Health and Human Services. (2000). *Healthy people 2010: Understanding and improving health.* (2nd ed.) Washington, DC: U.S. Government Printing Office, November 2000.

Department of Health and Human Services. (2009). *Healthy people 2020.* Washington, DC, Retrieved January 24, 2010, from http://www.healthypeople.gov/hp2020.

deTornyay, R. (1990). The curriculum revolution. *Journal of Nursing Education, 29,* 292.

Diekelmann, N. (1990). Nursing education: Caring, dialogue, and practice. *Journal of Nursing Education, 29,* 300–306.

Diekelmann, N. (2002). "She asked this simple question": Reflecting and the scholarship of teaching. *Journal of Nursing Education, 41*(9), 381–382.

Diekelmann, N., & Ironside, P.M. (2002). Developing a science of nursing education: Innovation with research. *Journal of Nursing Education, 41*(9), 379–380.

DiMaria-Ghalili, R.A., Ostrow, L., & Rodney, K. (2005). Webcasting: A new instructional technology in distance graduate nursing education. *Journal of Nursing Education, 44*(1), 11–18.

Dolgan, C.M. (2001). *The effects of cultural competency training on nurses' attitudes.* Unpublished master's thesis, Cleveland State University, Cleveland, OH.

Donnelly, P.J.L. (1992). The impact of culture on psychotherapy: Korean clients' expectations in psychotherapy, *Journal of the New York State Nurses Association, 23*(2), 12–19.

Donnelly, P.J.L. (2005). Mental health beliefs and help seeking behaviors of Korean American parents of adult children with schizophrenia. *Journal of Multicultural Nursing and Health, 11*(2), in press.

Dorrian, J., & Wache, D. (2008). Introduction of an online approach to flexible learning for on-campus and distance education students:

Lessons learned and ways forward. *Nurse Education Today, 29,* 157–167.

Douglas, M. (2000). The effect of globalization on health care: A double-edged sword. *Journal of Transcultural Nursing, 11*(2), 85–86.

Douglas, M.K., Uhl Pierce, J., Rosenkoetter, M., Clark Callister, L., Hattar-Pollara, M., Lauderdale, J., Miller, J., Milstead, J., Nardi, D.A., & Pacquiao, D. (2009). Standards of practice for culturally competent nursing care: A request for comments. *Journal of Transcultural Nursing, 20*(3), 257–269.

Drevdahl, D.J., Stackman, R.W., Purdy, J.M., & Louie, B.Y. (2002). Merging reflective inquiry and self-study as a framework for enhancing the scholarship of teaching. *Journal of Nursing Education, 41*(9), 413–418.

Duchscher, J.B. (2004). Transition to professional nursing practice: Emerging issues and initiatives. In M. Oermann & K. Heinrich (Eds.), *Annual Review of Nursing Education (Vol. II,* pp. 283–303). New York: Springer.

Edwards, H., Nash, R., Sacre, S., Courtney, M., & Abbey, J. (2007). Development of a virtual learning environment to enhance undergraduate nursing students' effectiveness and interest in working with older people. *Nurse Education Today, 28,* 672–679.

Elbow, P. (1997). High stakes and low stakes in assigning and responding to writing. *New Directions for Teaching and Learning, 69,* 5–13.

Ellerton, M-L., & Gregor, F. (2003). A study of transition: The new nurse graduate at 3 months. *Journal of Continuing Education in Nursing, 34*(3), 103–107.

Emerson, R.J., & Records, K. (2008). Today's challenge, tomorrow's excellence: The practice of evidence-based education. *Journal of Nursing Education, 47*(8), 359–370.

Eshleman, J., & Davidhizar, R.E. (2006). Strategies for developing cultural competency in an RN-BSN program. *Journal of Transcultural Nursing, 17*(2), 179–183.

Fadiman, A. (1997). *The spirit catches you and you fall down.* New York: Farrar, Straus and Giroux.

Farella, C. (2002). School of hard knocks: Is racism a fixture of nursing academia? *Nursing Spectrum, 14*(12) NY/NJ, 34–35.

Ferguson, L. (2004). External validity, generalizability, and knowledge utilization. *Journal of Nursing Scholarship, 36*(1), 16–22.

Ferketich, S. (1991). Aspects of item analysis. *Research in Nursing and Health, 14,* 165–168.

Flege, J.E. & Liu, S. (2001). The effects of experience on adults' acquisition of a second language. *Studies in Second Language Acquisition, 23*(4), 527–552.

Flinn, J.B. (2004). Teaching strategies used with success in the multicultural classroom *Nurse Educator, 29*(1), 10–12.

Foley, R., & Wurmser, T.A. (2004). Culture diversity/A mobile workforce command creative leadership, new partnerships, and innovative approaches to integration, *Nursing Administration Quarterly, 28*(2), 122–128.

Forbes, M.O., & Hickey, M.T. (2008). Podcasting: Implementation and evaluation in an undergraduate nursing program. *Nurse Educator, 33*(5), 224–227.

Ford, J.K., MacCallum, R.C., & Tait, M. (1986). The application of exploratory factor-analysis in applied psychology—a critical review and analysis. *Personnel Psychology, 39*(2), 291–314.

Forneris, S.G., & Campbell, S.E. (2009). Journeying beyond traditional lecture: Using stories to create context for critical thinking. In S.D. Bosher & M.D. Pharris (Eds.), *Transforming nursing education: The culturally inclusive environment* (pp. 129–153). New York: Springer.

Fortier, J.P., & Bishop, D. (2003). *Setting the agenda for research on cultural competence in health care: final report* (Ed.) C. Brach. Rockville, MD: U.S. Department of Health and Human Services Office of Minority Health and Agency for Healthcare Research and Quality.

Fuertes, J.N., & Westbrook, F.D. (1996). Using the social, attitudinal, familial, and environmental (S.A.F.E.) acculturation stress scale to assess the adjustment needs of Hispanic college students. *Measurement and Evaluation in Counseling and Development, 29*, 67–76.

Gaffney, K.F. (2000). Encouraging collaborative learning among culturally diverse students. *Nurse Educator, 25*(5), 219–221.

Garcia, M. (1987). *Community college persistence: A field application of the Tinto model, doctoral dissertation*. Unpublished manuscript, Teachers College, Columbia University.

Gasper, M.L. (2009). Building a community with your advisees. *Nurse Educator, 34*(2), 88–94.

Georges, C.A. (2004). African American nurse leadership: Pathways and opportunities. *Nursing Administration Quarterly, 28*(3), 170–172.

Gerstein, L.H., Heppner, P.P., Aegisdottir, S., Leung, S.-M.A., & Norsworthy, K.L. (2009). *International handbook of cross-cultural counseling: Cultural assumptions and practices worldwide*. Washington, DC: Sage.

Giger, J., Davidhizar, R.E., Purnell, L., Harden, J.T., Phillips, J., & Strickland, O. (2007). American Academy of Nursing Expert Panel Report: Developing cultural competence to eliminate health disparities in ethnic minorities and other vulnerable populations. *Journal of Transcultural Nursing, 18*(2), 95–102.

Giger, J.N., & Davidhizar, R.E. (2008). *Transcultural nursing: Assessment and intervention* (5th ed.). St. Louis, MD: Mosby.

Gigliotti, E. (1999). Women's multiple role stress: Testing Neuman's flexible line of defense. *Nursing Science Quarterly, 12*(1), 36–44.

Gigliotti, E. (2001). Development of the perceived multiple role stress scale (PMRS). *Journal of Nursing Measurement, 9*(2), 163–180.

Gilchrist, K.L., & Rector, C. (2007) Can you keep them? Strategies to attract and retain nursing students from diverse populations: Best practices in nursing education, *Journal of Transcultural Nursing, 18*, 277–285.

Gilley, W.F., & Uhlig, G.E. (1993). Factor analysis and ordinal data. *Education, 114*, 258–264.

Gist, M.E., & Mitchell, T.R. (1992). Self-efficacy: A theoretical analysis of its determinants and malleability. *Academy of Management Review, 17*, 183–211.

Glittenberg, J. (2004). A transdisciplinary, transcultural model for health care. *Journal of Transcultural Nursing, 15*(1), 6–10.

Gloria, A.M., & Kurpius, S.E.R. (1996). The validation of the cultural congruity scale and the university environment scale with Chicano/a students. *Hispanic Journal of Behavioral Sciences, 18*(4), 533–549.

Gomez, G.E., & White, M.J. (2002). An international educational experience. *Hispanic Health Care International, 1*(3), 124–127.

Goode C.J., Tanaka D.J., Krugman M., O'Connor P.A., Bailey C., Deutchman M., & Stolpman N.M. (2000). Outcomes from use of an evidence-based practice guideline. *Nursing Economics, 18*, 202–207.

Gorsuch, R.L. (1990). Common factor-analysis versus component analysis—some well and little known facts. *Multivariate Behavioral Research, 25*(1), 33–39.

Gorsuch, R.L. (1997). Exploratory factor analysis: Its role in item analysis. *Journal of Personality Assessment, 68*(3), 532–560.

Grainger-Mosen, & Haslett, J. (Producers) (2005). *Hold your Breath* [DVD]. (Available from Fanlight Productions, 4196 Washington Street, Boston, MA 02131.)

Greenhaus, J.H. & Beutell, N.J. (1985). Sources of conflict between work and family roles. *Academy of Management Review, 10*, 76–88.

Griffiths, M.J., & Tagliareni, M.E. (1999). Challenging traditional assumptions about minority students in nursing education. *Nursing & Health Care Perspectives, 20*, 290–295.

Grosset, J.M. (1991). Patterns of integration, commitment, and student characteristics and retention among younger and older students. *Research in Higher Education, 32* (2), 159–178.

Grossman, D., & Jorda, M.L. (2008). Transitioning foreign-educated physicians to nurses: The new Americans in nursing. *Journal of Nursing Education*, 47(12), 544–551.

Hackett, G. (1985). Role of mathematics self-efficacy in the choice of math-related majors of college women and men: A path analysis. *Journal of Counseling Psychology*, 32(1), 47–56.

Hall, C.C.I. (1992). Coloring outside the lines. In M.P.P. Root (Ed.), *Racially mixed people in America* (pp. 326–329). Newbury Park, CA: Sage.

Haloburdo, E.P., & Thompson, M.A. (1998). A comparison of international learning experiences for baccalaureate nursing students: Developed and developing countries. *Journal of Nursing Education*, 37(1), 13–21.

Hammer, V.R., & Craig, G.P. (2008). The experiences of inactive nurses returned to nursing after completing a refresher course. *Journal of Continuing Education in Nursing*, 39(8), 358–367.

Hammond, P.V., Davis, B.L., Hodges, G., & Warfield, M. (1997). Increasing retention rates of disadvantaged students through a faculty development program. *The Association of Black Nursing Faculty Journal*, 8(3), 51–53.

Hansen, G. (1988). Student retention in associate degree nursing education. In *nursing shortage: Strategies for nursing practice and education*. Washington, DC: Report for the National Invitation Workshop. (ERIC Document Reproduction Service No. ED 310 257).

Harden, J.K. (2003). Faculty and student experiences with web-based discussion groups in a large lecture setting. *Nurse Educator*, 28(1), 26–30.

Harper, M.G. (2008). *Evaluation of the antecedents of cultural competence, doctoral dissertation*. Unpublished manuscript, University of Central Florida, Orlando, FL.

Harrington, S.S., & Walker, B.L. (2004). The effects of computer-based training on immediate and residual learning of nursing facility staff. *Journal of Continuing Education in Nursing*, 35(4), 154–163.

Harrison, E. (2009). (Re)Visiting academic advisement. *Nurse Educator*, 34(2), 64–68.

Harrow, A.J. (1972). *A Taxonomy of the psychomotor domain*. New York: McKay.

Harvath, T.A. (2008). A culture of learning. *Journal of Nursing Education*, 47(12), 535–536.

Heater, B.S., Becker, A.M., & Olson, R.K. (1988). Nursing interventions and patient outcomes. *Nursing Research*, 37(5), 303–307.

Hegge, M.J., & Hallman, P.A. (2008). Changing nursing culture to welcome second-degree students: Herding and corralling sacred cows. *Journal of Nursing Education, 47*(12), 552–556.

Heller, B.R., Drenkard, K., Esposito-Herr, M.B., Romano, C., Tom, S., & Valentine, N. (2004). Educating nurses for leadership roles. *Journal of Continuing Education in Nursing, 35*(5), 203–210.

Heller, B.R., Oros, M.T., & Durney-Crowley, J. (2000). The future of nursing education: 10 trends to watch. *Nursing and Health Care Perspectives, 21*(1), 9–13.

Herndorn, J.B., Kaiser, J., & Creamer, D.G. (1996). Student preferences for advising style in community college environments. *Journal of College Student Development, 37*(6), 637–647.

Hesser, A., Pond, F., Lewis, L., & Abbott, B. (1996). Evaluation of a supplementary retention program for African-American baccalaureate nursing students. *Journal of Nursing Education, 35*(7), 304–309.

Hodge, M., Martin, C.T., Taveier, D., Perea-Ryan, M., & Alcala-Van Houten, L. (2008). *Nurse Educator, 33*(5), 210–214.

Holtz, C. (2008). *Global health care.* Boston: Jones and Bartlett.

Horsfall, J. & Cleary, M. (2008). Planning and facilitating workshops. *Journal of Continuing Education in Nursing,39*(11), 511–516.

Horton, J.O. (2005). *Slavery in New York (exhibit).* New York Historical Society, New York.

Hubbard, R., & Allen, S.J. (1987). A cautionary note on the use of principal components analysis: Supportive empirical evidence. *Sociological Methods and Research, 16*, 301–308.

Huff, C. (1997). Cooperative learning: A model for teaching. *Journal of Nursing Education, 36*(9), 434–436.

Huff, R.M., & Kline, M.V. (1999). *Promoting health in multicultural populations: A handbook for practitioners.* Thousand Oaks, CA: Sage.

Hughes, K.H., & Hood, L.J. (2007). Teaching methods and an outcome tool for measuring cultural sensitivity in undergraduate students. *Journal of Transcultural Nursing, 18*(1), 57–62.

Hunter, J.L. (2008). Applying constructivism to nursing education in cultural competence: A course that bears repeating. *Journal of Transcultural Nursing, 18*(4), 354–362.

International Council of Nurses. (1973). *Code for nurses.* Geneva, Switzerland: Author.

Ironside, P.M. (2005). Teaching thinking and reaching the limits of memorization: Enacting new pedagogies. *Journal of Nursing Education, 44*, 441–449.

Jalili-Grenier, F. & Chase, M.M. (1997). Retention of nursing students with English as a second language. *Journal of Advanced Nursing*, *25*, 199–203.

Jarrett, S., Horner, M., Center, D., & Kane, L.A. (2008). Curriculum for the development of staff nurses as clinical faculty and scholars. *Nurse Educator*, *33*(6), 268–272.

Jeffreys, M.R. (1991). Time out! Let's play charades. *Nurse Educator*, *16*(5), 12, 34.

Jeffreys, M.R. (1993). *The relationship of self-efficacy and select academic and environmental variables on academic achievement and retention, doctoral dissertation*. Unpublished manuscript. New York: Teachers College, Columbia University.

Jeffreys, M.R. (1994). *Transcultural self-efficacy tool (TSET)*. Unpublished manuscript. Instrument copyrighted by author.

Jeffreys, M.R. (2000). Development and psychometric evaluation of the Transcultural Self-Efficacy Tool: A synthesis of findings. *Journal of Transcultural Nursing*, *11*(2), 127–136.

Jeffreys, M.R. (2001). Evaluating enrichment program study groups: Academic outcomes, psychological outcomes, and variables influencing retention. *Nurse Educator*, *26*(3), 142–149.

Jeffreys, M.R. (2002a). Students' perceptions of variables influencing retention: A pretest and post-test approach. *Nurse Educator*, *27*(1), 16–19. [Erratum, 2002, 27(2), 64].

Jeffreys, M.R. (2002b). A transcultural core course in the clinical nurse specialist curriculum. *Clinical Nurse Specialist: The Journal for Advanced Nursing Practice*. *16*(4), 195–202.

Jeffreys, M.R. (2003). Strategies for promoting nontraditional student retention and success. In M. Oermann & K. Heinrich (Eds.), *Annual Review of Nursing Education* (*Vol. I*, pp. 61–90). New York: Springer.

Jeffreys, M.R. (2004). *Nursing student retention: Understanding the process and making a difference*. New York: Springer.

Jeffreys, M.R. (2005). Clinical nurse specialists as cultural brokers, change agents, and partners in meeting the needs of culturally diverse populations. *Journal of Multicultural Nursing and Health*, *11*(2), 41–48.

Jeffreys, M.R. (2006a). Cultural competence in clinical practice. *Imprint*, *53*(2), 36–41.

Jeffreys, M.R. (2006b). *Teaching cultural competence in nursing and health care: Inquiry, action, and innovation*. New York: Springer.

Jeffreys, M.R. (2008a). Dynamics of diversity: Becoming better nurses through diversity awareness. *Imprint*. *55*(5), 36–41.

Jeffreys, M.R. (2008b). *Advanced certificate program in cultural competence*. Unpublished manuscript.

Jeffreys, M.R., & Dogan, E. (2007). *Evaluating students' transcultural self-efficacy perceptions and cultural competence following an integrated approach to cultural competence education*. Research grant proposal. Unpublished manuscript.

Jeffreys, M.R. & Dogan, E. (2010). Factor analysis of the Transcultural Self-Efficacy Tool (TSET). Journal of Nursing Measurement, 18(2), accepted for publication. Unpublished manuscript.

Jeffreys, M.R., Massoni, M., O'Donnell, M., & Smodlaka, I. (1997). Student evaluation of courses: Determining the reliability and validity of three survey instruments. *Journal of Nursing Education, 36*(8), 397–400.

Jeffreys, M.R., & O'Donnell, M. (1997). Cultural discovery: An innovative philosophy for creative learning activities. *Journal of Transcultural Nursing, 8*(2), 17–22.

Jeffreys, M.R., & Smodlaka, I. (1996). Steps of the instrument-design process: An illustrative approach for nurse educators. *Nurse Educator, 21*(6), 47–52. [Erratum, 1997, 22(1), 49].

Jeffreys, M.R., & Smodlaka, I. (1998). Exploring the factorial composition of the Transcultural Self-Efficacy Tool. *International Journal of Nursing Studies, 35*, 217–225.

Jeffreys, M.R., & Smodlaka, I. (1999a). Changes in students' transcultural self-efficacy perceptions following an integrated approach to culture care. *Journal of Multicultural Nursing and Health, 5*(2), 6–12. [Erratum, 2000, 6(1), 20].

Jeffreys, M.R., & Smodlaka, I. (1999b). Construct validation of the Transcultural Self-Efficacy Tool. *Journal of Nursing Education, 38*, 222–227.

Jeffreys, M.R., & Zoucha, R. (2001). The invisible culture of the multiracial, multiethnic individual: A transcultural imperative. *Journal of Cultural Diversity, 8*(3), 79–83.

Joel, L.A., & Kelly, L.Y. (2002). *The nursing experience: Trends, challenges, and transitions*. New York: McGraw-Hill.

Johnson, S.A., & Johnson, L.J. (2008). Second-degree, entry-into-practice master's of nursing program: Lessons learned. *Nurse Educator, 33*(5), 228–232.

Johnson, T.P. et al. (1997). Dimensions of self-identification among multiracial and multiethnic respondents in survey interviews. *Evaluation Review, 21*(6), 671–687.

Joint Commission on Accreditation of Healthcare Organizations (JCAHO). (1995). *Comprehensive accreditation manual for hospitals*. Oakwood Terrace, IL: Author.

Joint Commission on Accreditation of Healthcare Organizations (JCAHO). (2002). *Health care at the crossroads: Strategies for addressing the evolving nursing crisis.* Author.

Joint Commission on Accreditation of Healthcare Organizations. (2008). *Developing culturally competent patient-centered care standards.* Retrieved August 16, 2009, from http: jointcommission.org/Patient Safety/HLC/HLC_Develop_Culturally_Competent_Pt_Centered_Stds. htm.

Jones-Schenk, J., & Yoder-Wise, P.S. (2002). Professional self-regulation: Another Enron casualty? *Journal of Continuing Education in Nursing, 33*(3), 100–101.

Kaiser Permanente. (2002). *Cultural issues in the clinical setting (Series A and B)* [videocassette}. Available from Kaiser Permanente National Video Communications and Media Services, 825 Colorado Blvd., Suite 301, Los Angeles, CA, 90041.

Kaiser Permanente. (2003). *The multicultural health series (Part 1)* [videocassette]. Available from Kaiser Permanente National Video Communications and Media Services, 825 Colorado Blvd., Suite 301, Los Angeles, CA, 90041.

Kaiser Permanente. (2004). *The multicultural health series (Part 2)* [videocassette]. Available from Kaiser Permanente National Video Communications and Media Services, 825 Colorado Blvd., Suite 301, Los Angeles, CA, 90041.

Kataoka-Yahiro, M.R. & Abriam-Yago, K. (1997). Culturally competent teaching strategies for Asian nursing students for whom English is a second language. *Journal of Cultural Diversity, 4*(3), 83–87.

Kavanagh, K.H. & Kennedy, P.H. (1992). *Promoting cultural diversity: Strategies for health care.* Newbury Park, CA: Sage.

Kazdin, A. (2008a). President's site: Broader initiatives. Retrieved May 10, 2008, from http://www.apa.org/about/president/themes.html.

Kazdin, A. (2008b). Kazdin Convention Video, May 2008.

Keane, M. (1993). Preferred learning styles and study strategies in a linguistically diverse baccalaureate nursing student population. *Journal of Nursing Education, 32*(5), 214–221.

Kelly, E. (1997). Development of strategies to identify the learning needs of baccalaureate nursing students. *Journal of Nursing Education, 36,* 156–162.

Keltner, B., Kelley, F.J., & Smith, D. (2004). Leadership to reduce health disparities: A model for nursing leadership in American Indian communities. *Nursing Administration Quarterly, 28*(3), 181–190.

Kennedy, H.P., Fisher, L., Fontaine, D., & Martin-Holland, J. (2008). Evaluating diversity in nursing education: A mixed method study. *Journal of Transcultural Nursing, 19*(4), 363–370.

Kessler, P.D. & Lund, C.H. (2004). Reflective journaling: developing an online journal for distance education. *Nurse Educator, 29*(1), 20–24.

Khoiny, F.E. (1995). Factors that contribute to computer-assisted instruction effectiveness. *Computers in Nursing, 13*(4), 165–168.

Kim, J., & Mueller, C.W. (1978). *Factor analysis: Statistical methods and practical issues.* Newbury Park, CA: Sage.

Kimball, B., & O'Neil, E. (2002). *Health care's human crisis: The American nursing shortage.* Princeton, NJ: Robert Wood Johnson.

King, P.A. (1993). A teaching strategy for identifying values: A clinical experience with the homeless. *Nurse Educator, 18* (4), 17–20.

Kirkland, M.L.S. (1998). Stressors and coping strategies among successful female African American baccalaureate nursing students. *Journal of Nursing Education, 37*(1), 5–12.

Kirkpatrick, M.K., & Koldjeski, D. (1997). Career planning: The nurse educator as facilitator and career counselor. *Nurse Educator, 27*(3), 17–20.

Kirst, M.W. (2008). Secondary schools and colleges must work together. *Thought and Action, 24,* 111–122.

Kitson, A. (2000). Toward evidence-based quality improvement: Perspectives from nursing practice. *International Journal for Quality in Health Care, 12*(6), 459–464.

Knapp, T.R. (1990). Treating ordinal scales as interval scales: An attempt to resolve the controversy. *Nursing Research, 39*(2), 121–123.

Knapp, T.R. (1993). Treating ordinal scales as ordinal scales. *Nursing Research, 42*(3), 184–186.

Knowles, M. (1984). *The adult learner: A neglected species.* Houston, TX: Gulf.

Koeckeritz, J., Malkiewicz, J., & Henderson, A. (2002). The seven principles of good practice: Applications for online education in nursing. *Nurse Educator, 27*(6), 283–287.

Koenig, J.M., & Zorn, C.R. (2002). Using storytelling as an approach to teaching and learning with diverse students. *Journal of Nursing Education, 41*(9), 393–399.

Kollar, S.J., & Ailinger, R.L. (2002). International clinical experiences: Long-term impact on students. *Nurse Educator, 27*(1), 28–31.

Kosoko-Lasaki, S., Cook, C.T., & O'Brien, R.L. (2009). *Cultural proficiency in addressing health disparities.* Boston: Jones and Bartlett.

Kramer, N. (1995). Using games for learning. *Journal of Continuing Education in Nursing, 26,* 40–42.

Krathwohl, D.R., Bloom, B.S., & Masia, B. (Eds.). (1964). *Taxonomy of educational objectives: Handbook II, affective domain.* New York: McKay.

Krentzman, A.R. & Townsend, A.L. (2008). Review of multidisciplinary measures of cultural competence for use in social work education. *Journal of Social Work Education, 44*(2), 1–25.

Kubsch, S., Henniges, A., Lorenzoni, N., Eckardt, S., & Oleniczak, S. (2003). Factors influencing accruement of contact hours for nurses. *Journal of Continuing Education in Nursing, 34*(5), 205–212.

Kuh, G.D. (2001). Organizational culture and student persistence: Prospects and puzzles. *Journal of College Student Retention: Research, Theory, & Practice, 3*(1), 23–40.

Kuh, G.D. & Love, P.G. (2000). A cultural perspective on student departure. In J.M. Braxton (Ed.) *Reworking the student departure puzzle* (pp. 196–212). Nashville, TN: Vanderbilt University Press.

Kurz, J.M. (1993). The adult ESL baccalaureate nursing student. *Journal of Nursing Education, 32* (5), 227–229.

Labun, E. (2002). The Red River College Model: Enhancing success for native Canadian and other nursing students from disenfranchised groups. *Journal of Transcultural Nursing, 13*(4), 311–317.

Lambert, V.A. & Nugent, K.E. (1994). Addressing the academic progression of students encountering mental health problems. *Nurse Educator, 19*(5), 33–39.

Lasater, K., & Nielsen, A. (2009). Reflective journaling for clinical judgment development. *Journal of Nursing Education, 48*(1), 40–44.

Lattanzi, J.B., & Purnell, L.D. (2006). *Developing cultural competence in physical therapy practice*. Philadelphia, PA: FA Davis.

Lavoie-Tremblay, M., Wright, D., Desforges, N., Gelinas, C., Marchionni, C., & Drevniok, U. (2008). Creating a healthy workplace for new-generation nurses. *Journal of Nursing Scholarship, 40*(3), 290–297.

Ledesma, R.D., & Valero-Mora, P. (2007). Determining the number of factors to retain in EFA: An easy-to-use computer program for carrying out parallel analysis. *Practical Assessment, Research & Evaluation, 12*(2). Retrieved January 24, 2010, from http://pareonline.net/genpare.asp?wh = 4 = ledesma

Lee, C., & Bobko, P. (1994). Self-efficacy beliefs: Comparison of five measures. *Journal of Applied Psychology, 79*(3), 364–369.

Lee, S.M., & Fernandez, M. (1998). Trends in Asian American racial/ethnic intermarriage: A comparison of 1980 and 1990 census data. *Sociological Perspectives, 41*(2), 323–342.

Lehna, C., Jackonen, S., & Wilson, L. (1996). Navigating a nursing curriculum: Bridges and barriers. *Association of Black Nursing Faculty Journal, 7*(July/August), 98–103.

Leininger, M.M. (1978). *Transcultural nursing: Theories, concepts, and practices*. New York: John Wiley & Sons.

Leininger, M. (1988). Leininger's theory of nursing: Cultural care diversity and universality. *Nursing Science Quarterly, 1* (4), 152–160.

Leininger, M.M. (1989). Transcultural nurse specialists and generalists: New practitioners in nursing. *Journal of Transcultural Nursing, 1,* 4–16.

Leininger, M.M. (1991a). *Culture Care Diversity and Universality: A theory of nursing.* New York: National League for Nursing.

Leininger, M. (1991b). Transcultural care principles, human rights, and ethical considerations, *Journal of Transcultural Nursing, 3*(1), 21–23.

Leininger, M. (1991c). *Transcultural nursing: Cultural care assessment of an American Polish client [film].* (Available from Madonna University, Livonia, MI).

Leininger, M.M. (1994a). *Transcultural nursing: Concepts, theories, and practices.* Columbus, OH: Greyden Press.

Leininger, M. (1994b). Are nurses prepared to function worldwide? *Journal of Transcultural Nursing, 5*(2), 2–4.

Leininger, M.M. (1995a). *Transcultural nursing: Concepts, theories, research, and practice.* Blacklick, OH: McGraw-Hill College Custom Services.

Leininger, M.M. (1995b). Teaching transcultural nursing in undergraduate and graduate programs. *Journal of Transcultural Nursing, 6*(2), 10–26.

Leininger, M.M. (2002a). Essential transcultural nursing care concepts, principles, examples, and policy statements. In Leininger, M.M. & McFarland, M.R. (Eds.), *Transcultural Nursing: Concepts, Theories, Research, and Practice* (3rd ed., pp. 45–69). New York: McGraw-Hill.

Leininger, M.M. (2002b). The future of transcultural nursing: A global perspective. In M.M. Leininger & M.R. McFarland (Eds.), *Transcultural Nursing: Concepts, Theories, Research, and Practice* (3rd ed., pp. 585–586). New York: McGraw-Hill.

Leininger, M.M. (2002c). Transcultural food functions, beliefs, and practices. In M.M. Leininger & M.R. McFarland (Eds.), *Transcultural nursing: Concepts, theories, research, and practice* (3rd ed., pp. 205–216). New York: McGraw-Hill.

Leininger, M.M. (2002d). Part I. The theory of culture care and the ethnonursing research method. In M.M. Leininger & M.R. McFarland (Eds.), *Transcultural nursing: Concepts, theories, research, and practice* (3rd ed., pp. 71–98). New York: McGraw-Hill.

Leininger, M.M., & McFarland, M.R. (2002). *Transcultural nursing: Concepts, theories, research, and practice* (3rd ed.). New York: McGraw-Hill.

Leininger, M.M., & McFarland, M.R. (2006). *Culture Care Diversity and Universality: A worldwide nursing theory* (2nd ed.). Boston, MA: Jones and Bartlett.

Lent, R.W., Brown, S.D., & Gore, P.A. (1997). Discriminant and predictive validity of academic self-concept, academic self-efficacy, and mathematics-specific self-efficacy. *Journal of Counseling Psychology*, 44(3), 307–315.

Lent, R.W., Brown, S.D., & Larkin, K.C. (1986). Self-efficacy in prediction of academic performance and career options. *Journal of Counseling Psychology*, 33(3), 265–269.

Lent, R.W., Brown, S.D., & Larkin, K.C. (1987). Comparison of three theoretically derived variables in predicting career and academic behavior: Self-efficacy, interest congruence, and consequence thinking. *Journal of Counseling Psychology*, 34(3), 293–298.

Lent, R.W., Lopez, F.G., & Bieschke, K.J. (1993). Predicting mathematics-related choice and success behaviors: Test of an expanded social cognitive model. *Journal of Vocational Behavior*, 42, 223–236.

Lim, J., Downie, J., & Nathan, P. (2004). Nursing students' self-efficacy in providing transcultural care. *Nurse Education Today*, 24(6), 428–234.

Lin, H.F. (2007). Effects of extrinsic and intrinsic motivation on employee knowledge sharing intentions. *Journal of Information Science*, 33(2), 135–149.

Lipson, J.G., & DeSantis, L.A. (2007). Current approaches to integrating elements of cultural competence in nursing education. *Journal of Transcultural Nursing, Supplement to Vol. 18* (1), 10S–20S.

LoBiondo-Wood, G., & Haber, J. (1998). *Nursing research: Methods, critical appraisal, and utilization* (4th ed.). New York: Mosby.

Loerch, K.J.; Russell, J.E.A.; & Rush, M.C. (1989). The relationships among family domain variables and work-family conflict for men and women. *Journal of Vocational Behavior*, 35, 288–308.

Lubinski, R., & Matteliano, M.A. (2008). *A guide to cultural competence in the curriculum: Speech-language pathology.* Buffalo, NY: Center for International Rehabilitation Research Information and Exchange.

Lundquist, C., Spalding, R.J., & Landrum, R.E. (2002). College student's thoughts about leaving the university: The impact of faculty attitudes and behaviors. *Journal of College Student Retention: Research, Theory, and Practice*, 4(2), 123–134.

Luthy, K.E., Perterson, N.E., Lassetter, J.H., & Callister, L.C. (2009). Successfully incorporating writing across the curriculum with advanced writing in nursing. *Journal of Nursing Education*, 48(1), 54–59.

MacIntosh, J., MacKay, E., Mallet-Boucher, M., & Wiggins, N. (2002). Discovering co-learning with students in distance education sites. *Nurse Educator*, 27(4), 182–186.

MacQuarrie, D. (2004). *Assessment of student nurses' transcultural self-efficacy perceptions (confidence) when caring for culturally diverse clients*. Unpublished doctoral dissertation, McMaster University, Hamilton, Ontario, Canada.

Madorin, S., & Iwasiw, C. (1999). The effects of computer-assisted instruction on the self-efficacy of baccalaureate nursing students. *Journal of Nursing Education*, 38(6), 282–285.

Maddux, J.E. (1995). *Self-efficacy, adaptation, and adjustment: Theory, research, and application*. New York: Plenum Press.

Majumdar, B., Browne, G., Roberts, J., & Carpio, B. (2004). Effects of cultural sensitivity training on health care provider attitudes and patient outcomes. *Journal of Nursing Scholarship*, 36(2), 161–166.

Management Sciences for Health. (2005). *Providers guide to quality and culture*. Retrieved January 30, 2005, from http://erc.msh.org/mainpage.cfm?file.

Manifold, C. & Rambur, B. (2001). Predictors of attrition in American Indian nursing students. *Journal of Nursing Education*, 40(6), 279–281.

Mateo, M.A., & McMyler, E. (2004). The nurse educator role in staff competency. In M. Oermann, & K. Heinrich (Eds.), *Annual Review of Nursing Education* (Vol. II, pp. 305–325, New York: Springer.

Mathews, M.B. (2003). Resourcing nursing education through collaboration. *Journal of Continuing Education in Nursing*, 34(6), 251–257.

Matzo, M.L., Sherman, D.W., Mazanec, P., Barber, M.A., Virani, R., & McLaughlin, M.M. (2002). Teaching cultural considerations at the end of life: End of life nursing education consortium program recommendations. *Journal of Continuing Education in Nursing*, 33(6), 270–278.

Maville, J. & Huerta, C.G. (1997). Stress and social support among Hispanic student nurses: Implications for academic achievement. *Journal of Cultural Diversity*, 4(1), 18–25.

McArdle, J.J. (1990). Principles versus principals of structural factor-analyses. *Multivariate Behavioral Research*, 25(1), 81–87.

McDonald, R.P. (1985). *Factor analysis and related methods*. Hillsdale, NJ: Erlbaum.

Medley, C.F., & Horne, C. (2005). Using simulation technology for undergraduate nursing education. *Journal of Nursing Education*, 44(1), 31–34.

Merril, E.B., Reinckens, T., Yarborough, M., & Robinson, V.I. (2006). Retaining and assisting nontraditional nursing student in a baccalaureate nursing program utilizing blackboard and integrity technolgies. *The ABNF Journal (summer)*, 107–110.

Mertig, R.G. (2003). *Teaching nursing in an associate degree program.* New York: Springer.

Miller, J. (1997). Politics and care: A study of Czech Americans within Leininger's Theory of Culture Care Diversity and Universality. *Journal of Transcultural Nursing*, 9(1), 3–13.

Miller, J., Koyanagi, M.L.S., & Morgan, K.J. (2005). Faculty as a community engaged with ongoing curricular development: Use of groupware and electronic resources. *Journal of Nursing Education*, 44(1), 27–30.

Miller, L.C., Devaney, S.W., Kelly, G.L., & Kuehn, A.F. (2008). E-mentoring in public health nursing practice. *The Journal of Continuing Education in Nursing*, 39(9), 394–399.

Moccia, P. (1989). 1989: Shaping a human agenda for the nineties, trends that demand our attention as managed care prevails. *Nursing and Health Care*, 10, 15–17.

Moch, S.D., Long, G.L., Jones, J.W., Shadlick, K., & Solheim, K. (1999). Faculty and student cross-cultural learning through teaching health promotion in the community. *Journal of Nursing Education*, 38(5), 238–240.

Mone, M.A., Baker, D.D., & Jeffries, F. (1995). Predictive validity and time dependency of self-efficacy, self-esteem, personal goals, and academic performance. *Educational and Psychological Measurement*, 55(5), 716–727.

Montag, M.L., & Gotkin, L.G. (1959). *Community college education for nursing.* New York: McGraw-Hill.

Morton, P.G., & Rauen, C.A. (2004). Using simulation in nursing education: The University of Maryland and Georgetown University experiences. In M. Oermann & K. Heinrich, (Eds.) *Annual Review of Nursing Education* (Vol. II, pp. 139–161). New York: Springer.

Mueller, S.S., Pullen, R.L., & McGee, K.S. (2002). A model nursing computer resource center. *Nurse Educator*, 27(3), 115–117.

Mulaik, Stanley A. (1990). Blurring the distinctions between component analysis and common factor analysis. *Multivariate Behavioral Research*, 25(1), 53–59.

Multon, K.D., Brown, S.D., & Lent, R.W. (1991). Relation of self-efficacy beliefs to academic outcomes: A meta-analytic investigation. *Journal of Counseling Psychology*, 38(1), 30–38.

Munoz, C., & Hilgenberg, C. (2005). Ethnopharmacology. *American Journal of Nursing*, 105(8), 40–49.

Munro, B.H. (2005). *Statistical methods for health care research (Fifth edition)*, New York: Lippincott, Williams, and Wilkins.

Nash, G.B. (1995). The hidden history of mestizo in America. *Journal of American history, 82*(3), 941–962.

National Association of Clinical Nurse Specialists. (2005). *Statement on clinical nurse specialist practice and education.* Glenview, IL: National Association of Clinical Nurse Specialists.

National Association of School Nurses. (2002), *Code of Ethics.* Silver Spring, MD: Author.

National Association of Social Workers. (2001). *Standards for cultural competence in social work practice.* Washington, DC: Author.

National Association of Social Workers. (2007). *Indicators for the achievement of the NASW standards for cultural competence in social work practice.* Washington, DC: Author.

National Association of Social Workers. (2009). *Code of ethics.* Washington, DC: Author.

National League for Nursing. (2002a). *Nursing Education Research, Technology, and Information Management Advisory Council (NERTIMAC).* Retrieved April 2, 2003, from http://nln.org/aboutnln/nertimac.htm.

National League for Nursing. (2002b). *Nursing education research priorities.* Retrieved April 2, 2003, from http://nln.org/aboutnln/research.htm.

National League for Nursing (2009) A Commitment to Diversity in Nursing and Nursing Education. Retrieved January 24, 2010, from http://www.nln.org/aboutnln/reflection_dialogue/refl_dial_3.htm

National League for Nursing Accrediting Commission, Inc. (2008a). NLNAC Standards and Criteria: Clinical Doctorate Degree Programs in Nursing. New York: Author.

National League for Nursing Accrediting Commission, Inc. (2008b). NLNAC Standards and Criteria: Master's/Post-Masters Certificate Programs in Nursing. New York: Author.

National League for Nursing Accrediting Commission, Inc. (2008c). NLNAC Standards and Criteria: Baccalaureate Degree Programs in Nursing. New York: Author.

National League for Nursing Accrediting Commission, Inc. (2008d). NLNAC Standards and Criteria: Associate Degree Programs in Nursing. New York: Author.

National League for Nursing Accrediting Commission, Inc. (2008e). NLNAC Standards and Criteria: Diploma Programs in Nursing. New York: Author.

Nehring, W.M., & Lashley, F.R. (2004). Using the human patient simulator in nursing education. In M. Oermann & K. Heinrich, (Eds.)

Annual review of nursing education (Vol. II, pp. 163–181). New York: Springer.

Neumann, J.A., & Forsyth, D. (2008). Teaching in the affective domain for institutional values. *The Journal of Continuing Education in Nursing, 39*(6), 248–252.

Nochajski, S.M., & Matteliano, M.A. (2008). *A guide to cultural competence in the curriculum: Occupational therapy*. Buffalo, NY: Center for International Rehabilitation Research Information and Exchange.

Nora, A. (1987). Determinants of retention among Chicano college students: A structural model. *Research in Higher Education, 26*(1), 31–60.

Nora, A. (2001). The depiction of significant others in Tinto's "Rites of Passage": A reconceptualization of the influence of family and community in the persistence process. *Journal of College Student Retention: Research, Theory, & Practice, 3*(1), 41–56.

Nunnally, J.C., & Bernstein, I.H. (1994). *Psychometric theory*. New York: McGraw-Hill.

Nurmi, J-E., & Aunola, K. (2001). How does academic achievement come about: Cross-cultural and methodological notes. *International Journal of Educational Research, 35*, 403–409.

Oermann, M.H., & Gaberson, K.B. (2009). *Evaluation and testing in nursing education*. New York: Springer.

Office of Minority Health. (2001). *National standards for culturally and linguistically appropriate services in health care*. Washington, DC: U.S. Department of Health and Human Services.

Office of Minority Health. (2005). *Potential measures/indicators of cultural competence*. Retrieved January 30, 2005, from http://www.hrsa.gov/OMH/cultural/attachment3.htm.

Olenchak, F.R. & Hebert, T.P. (2002). Endangered academic talent: Lessons learned from gifted first-generation college males. *Journal of College Student Development, 43*(2), 195–212.

O'Neill, C.A., Fisher, C.A., & Newbold, S.K. (2009). *Developing online learning environments in nursing education*. New York: Springer.

Ostrow, L. & DiMaria-Ghalili, R.A. (2005). Distance education for graduate nursing: One state school's experience. *Journal of Nursing Education, 44*(1), 5–10.

Pacquiao, D.F. (2004). President's message: Building collaborative influence. *Journal of Transcultural Nursing, 15*(2), 155.

Padilla, R.V. (1999). College student retention: Focus on success. *Journal of College Student Retention: Research, Theory, and Practice, 1*(2), 131–146.

Panzarella, K.J., & Matteliano, M.A. (2008). *A guide to cultural competence in the curriculum: Physical therapy.* Buffalo, NY: Center for International Rehabilitation Research Information and Exchange.

Pascoe, P. (1996). Miscegenation law, court cases, and ideologies of "race" in twentieth-century America. *Journal of American history, 83*(1), 44–69.

Pastuszak, J., & Rodowicz, M.O. (2002). Internal e-mail: An avenue of educational opportunity. *Journal of Continuing Education in Nursing, 33*(4), 164–167.

Patterson, B.J. & Morin, K.H. (2002). Perceptions of the maternal-child clinical rotation: The male student nurse experience. *Journal of Nursing Education, 41*(6), 266–272.

Pender, N.J., Murdaugh, C., & Parsons, M.A. (2006). *Health Promotion in Nursing Practice,* 5th edition. Upper Saddle River, NJ: Prentice-Hall Health.

Penprase, B., & Koczara, S. (2009). Understanding the experiences of accelerated second-degree nursing students and graduates: A review of the literature. *Journal of Continuing Education in Nursing, 40*(2), 74–78.

Perlmann, J. (1997). Multiracials, intermarriage, and ethnicity. *Society, 6,* 20–23.

Phinney, J.S. (1996). Understanding ethnic diversity. *American Behavioral Scientist, 40*(2), 143–152.

Pickerell, K.D. (2001). A cross-cultural nursing experience on the Rosebud reservation. *Nurse Educator, 26*(3), 128–131.

Piercy, E.C. (2004). Using WebQuests to promote active learning. *Journal of Continuing Education in Nursing, 35*(5), 200–201.

Pimple, C., Schmidt, L., & Tidwell, S. (2003). Achieving excellence in end-of-life care. *Nurse Educator, 28*(1), 40–43.

Pinderhughes, E. (1995). Biracial identity—asset or handicap? In H. W. Harris, C. Blue, & E. E. H. Griffith, *Racial and ethnic identity: Psychological development and creative expression.* (pp. 73–93), New York: Routledge.

Pinkerton, S.E. (2004). The financial return on education programs. *Journal of Continuing Education in Nursing, 35*(6), 244–245.

Pintrich, P.R., & Garcia, T. (1994). Self-regulated learning in college students: Knowledge, strategies, and motivation. In P.R. Pintrich, D.R. Brown, & C.E. Weinstein, (Eds.), *Student motivation, cognition, and learning: Essays in honor of Wilbert J. McKeachie.* (pp. 113–133). Hillsdale, NJ: Lawrence Erlbaum Associates.

Platter, B. (2005, October). *Clinical nurse cultural competency pre and post transcultural nursing education.* Paper presented at the annual conference of the Trancultural Nursing Society, New York.

Polit, D.F., & Beck, C.T. (2004). *Nursing research: Principles and methods*. New York: Lippincott, Williams, and Wilkins.

Polit, D.F., & Hungler, B.P. (1997). *Essentials in nursing research— Methods, appraisal, and utilization*. New York: Lippincott.

Ponterotto, J.G., Cassas, J.M., Suzuki, L.A., & Alexander, C.M. (2010). *Handbook of multicultural counseling* (3rd ed.). Washington, DC: Sage.

Poorman, S.G., Webb, C.A., & Mastorovich, M.L. (2002). Students' stories: How faculty help and hinder students at risk. *Nurse Educator*, 27(3), 126–131.

Porter, C.P. & Barbee, E. (2004). Race and racism in nursing research: Past, present, and future. In L. Fitzpatrick (Ed.), *Annual review of nursing research, Vol. 22*, pp. 9–38.

Pressler, J.L., & Kenner, C. (2009). Embracing new directions in curricula and teaching. *Nurse Educator, 34*(2), 49–50.

Pullen, R.L., Murray, P.H., & McGee, K.S. (2001). Care groups: A model to mentor novice nursing students. *Nurse Educator, 26*, 283–288.

Pullen, R.L., Murray, P.H., & McGee, K.S. (2003). Using care groups to mentor novice nursing students. (In: Oermann, M. & Heinrich, K. ed.) *Annual Review of Nursing Education* (*Vol. I*, pp. 147–161). New York: Springer.

Purnell, L.D. (2008). Purnell's model for cultural competence. In Purnell & Paulanka (Eds.), *Transcultural health care: A culturally competent approach* (3rd ed.) Philadelphia, PA: FA Davis, 19–55.

Purnell, L.D., & Paulanka, B.J. (2003). *Transcultural health care: A culturally competent approach* (2nd ed.). Philadelphia, PA: FA Davis.

Purnell, L.D., & Paulanka, B.J. (2008). *Transcultural health care: A culturally competent approach* (3rd ed.). Philadelphia, PA: FA Davis.

Quintilian, E.M. (1985). Influential factors in recruitment and retention of minority students in a community college. *Journal of Allied Health, 14*(1), 63–70.

Ramirez, C. (2009). Latino nursing career opportunity program: A project designed to increase the number of Latino nurses. In S. D. Bosher & M. D. Pharris (Ed). *Transforming nursing education: The culturally inclusive environment* (pp. 313–327). New York: Springer.

Ransdell, S. (2001a). Predicting college success: The importance of ability and non-cognitive variables. *International Journal of Educational Research, 35*, 357–364.

Ransdell, S. (2001b). Discussion and implications. *International Journal of Educational Research, 35*, 391–395.

Ransdell, S., Hawkins, C., & Adams, R. (2001a). Models, modeling, and the design of the study. *International Journal of Educational Research, 35*, 365–372.

Ransdell, S., Hawkins, C., & Adams, R. (2001b). Results of the study. *International Journal of Educational Research, 35*, 373–389.

Rash, E.M. (2008). A problem-based learning hybrid in a women's health course. *Journal of Nursing Education, 47*(10), 477–479.

Rashotte, J. & Thomas, M. (2002). Incorporating educational theory into critical care orientation. *Journal of Continuing Education in Nursing, 33*(3), 131–137.

Rattray, J., & Jones, M.C. (2007). Essential elements of question-naire design and development. *Journal of Clinical Nursing, 16*, 234–243.

Rauen, C. (2001). Using simulation to teach critical thinking skills: You can't just throw the book at them. *Critical Care Nursing Clinics of North America, 13*, 93–103.

Ravert, P. (2008). Patient simulator sessions and critical thinking. *Journal of Nursing Education, 47*(12), 557–562.

Reeves, J.S. (2001). Weaving a transcultural thread. *Journal of Transcultural Nursing, 12*(2), 140–145.

Rendon, L.I. (1994). Validating culturally diverse students: Toward a new model of learning & student development. *Innovative Higher Education, 19*(1), 23–32.

Rendon, L.I., Jalomo, R.E., & Nora, A. (2000). Theoretical consider-ations in the study of minority student retention in higher educa-tion. In J.M. Braxton (Ed.), *Reworking the tudent departure puzzle* (pp. 127–156). Nashville, TN: Vanderbilt University Press.

Rew, L. (1996). Affirming cultural diversity: A pathways model for nurs-ing faculty. *Journal of Nursing Education, 35*(7), 310–314.

Richardson, A., Miller, M., & Potter, H. (2002). Developing, delivering, and evaluating cancer nursing services: Searching for a United King-dom evidence base for practice. *Cancer Nursing, 25*(5), 404–415.

Riley, J.M., Beal, J., Levi, P., & McCausland, M.P. (2002). Revisioning nursing scholarship. *Journal of Nursing Scholarship, 34*(4), 383–389.

Rizzolo, M.A. (2002). Where have all the teachers gone? Long time pass-ing. . . . *Shaping the Future, 1*(1), 2–4.

Root, M.P.P. (1992). Within, between, and beyond race. In M.P.P. Root (Ed.), *Racially mixed people in America* (pp. 3–11). Newbury Park, CA: Sage.

Root, M.P.P. (1997). Multiracial Asians: Models of ethnic identity. *Ameriasia Journal, 23*(1), 29–41.

Rosal, M.C., & Bodentos, J.S. (2009). Culture and health-related behav-ior. In: Shumaker, S.A., Ockene, J.K., & Riekert, K.A. (Eds.) *The handbook of health behavior change* (3rd ed.) (pp. 39–58). New York: Springer.

Rosenfeld, P., Duthie, E., Bier, J., Bower-Ferres, S., Fulmer, T., Iervolino, L., et al. (2000). Engaging staff in evidence-based research to identify nursing practice problems and solutions. *Applied Nursing Research*, *13*(4), 197–203.

Rosenkoetter, M.M., & Nardi, D.A. (2007). American Academy of Nursing Expert Panel on Global Nursing and Health: White paper on global nursing and health. *Journal of Transcultural Nursing*, *18*(4), 305–315.

Roufs, A. (2007). In theory, advising matters. In: P. Fulson (Ed.), *The new advisor guidebook: Mastering the art of advising through the first year and beyond* (pp. 33–37). Kansas, MO: NACADA.

Rubini, S. (1988). *The community college role in the education of professional nurses.* (ERIC Document Reproduction Service No. ED 293 587).

Ruth-Sahd, L.A. (2003). Reflective practice: A critical analysis of data-based studies and implications for nursing education. *Journal of Nursing Education*, *42*, 488–497.

Ryan, M., Carlton, K.H., & Ali, N. (2000). Transcultural nursing concepts and experiences in nursing curricula. *Journal of Transcultural Nursing*, *11*(4), 300–307.

Ryan, M., Twibell, R., Brigham, C., & Bennett, P. (2000). Learning to care for clients in their world, not mine. *Journal of Nursing Education*, *39*(9), 401–408.

Saks, A.M. (1995). Longitudinal field investigation of the moderating and mediating effects of self-efficacy on the relationship between training and newcomer adjustment. *Journal of Applied Psychology*, *80*, 211–225.

Sandin, I., Grahn, K., & Kronvall, E. (2004). Outcomes of Swedish nursing students' field experiences in a hospital in Tanzania. *Journal of Transcultural Nursing*, *15*(3), 225–230.

Sands, N., & Schuh, J.H. (2004). Identifying interventions to improve the retention of biracial students: A case study. *Journal of College Student Retention: Research, Theory, and Practice*, *5*(4), 349–363.

Schim, S.M., Doorenbos, A., Benkert, R., & Miller, J. (2007). Culturally congruent care: Putting the puzzle together. *Journal of Transcultural Nursing*, *18*(2), 103–110.

Schmidt, L.A. (2004a). Psychometric evaluation of the writing-to-learn attitude survey. *Journal of Nursing Education*, *43*(10), 458–465.

Schmidt, L.A. (2004b). Evaluating the writing-to-learn strategy with undergraduate nursing students. *Journal of Nursing Education*, *43*(10), 466–473.

Schön, D. (1987). *Educating the reflective practitioner*. San Franscisco, CA: Jossey-Bass.

Schoolcraft, V., & Novotny, J. (2000). *A nuts and bolts approach to teaching nursing*. New York: Springer.

Schultz, E.D. (1998). Academic advising from a nursing theory perspective. *Nurse Educator, 22*(2), 22–25.

Schumacher, G., Risco, K., & Conway, A. (2008). The Schumacher model: Fostering scholarship and excellence in nursing and for recruiting and grooming new faculty. *Journal of Nursing Education, 47*(12), 571–575.

Schunk, D. (1995). Self-efficacy and education and instruction. In J.E. Maddux (Ed.), *Self-efficacy, adaptation, and adjustment: Theory, research, and application* (pp. 281–304). New York: Plenum Press.

Schunk, D. (1987). *Self-efficacy and cognitive achievemnt*. Paper presented at the Annual Meeting of the American Psychological Association (New York, August 28–Septmeber 1, 1987). In (ERIC Document Reproduction Service No. ED 287 880).

Scisney-Matlock, M., McCloud, P.K., & Barnard, R.M. (2001). Systematic assessment and evaluation of diversity content presented in classroom lectures: The FRDC tool. *Journal of Cultural Diversity, 8*(3), 85–93.

Seidman, A. (2005). *College student retention: Formula for student success*. Westport, CT: Praeger.

Seidman, A. (2007). *Minority student retention: The best of the Journal of College Student Retention: Research, Theory, and Practice*. Amityville, NY: Bayood.

Selig, C. (2000). Sexual assault nurse examiner and sexual assault response team (SANE/SART) program. *Nursing Clinics of North America, 32*(5), 311–319.

Sevean, P.A., Poole, K., & Shane Strickland, D. (2005). Actualizing scholarship in senior baccalaureate students. *Journal of Nursing Education, 44*, 473–476.

Shadbolt, A. (2004). (Personal communication, October 29, 2004), Professional Development Officer, RACGP Project, Royal Australian College of General Practitioners, South Melbourne, Victoria 3205, Australia.

Shell, D.F., Murphy, C.C., & Bruning, R.H. (1989). Self-efficacy and outcome expectancy mechanisms in reading and writing achievement. *Journal of Educational Psychology, 81*, 91–100.

Sherman, R.O., & Eggenberger, T. (2008). Transitioning internationally recruited nurses into clinical settings. *Journal of Continuing Education in Nursing, 39*(12), 535–544.

Sherrod, R.A. & Harrison, L. (1994). Evaluation of a comprehensive advisement program designed to enhance student retention. *Nurse Educator, 19*(6), 29–33.

Shinn, L.J. (1998). Contemporary issues in professional organizations. In D.J. Mason & J.K. Leavitt, (Eds.), *Policy and politics in nursing and health care* (3rd ed., pp. 525–534). New York: WB Saunders.

Simpson, R.L. (2004). Recruit, retain, assess: Technology's role in diversity. *Nursing Administration Quarterly, 28*(3), 217–220.

Siu, H.M., Spence Laschinger, H.K., & Vingilis, E. (2005). The effect of problem-based learning on nursing students' perceptions of empowerment. *Journal of Nursing Education, 44*, 459–469.

Skaggs, B.J., & DeVries, C.M. (1998). You and your professional organization. In D.J. Mason & J.K. Leavitt, (Eds.), *Policy and politics in nursing and health care* (3rd ed., pp. 535–545). New York: WB Saunders.

Smart, J.F. & Smart, D.W. (1995). Acculturative stress: the experience of the Hispanic immigrant. *The Counseling Psychologist, 23*, 25–42.

Sommer, S. (2001). Multicultural nursing education. *Journal of Nursing Education, 40*(6), 276–278.

Spanard, J.-M.A. (1990). Beyond intent: Reentering college to complete the degree. *Review of Educational Research, 30*, 309–344.

Spector, R.E. (2009). *Cultural Diversity in Health and Illness.* (7th Edition). Upper Saddle River, NJ: Pearson, Prentice Hall.

Spence, D.G. (2005). Hermeneutic notions augment cultural safety education. *Journal of Nursing Education, 44*, 409–414.

Spickard, P.R. (1997). What must I be? Asian Americans and the question of multiethnic identity. *Ameriasia Journal, 23*(1), 43–60.

Spickard, P.R., & Fong, R. (1995). Pacific Islander Americans and the question of multiethnicity: A vision of America's future? *Social Forces, 73*(4), 1365–1383.

Squires, A. (2002). New graduate orientation in the rural community hospital. *Journal of Continuing Education in Nursing, 33*(5), 203–209.

Stage, F.K., & Hossler, D. (2000). Where is the student? Linking student behaviors, college choice, and college persistence. In J. Braxton (Ed.), *Reworking the student departure puzzle* (pp. 170–195). Nashville, TN: Vanderbilt University.

Sternberger, C.S. (2002). Embedding a pedagogical model in the design of an online course. *Nurse Educator, 27*(4), 170–173.

Stevens, G.L. (1998). Experience the culture. *Journal of Nursing Education, 37*(1), 30–33.

Stevenson, E.L. (2003). Future trends in nursing employment. *American Journal of Nursing Career Guide 2003*, 19–25.

Stigler, J.W. & Hiebert, J. (1998). Teaching is a cultural activity. *American Educator, (Winter)*, 4–11.

Stolder, M.E., Hydo, S.K., Zorn, C.R., & Bottoms, M.S. (2007). Fire, wind, earth, and water: Raising the education threshold through teacher self-awareness. *Journal of Transcultural Nursing, 18*(3), 265–270.

Storch, J. & Gamroth, L. (2002). Scholarship revisited: A collaborative nursing education program's journey. *Journal of Nursing Education, 41*(12), 524–530.

Strauss, S.E., Richardson, W.S., Glasziou, P., & Haynes, R.B. (2005). *Evidence-based medicine: How to practice and teach EBM* (3rd ed.). Edinburgh: Elsevier.

Streubert, H.J. (1994). Male nursing students' perceptions of clinical experience. *Nurse Educator, 19*(5), 28–32.

St. Clair, A., & McKenry, L. (1999). Preparing culturally competent practitioners. *Journal of Nursing Education, 38*(5), 228–234.

St. Hill, P., Lipson, J.G., & Meleis, A.I. (2003). *Caring for women cross-culturally*. Philadelphia: Davis.

Sudman, S., & Bradburn, N.M. (1991). *Asking questions*. San Francisco, CA: Jossey-Bass.

Suh, E.E. (2004). The model of cultural competence through an evolutionary concept analysis. *Journal of Transcultural Nursing, 15*(4), 93–102.

Swanson, J.W. (2004). Diversity: Creating an environment of inclusiveness. *Nursing Education Quarterly, 28*(3), 207–211.

Sweeney, N.M., Saarmann, L., Flagg, J., & Seidman, R. (2008). The keys to successful online continuing education programs for nurses. *The Journal of Continuing Education in Nursing, 39*(1), 34–41.

Sweet, S., & Fusner, S. (2008). Social integration of the advanced placement LPN: A peer mentoring program. *Nurse Educator, 33*(5), 202–205.

Tabi, M.M., & Mukherjee, S. (2003). Nursing in a global community: A study abroad program. *Journal of Transcultural Nursing, 14*(2), 134–138.

Tagliareni, M.E. (2008). Quoted in Sapers, J. Shaping the future of nursing, *TC Today, 33*(1), 13–17.

Tanner, C. (1990). Reflections on the curriculum revolution. *Journal of Nursing Education, 29*, 295–299.

Tanner, C.A. (2002). Learning to teach: An introduction to "Teacher talk: New Pedagogies for Nursing." *Journal of Nursing Education, 41*(3), 95–96.

Tayebi, K., Moore-Jazayeri, M., & Maynard, T. (1998). From the borders: Reforming the curriculum for the at-risk student. *Journal of Cultural Diversity, 5*(3), 101–109.

Thede, L.Q., Taft, S., & Coeling, H. (1994). Computer-assisted instruction: A learner's viewpoint. *Journal of Nursing Education, 33*(7), 299–305.

Thompson, P.A. (2004). Leadership from an international perspective. *Nursing Administration Quarterly, 28*(3), 191–198.

Thorpe, K., & Loo, R. (2003). The values profile of nursing undergraduate students: Implications for education and professional development. *Journal of Nursing Education, 42*(2), 83–90.

Thurber, F., Hollingsworth, A., Brown, L., & Whitaker, S. (1989). The faculty advisor role: An imperative for student retention. *Nurse Educator, 13*(3), 27–33.

Tomey, A.M. (2003). Learning with cases. *Journal of Continuing Education in Nursing, 34*(1), 34–38.

Toney, D. (2004). *Exploring the relationship between levels of cultural competence and the perceived level of quality care among registered nurses caring for culturally diverse patients*, doctoral dissertation. Unpublished manuscript. Capella University.

Trent, B.A. (1997). Student perceptions of academic advising in an RN-to-BSN program. *Journal of Continuing Education in Nursing, 28*(6), 276–283.

Tuck, I., & Harris, L.H. (1988). Teaching students transcultural concepts. *Nurse Educator, 13* (3), 336–339.

Tucker-Allen, S., & Long, E. (1999). *Recruitment and Retention of Minority Students: Stories of Success*. Lisle, IL: Tucker Publications.

Ulrich, D.L. & Glendon, K.J. (1999). *Interactive group learning: Strategies for nurse educators*. New York: Springer.

United Nations (1948). *Universal Declaration of Human Rights*. Author.

Upton, T.A. & Lee-Thompson, L-C. (2001). The role of the first language in second language reading. *Studies in Second Language Acquisition, 23*(4), 469–495.

U.S. Census Bureau. (2002). *United States Census 2000*. Retrieved February 17, 2006, from http://census.gov/main/www/cen2000.html.

U.S. Department of Health and Human Services Office of Minority Health, (2001). *National standards for culturally and linguistically appropriate services in health care*. Retrieved January 24, 2010, from http://minorityhealth.hhs.gov/templates/content.aspx?ID = 87

Vance, C., & Olson, R.K. (1998). *The mentor connection in nursing*. New York: Springer.

Van Ginkel, J.R., Van der Ark, L.A., & Sijtsma, K. (2007). Multiple imputation for item scores when test data are factorially complex.

British Journal of Mathematical and Statistical Psychology, 60, 315–337.

Velez, J. (2005). *The effects of cultural competency training using self-instruction on obstetrical nurses' awareness, knowledge, and attitudes.* Unpublished master's thesis, Cleveland State University, Cleveland, OH.

Velicer, W.F., & Jackson, D.N. (1990). Component analysis versus common factor analysis: Some issues in selecting an appropriate procedure. *Multivariate Behavioral Research, 25*, 1–28.

Villaruel, A.M., Canales, M., & Torres, S. (2001). Bridges and barriers: Educational mobility of Hispanic nurses. *Journal of Nursing Education, 40*(6), 245–251.

Villarruel, A.M., & Peragallo, N. (2004). Leadership development of Hispanic nurses. *Nursing Administration Quarterly, 28*(3), 173–180.

Voorhees, R.A. (1987). Toward building models of community college persistence: A logit analysis. *Research in Higher Education, 26,* (2), 115–129.

Waltz, C.F. (1988). *Survey of schools.* In Hart, S.C. & Waltz, C.F. *Educational outcomes: Assessment of quality.* State of the Art and Future Directions. Helene Fuld Trust Accreditation Project (pp. 67–89). New York: National League for Nursing.

Waltz, C.F., Strickland, O.L., & Lenz, E.R. (2005). *Measurement in nursing research.* Philadelphia: Davis.

Washington, D., Erickson, J.I., & Ditomassi, M. (2004). Mentoring the minority leader of tomorrow. *Nursing Administration Quarterly, 28*(3), 165–169.

Waters, V. (1990). Associate degree nursing and curriculum revolution II. *Journal of Nursing Education, 29*, 322–325.

Waters, C.M. (2007). Commentary on community-based approaches to strengthen cultural competence in nursing education and practice. *Journal of Transcultural Nursing, Supplement to Vol. 18*, 66S–67S.

Weaver, H.N. (2001). Indigenous nurses and professional education: Friends or foes? *Journal of Nursing Education, 40*(6), 252–258.

Weis, P.A., & Guyton-Simmons. (1998). A computer simulation for teaching critical thinking. *Nurse Educator, 23*(2), 30–33.

White, M.J., Amos, E., & Kouzekanani, K. (1999). Problem-based learning: An outcomes student. *Nurse Educator, 24*(2), 33–36.

Whitt-Glover, M.C., Beech, B.M., Bell, R.A., Jackson, S.A., Loftin-Bell, K.A., & Mount, D.L. (2009). In S.A. Shumaker, J.K. Ockene, & K.A. Riekert (Eds.), *The handbook of health behavior change (3rd Edition)* (pp. 589–606). New York: Springer.

Williams, M.E., & Jones, J.J. (2004). Creating staff-friendly continuing education: The tidbits and niblets program. *Journal of Continuing Education in Nursing, 35*(6), 248–249.

Williams, R.P., & Calvillo, E.R. (2002). Maximizing learning among students from culturally diverse backgrounds. *Nurse Educator, 27*(5), 222–226.

Wilson, D.W. (2007). From their own voices: The lived experience of African American registered nurses. *Journal of Transcultural Nursing, 18*(2), 142–149.

Wilson, L., & Houghtaling, S. (2001). Report on a study of cultural competence teaching in California medical and dental schools.

Winch, S., Creedy, D., & Chaboyer, A.W. (2002). Governing nursing conduct: the rise of evidence-based practice. *Nursing Inquiry, 9*(3).

Wink, D. (2009). Teaching with technology: Finding information on the Internet. *Nurse Educator, 34*(2), 51–53.

Winters, C. (1990). Excellence in advisement: A strategy for declining nursing enrollments. *Journal of Nursing Education, 29*(5), 233–234.

Winters, C., & Owens, R. (1993). Alternative teaching strategies: Using a health fair to meet tribal college and nursing program needs. *Journal of Nursing Education, 32*(5), 237–238.

Woloshin, R.S. (1981). *Improving the prediction of academic persistence in community college for minority students by the addition of nonintellective variables to traditional intellective variables*, doctoral dissertation. Unpublished manuscript, The Graduate School of Arts and Sciences, Columbia University.

World Health Organization (2002). 25 Questions and answers on health and human rights, *Health and human rights publication series*, Issue 1, Author.

World Health Organization (2006). *Constitution of the World Health Organization, Basic Documents*, 45th edition, Supplement, October 2006, Author.

Xiao, J. (2005). Resources in transcultural nursing: A library orientation program for nursing students. *Journal of Multicultural Nursing and Health, 11*(2), 56–63.

Yearwood, E., Brown, D.L., & Karlik, E.C. (2002). Cultural diversity: Students' perspectives. *Journal of Transcultural Nursing, 13*(3), 237–240.

Yoder, M.K. (1996). Instructional responses to ethnically diverse nursing students. *Journal of Nursing Education, 35*(7), 315–321.

Yoder, M.K. (2001). The bridging approach: Effective strategies for teaching ethnically diverse nursing students. *Journal of Transcultural Nursing, 12*, 319–325.

Yoder, M.K. & Saylor, C. (2002). Student and teacher roles: Mismatched expectations. *Nurse Educator*, 27(5), 201–203.

Yoder-Wise, P.S. (2009). State and certifying boards/associations: CE and competency requirements. *Journal of Continuing Education in Nursing*, 40(1), 3–11.

Young, P., & Diekelmann, N. (2002). Learning to lecture: Exploring the skills, strategies, and practices of new teachers in nursing education. *Journal of Nursing Education*, 41(9), 405–412.

Yurkovich, E.E. (2001). Working with American Indians toward educational success. *Journal of Nursing Education*, 40(6), 259–269.

Zalon, M.L. (2008). Using technology to build community in professional associations. *The Journal of Continuing Education in Nursing*, 39(5), 235–240.

Zimmerman, B.J. (1995). Self-efficacy and educational development. In A. Bandura (Ed.), *Self-efficacy in changing societies* (pp. 202–231). New York: Cambridge University Press.

Zimmerman, B.J. (1996). Enhancing student academic and health functioning: A self-regulatory perspective. *School Psychology Quarterly*, 11(1), 47–66.

Zinatelli, M., Dube, M.A., & Jovanovic, R. (2002). Computer-based study skills training: The role of technology in improving performance and retention. *Journal of College Student Retention: Research, Theory, & Practice*, 4(1), 67–78.

Zizzo, K.A., & Xu, Y. (2009). Post-hire transitional programs for international nurses: A systematic review. *Journal of Continuing Education in Nursing*, 40(2), 57–64.

Zwick, W.R., & Velicer, W.F. (1986). Comparison of five rules for determining the number of components to retain. *Psychological Bulletin*, 99, 432–442.

Index

Page numbers followed by *f* indicate figure; those followed by *t* indicate table; those followed by *b* indicate box.